Th

P

Vc

Evolve Learning Resources for Students and Lecturers.
See the instructions *and PIN code panel* on the inside cover
for access to the web site.

Think outside the book ... **evolve**

Commissioning Editor: Rita Demetriou-Swanwick
Development Editor: Catherine Jackson
Project Manager: Maggie Johnson
Designer/Design Direction: Miles Hitchin
Illustration Manager: Tim Ainslie

The Concise Guide to
Physiotherapy
Volume Two – Treatment

Edited by

Tim Ainslie MSc GradDipPhys MCSP MMACP
Clinical Education Co-ordinator/Senior Lecturer, Physiotherapy Programme,
Oxford Brookes University, Oxford, UK

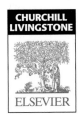

Edinburgh London New York Oxford Philadelphia St Louis Sydney Toronto 2012

CHURCHILL LIVINGSTONE
ELSEVIER

© 2012 Elsevier Ltd. All rights reserved.

No part of this publication may be reproduced or transmitted in any form or by any means, electronic or mechanical, including photocopying, recording, or any information storage and retrieval system, without permission in writing from the publisher. Details on how to seek permission, further information about the Publisher's permissions policies and our arrangements with organisation such as the Copyright Clearance Center and the Copyright Licensing Agency, can be found at our website: www.elsevier.com/permissions.

This book and the individual contributions contained in it are protected under copyright by the Publisher (other than as may be noted herein).

ISBN 978 0 7020 4049 8

ISBN of Vol 1 978 0 7020 35552 4
ISBN of 2-Vol Set 978 0 7020 4048 1

British Library Cataloguing in Publication Data
A catalogue record for this book is available from the British Library

Library of Congress Cataloging in Publication Data
A catalog record for this book is available from the Library of Congress

Notices
Knowledge and best practice in this field are constantly changing. As new research and experience broaden our understanding, changes in research methods, professional practices, or medical treatment may become necessary.

Practitioners and researchers must always rely on their own experience and knowledge in evaluating and using any information, methods, compounds, or experiments described herein. In using such information or methods they should be mindful of their own safety and the safety of others, including parties for whom they have a professional responsibility.

With respect to any drug or pharmaceutical products identified, readers are advised to check the most current information provided (i) on procedures featured or (ii) by the manufacturer of each product to be administered, to verify the recommended dose or formula, the method and duration of administration, and contraindications. It is the responsibility of practitioners, relying on their own experience and knowledge of their patients, to make diagnoses, to determine dosages and the best treatment for each individual patient, and to take all appropriate safety precautions.

To the fullest extent of the law, neither the Publisher nor the authors, contributors, or editors, assume any liability for any injury and/or damage to persons or property as a matter of products liability, negligence or otherwise, or from any use or operation of any methods, products, instructions, or ideas contained in the material herein.

ELSEVIER your source for books, journals and multimedia in the health sciences
www.elsevierhealth.com

Working together to grow libraries in developing countries
www.elsevier.com | www.bookaid.org | www.sabre.org
ELSEVIER   BOOK AID International   Sabre Foundation

The publisher's policy is to use paper manufactured from sustainable forests

Printed in China

Contents

Anne Alexander MSc BSc(Hons) MCSP MMACP
Clinical Specialist Physiotherapist, Hand Therapy and Plastic Surgery Department, John Radcliffe Hospital, Oxford
Chapter 4 – Burns and plastic surgery

Rebecca Aston MA MCSP
Specialist Women's Health Physiotherapist, Community PFD Service Team Lead, Homerton Hospital, London
Chapter 11 – Obstetrics and gynaecology

Kate Baker BSc(Hons) MCSP
Macmillan Cancer Lead Physiotherapist, Velindre Cancer Centre, Cardiff
Chapter 12 – Oncology and palliative care

Louise Briggs MSc BSc(Hons) MCSP
AHP Therapy Consultant – Acute Rehabilitation St George's Health Care NHS Trust, London
Chapter 7 – Gerontology

Joanna Camp BSc(Hons) MCSP
Specialist Physiotherapist, National Spinal Injuries Unit, Stoke Mandeville Hospital, Buckinghamshire Healthcare NHS Trust
Chapter 16 – Spinal cord injuries

Maureen Carter BA MCSP
Retired Senior Physiotherapist in Community and Intermediate Care, Croydon, Surrey
Chapter 6 – Community physiotherapy

Jackie Clifford MSc BA Cert. Management GradDipPhys MCSP
Self Employed Rehabilitation Consultant Worthing, West Sussex
Chapter 10 – Mental health

Mary Jane Cole MSc GradDipPhys MCSP ACE
Senior Lecturer, Practice Education, Kingston University and St George's University, London
Chapter 2 – Amputee rehabilitation

Karen Edwards MSc MCSP
Clinical Specialist Physiotherapist Great Ormond Street Hospital, London
Chapter 5 – Community paediatrics

Carole Fruin GradDipPhys Cert. Rheum. Practice MCSP
Clinical Specialist Physiotherapist – Rheumatology, South London Healthcare NHS Trust, London
Chapter 15 – Rheumatology

Kerry Gibson BSc(Hons) MCSP
Senior Physiotherapist Birmingham & Solihull Mental Health NHS Foundation Trust, Birmingham
Chapter 10 – Mental health

Susie Grady MSc BSc(Hons) MCSP
Aquatic Therapy Team Leader, The Gardens and Jacob Centres, Hertfordshire
Chapter 3 – Aquatic physiotherapy

Beverley Greensitt BSc(Hons) MCSP
Senior Physiotherapist, John Radcliffe Hospital, Oxford
Chapter 9 – Medicine

Caroline Griffiths GradDipPhys MCSP
Professional Lead, Physiotherapy, Oxford Health NHS Foundation Trust, Oxford
Chapter 10 – Mental health

Vicki Harding PhD MCSP
Research and Clinical Specialist Physiotherapist, INPUT Pain Management Programme, St Thomas' Hospital, London
Chapter 13 – Pain management

Nicola Harmer GradDipPhys MCSP
Highly Specialist Physiotherapist/Directorate Manual Handling Advisor Directorate of Learning Disability Services, Abertawe Bro Morgannwg University Health Board
Chapter 8 – Learning disabilities

Scott Hawthorne BAppSc MCSP MAPA
Band 7 Physiotherapist, Acute Spinal Injuries Physiotherapy Lead, national Spinal injuries Centre, Stoke Mandeville Hospital, Buckinghamshire Healthcare NHS Trust
Chapter 16 – Spinal cord injuries

Andrea Hounsell MSc BSc(Hons) MCSP
Physiotherapy Team Leader, Directorate of Learning Disability services, Abertawe Bro Morgannwg University Health Board
Chapter 8 – Learning disabilities

Julia Hyde MCSP BSc(Hons)
Children's Community Physiotherapist, Oxford Health NHS Foundation Trust, Oxford
Chapter 5 – Community paediatrics

Anne Jackson PhD MSc BA(Hons) MCSP
English Networks Programme Manager, Chartered Society of Physiotherapy, London
Chapter 3 – Aquatic physiotherapy

Deborah Jackson MSc BSc(Hons) MCSP
Clinical Specialist Physiotherapist, Great Ormond Street Hospital, London
Chapter 1 – Acute paediatrics

Contributors

Captain Mark Jenkins MSc BSc(Hons) MCSP RAMC
Officer in Command, Primary Care Rehabilitation Facility, Wellington Barracks, London
Chapter 14 – Rehabilitation

Lesley Katchburian MSc MCSP
Clinical Specialist Physiotherapist (Neurodisability), The Wolfson Neurodisability Service, Great Ormond Street Hospital, London
Chapter 1 – Acute paediatrics

Jane Leathwood GradDipPhys MCSP
Senior Physiotherapist Stoke Mandeville Hospital, Buckinghamshire Healthcare NHS Trust
Chapter 4 – Burns and plastic surgery

Karen Livingstone MCSP GradDipPhys
Clinical Specialist Physiotherapist in Oncology and Palliative Care, St Ann's Hospice, Neil Cliffe Centre, Wythenshawe Hospital, Manchester
Chapter 12 – Oncology and palliative care

Marion Main MA MCSP
Dubowitz Neuromuscular Centre, Great Ormond Street Hospital, London
Chapter 1 – Acute paediatrics

Mike Maynard GradDipPhys HT
Clinical Lead in Aquatic Physiotherapy, United Lincolnshire Hospitals
Chapter 3 – Aquatic physiotherapy

Aileen McCartney MSc BSc(Hons) MCSP
Senior Physiotherapist, Specialist Palliative Care, Wisdom Hospital, Rochester, Kent
Chapter 12 – Oncology and palliative care

Doreen McClurg PhD MCSP
Reader, NMAHP Research Unit, Glasgow Caledonian University, Glasgow
Chapter 11 – Obstetrics and gynaecology

Lorraine Moores MSc GradDipPhys MCSP
Principal Physiotherapist, Manchester and Salford Pain Centre, Salford Royal Hospital NHS Foundation Trust, Salford
Chapter 13 – Pain management

Venkataramanan Narayanan MSc BSc(Hons) MCSP
Senior Physiotherapist, Oxford Health NHS Foundation Trust, Oxford
Chapter 10 – Mental health

Clare Nickols MSc BSc(Hons) MCSP
In-Patient Team Leader/ Deputy Physiotherapy Manager, Heatherwood Hospital, Ascot, Berkshire
Chapter 9 – Medicine

Jayne R. Nixon BSc(Hons) Dip Sport Ex Med MCSP
Clinical Specialist and Clinical Lead – Lower Limbs Team, Defence Medical Rehabilitation Centre, Headley Court, Epsom, Surrey
Chapter 14 – Rehabilitation

Pauline Norris MCSP
Senior Children's Physiotherapist OxfordHealth NHS Foundation Trust, Oxford
Chapter 5 – Community paediatrics

Siobhan O'Mahony PGDip Health Services Management GradDipPhys MCSP
Physiotherapy Manager, St Patrick's Hospital (cork) Ltd, Cork, Ireland
Chapter 12 – Oncology and palliative care

Ankie Postma GradDipPhys
Band 7 Amputee Rehabilitation, Aquatic Physiotherapy and Ankylosing Spondylitis Basildon Hospital, Essex
Chapter 3 – Aquatic physiotherapy

Davina Richardson MSc BSc(Hons) MCSP
Clinical Lead Therapist, Neurosciences, Imperial College Healthcare NHS Trust, London
Chapter 14 – Rehabilitation

Karen A J Rix MSCP GradDipPhys
Clinical Team Leader, Community Intermediate Care Servie, London
Chapter 6 – Community physiotherapy

Andrew Rolls MSC BSC(Hons) MCSP
Head of Sports Medicine, West Ham United Football Club, London
Chapter 14 – Rehabilitation

Josie Scerri BSc(Hons) MCSP
Senior Physiotherapist, Neurodisability Service, Great Ormond Street Hospital, London
Chapter 1 – Acute paediatrics

Warren Sheehan BPhty MCSP
Senior Physiotherapist, John Radcliffe Hospital, Oxford
Chapter 14 – Trauma orthopaedics

Contributors

Alison Skinner FCSP Dip TP HT BA
Consultant Aquatic Physiotherapist/
Physiotherapy Educator, London
Chapter 3 – Aquatic physiotherapy

Sara Smith GradDipPhys PGCertClinEd
MCSP
Amputee Therapy Team Leader,
Rehabilitation Gym, Douglas Bader Centre,
Queen Mary's Hospital, London
Chapter 2 – Amputee rehabilitation

Sue Standing MSc MCSP
Lead Physiotherapist, Hampshire
Partnership Foundation Trust, Southampton
Chapter 8 – Learning disabilities

Robyn Stiger MSc BSc(Hons) MCSP
Associate Lecturer, Oxford Brookes
University, Oxford
Chapter 1 – Acute paediatrics

Catherine Stringer BSc(Hons) BEd
MCSP
Senior Musculoskeletal Physiotherapist/
Hydrotherapy, Physiotherapy
Department, Good Hope Hospital,
West Midlands
Chapter 3 – Aquatic physiotherapy

Anna Vines BSC(Hons) MCSP
Senior Physiotherapist, John Radcliffe
Hospital, Oxford
Chapter 17 – Trauma orthopaedics

Yvonne Wren GradDipPhys
Retired Clinical Therapy Lead
for Intermediate Care, Southward,
London; Retired Specialist Lecturer,
University of East London,
London
Chapter 6 – Community physiotherapy

Contributors

Preface

Students and graduate physiotherapists report feeling underprepared when entering an unfamiliar practice area for the first time. The core areas of musculoskeletal, neurology and cardio-respiratory tend to be covered in depth in the university as students are prepared for practice placements and it is often the 'non-core' areas such as burns and plastic surgery or palliative care that can cause a student to feel anxious and underprepared. Written by specialists from the 'non-core' areas of practice the two volumes of this book aim to provide the student or graduate with an insight into the philosophy of approach that needs to be taken in either the assessment (volume 1) or the treatment (volume 2) of the individual in these placement areas. The material provides an entry level of knowledge with the expectation that the reader will access more 'in-depth' information, in order to supplement the material provided in the two volumes and on-line resources.

Tim Ainslie

Preface

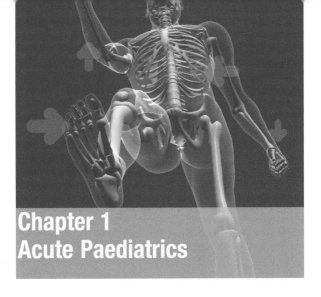

Chapter 1
Acute Paediatrics

Neuromuscular disorders

Treatment of children with neuromuscular disorders must be considered in the context of the child, the disorder and the family. These are life-long and many, life-limiting conditions, most of which will deteriorate over time. Many weak children will be prone to respiratory problems and repeated chest infections. Night time, sometimes day and night time ventilation, usually with BiPAP may be needed for survival.

The aims of management are

- Maximise useful function
- Improve or maintain quality of life
- Reduce the burden of care on parents and carers.

It is helpful to know the diagnosis to be able to anticipate problems but with the above aims in mind, treatment plans can be affected without a diagnosis if a neuromuscular disorder is suspected. Before being able to treat, an underlying knowledge of the major conditions is needed.

The most common neuromuscular disorders

- The largest group of neuromuscular disorders is the progressive muscular dystrophies: Duchenne muscular dystrophy (DMD), Becker muscular dystrophy (BMD, a milder form of DMD) and a group of childhood limb girdle dystrophies. The main features of these disorders are that ambulation is achieved in childhood but a large proportion of children will lose it before adulthood.

- Congenital muscular dystrophies (CMD): a wide spectrum of disorders characterised by weakness and severe and progressive contractures, which are a major cause of functional limitation. Depending on severity of the disorder, children may or may never walk, and those who walk may lose ambulation.

- The congenital myopathies: another diverse group of conditions, while there can be quite severe respiratory involvement in some types, they are much more slowly progressive than the dystrophies. Walking ability is variable as above.

- Spinal muscular atrophy (SMA) is a neurogenic disorder; a problem of the nerve impulses not reaching muscles. It is not considered progressive in childhood, but growth greatly affects function and development of scoliosis in non-ambulant children. Children with SMA are grouped into those with severe SMA (type 1) who never achieve independent sitting; moderate or type 2 SMA, who achieve independent sitting but not independent walking; type 3, mild SMA, who do walk, but may lose the ability before adulthood.

- Peripheral neuropathies: including the largest group, Charcot–Marie–Tooth syndrome, are slowly progressive disorders primarily affecting nerves and nerve sheaths and can interfere with lower arm and hand and lower leg and foot function. Almost all will walk into adulthood but need foot orthotics and possibly foot surgery. Foot pain is common. They tend to have weak hands and fatigue with writing.

- Arthrogryposis is the term used to describe children born with joint contractures. There are several causes, some with underlying neurogenic or neuromuscular origins. In some forms of CMD babies are born with contractures.

- Congenital myotonic dystrophy (DM1) is a relatively common disorder characterised by mild weakness, developmental delay, fatigue, and learning difficulties. The children have frequent incidence of talipes. The children should achieve ambulation.

Priorities of physiotherapy management

The priorities of management will depend on diagnosis and presentation of the varying disorders. Each disorder has a spectrum of disease with some children having more severe, rapidly progressive problems than others.

NB: in all cases, for children who have respiratory involvement, the primary aim of physiotherapy will be maintaining clear airways. When necessary, parents will be taught chest physiotherapy and secretion clearance techniques.

In some conditions, e.g. DMD, the course can be more predictable and therefore some problems, such as the development of contractures, can be anticipated and preventative measures tried.

Regular, comprehensive assessment is needed to assess the priorities of management at different stages as they will differ according to disorder, age, and difficulties.

When determining physiotherapy priorities it must be remembered that the family situation must be considered. Physiotherapy is only one small part of what the child needs and parents can do. Any programme must be given in context of the family as a whole. Medical considerations (medication, possible management of ventilation and/or gastrostomy), siblings, affected siblings and affected parents, school/nursery, housing/social problems all have to be taken into account.

It is not useful to assume that management strategies for DMD will work in SMA or Charcot–Marie–Tooth syndrome. Similarly it is not possible to extrapolate to neuromuscular disorders from neurological or musculoskeletal conditions.

Treatment objectives
- Maintain respiratory viability
- Improve or maintain power where possible

- Prevent or reduce contractures
- Encourage and maintain mobility
- Maintain symmetrical posture, where possible
- Prevent or reduce pain.

Respiratory management of the child with neuromuscular disorders

This is part of respiratory therapy and therefore not covered. It is important, however, when working with these children, in hospital or in the community to have knowledge of current respiratory management, appropriate positioning, contraindications to treatment, the use of equipment; ventilators (mostly Bipap), suction and cough-assist when necessary. Advice from a physiotherapist experienced in these areas is essential.

Improve or maintain power

The major problem in neuromuscular disorders is weakness. In some cases the muscle fibres or nerves are deteriorating so the weakness is progressive. In some conditions, the weakness is masked by increasing contractures, and in some the weakness does not increase but increases in height and weight will increase functional difficulties.

Weakness caused by deteriorating conditions cannot be improved, but in many cases, a proportion of weakness is caused by disuse atrophy; which can and should be treated.

- In the muscular dystrophies, increased muscle damage can be caused by using weights or repeated eccentric muscle work.
- Open chain exercise cannot be easily achieved by non-ambulant children.
- Asymmetry of power is extremely common; it is important to ensure exercise is tailored to produce symmetrical work.
- Muscle imbalance can be increased, with resultant increase in contractures if the exercise programmes do not target the correct muscle groups.

The weakest muscles

In many disorders the knee extensors, hip extensors and neck and trunk flexors are weak (Figure 1.1).

The knee and hip extensors weakness causes the hyper-lordotic posture seen in DMD and other conditions (Figure 1.2a, b).

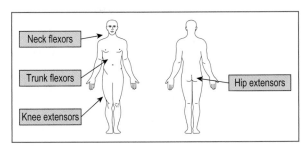

Figure 1.1 The weakest muscle groups.

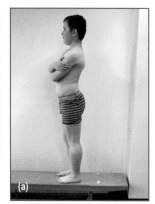 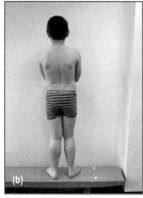

Figure 1.2 (a and b) Hyperlordosis caused by hip extensor weakness.

Due to the weakness of hip extensors, the hamstrings act as hip extensors and help to maintain the stability of the pelvis.

For this reason, hamstring stretches have no place in the management of most neuromuscular conditions.

Exercise and exercise programmes

Exercise programmes are frequently boring and rarely followed over time. Giving repetitive exercises to children will not be effective unless they are fun, varied and are seen to make a difference. In neuromuscular disorders it is frequently hard to see improvement, but it must be impressed on parents, carers and older children that no deterioration, particularly through growth spurts, is positive.

Exercises must be functional – they must target groups that make a difference. It is no good exercising stronger groups, increasing asymmetry or working on groups that ultimately are effective at increasing strength, but have no functional benefit.

Ideally, exercise should become part of daily routine like stretches. They must fit into daily activities, must be inexpensive and achievable. Aquatic physiotherapy, swimming (or playing in the water), bicycling/tricycling, horse riding, martial arts, non-contact sports and wheelchair sports should all be encouraged.

Trampolining, scooters, gymnastics, rugby and weights (in most cases) are not advised.

Prevent or reduce contractures

Contractures are caused by lack of movement, increasing fibrosis of muscle, persistent poor positioning and muscle imbalance. They will not go away on their own! Contractures interfere with function, can prevent or reduce the attainment of the upright posture and therefore walking, can cause pain and make positioning still more difficult. Scoliosis is a form of contracture which can also limit chest expansion and further reduce the ability of the chest to expand on inspiration.

Contractures can happen at any joint including the jaw and neck but in many disorders they are common patterns of contractures or predictable development of tightness.

Stretches must be targeted only at those groups where the contractures interfere with function. There is no value in stretching hypermobile joints or joints where very mild contractures do not and will not cause difficulty.

The management of contractures can be effected in the following ways.

Stretching

Stretching should never be painful.

Stretches will not be effective if they are not done regularly, for a long enough time and if there is no way of supporting or maintaining the range of movement or increase gained.

Stretches should be active assisted where possible, should be done daily (or six times per week) and should be held long enough for the stretch to be effective. Stretches coupled with splinting are proven to be more effective than stretching alone.

NB, it is very easy to sprain the ankles of non-ambulant children with SMA when doing stretches and therefore caution is needed to prevent this happening.

Positioning

The use of positioning for stretch is highly effective, the most useful position being standing as it will stretch all lower limb joints. Standing is of no benefit if it increases asymmetry of posture.

Prone lying in a symmetrical position without the feet being compromised and long sitting (with gaiters in some conditions) are also effective.

Splinting

Night time Ankle Foot Orthoses (AFO) to maintain ankle range have been shown, when used with stretching, to be most effective at maintaining range. They also help to prevent long-term foot deformities in non-ambulant children (Figure 1.3).

Knee splints and elbow splints can be used to maintain range during the day or at night. The use of splinting must be considered carefully and not cause functional limitation. Only one elbow splint at a time should be worn at night. Knee splints should not be worn with ankle splints.

The use of any splint worn at night which disturbs sleep or parents' sleep needs to be carefully evaluated. It must be remembered; a number of children will be using night-time ventilation and a few will wear spinal jackets at night. The use of other splints may not be possible and will need to be worn for periods during the day instead. Flexibility in approach is needed and discussion with parents and children as to how the differing demands can be best managed.

Serial casting

Serial casting is effective at improving range. It is important, however, that the following rules are followed.

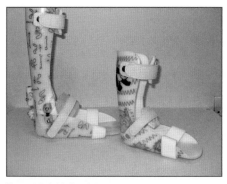

Figure 1.3 Ankle foot Orthoses.

1. Serial casting should never last more than 15 days.

2. Casting should never be painful.

3. The first cast is a resting splint, and will be the most effective.

4. When casting ankles in an ambulant child, both ankles must be cast, irrespective of whether both ankles are tight.

5. Ambulant children should always be able to walk in the casts.

6. Removable splints will need to be considered for elbows and knees if the casting interferes with function, sleep or mobility.

Surgery

In some cases the only way to reduce contractures will be to have surgical release. They must be considered very carefully with the whole team. The postoperative splinting needs to be carefully considered and ambulant children must be able to walk in plasters or be off their feet for no longer than 2 weeks.

Hip flexor releases will not last and recur within 9–12 months.

It is rarely useful to perform bony hip surgery on children with neuromuscular disorders. Dislocated hips are common and unless painful, causing problems with seating or preventing independent ambulation, surgery should not be considered.

Encourage and maintain mobility

The weaker the child, the less function they will have, but there are weak children who maintain ambulation and relatively weaker ones who are unable to walk.

Mobility needs to be considered as a whole and includes walking, independently or with splints/orthoses, manual and electric wheelchair mobility, dynamic standers, electric scooter, and bicycles/tricycles.

Some children will never achieve ambulation, some will achieve it and lose it, but the most important thing for the child is, whether they can walk or not, that they are able to move around and explore their environment, fully access their home, nursery/school and leisure facilities and if wheelchair-dependent, ensure transport for their wheelchair where needed.

The use of orthoses is common in neuromuscular disorders to achieve or maintain ambulation.

Maintain symmetrical posture

Almost all non-ambulant children with neuromuscular disorders will develop scoliosis. The age of onset, how severe and how rapidly it progresses varies in different disorders and different children. All children with type 2 SMA will develop scoliosis; many boys with DMD who lose ambulation will develop asymmetry.

Physiotherapy can help, along with other management strategies, to slow down the rate of progression by encouraging ambulation, through positioning, maintaining symmetry through exercise and stretches and ensuring good posture throughout the day.

As the deformity in neuromuscular disorders is caused by weakness, the children rarely need to have postural control when in bed.

Prevent or reduce pain

Direct pain is uncommon in children with neuromuscular disorders, although often reported as a symptom in adults. Pain is most frequently caused by injury, badly fitting splints, poor posture or seating, immobility causing stiffness or pressure, and stiff joints.

Boys with DMD who are taking steroids may complain of back pain. It may be persistent or caused by sudden or specific movements. This must always be taken seriously and the child referred to their paediatrician or GP.

Most pain can be prevented. The treatment of pain in these children is the same as in any other – first, remove the cause. Second, prevent it recurring.

Parental pain from poor manual handling or lack of equipment must also be considered as a major problem in the home.

Revision

The aims of physiotherapy in these children are:

1. To maintain maximum useful function – including respiratory function.
2. Ensure no physiotherapy is painful.
3. Physiotherapy should be targeted and specific – it should be made to fit with daily routine, must be fun and seen to be beneficial.
4. It must not increase the burden of care.
5. Ensure that any care is done in the context of the family.

Musculoskeletal

- Most young children are unlikely to co-operate with a formalised exercise programme so the creative use of toys and play is needed to encourage the child to move and maintain their interest.
- The physiotherapist should spend more time teaching parents, carers and teaching assistants how to handle and position their child so that they can continue therapy outside the physiotherapy sessions.
- Support, reassurance, gaining consent to carry out treatment and dealing sensitively with often highly anxious parents all play a central role in paediatric physiotherapy.
- Being aware of wider influences such as religious beliefs, past experiences, as well as individual coping abilities is all part of successfully managing the child and their family.
- Young skeletons have the potential to heal and remodel rapidly, but muscle imbalance, injury to growth plate through trauma or infections (e.g. meningococcal septicaemia), and certain conditions (e.g. Blount's disease) may lead to asymmetrical growth and progressive deformity as the child grows.
- The treatment of common conditions, such as developmental dysplasia of the hip (DDH) and congenital talipes equinovarus (CTEV), combines this remodeling ability of the growing skeleton with an understanding of the laws governing the remodeling of bone, which state that by improving the biomechanical environment, abnormal growth patterns may be reversed– Heuter–Volkmann law (Rauch 2005).

Normal variants

- If the presenting problem is symmetrical, symptom-free, without stiffness or systemic involvement and there is no skeletal dysplasia (refer to 5 'S's' in assessment volume), it is probably a normal variant and requires no intervention.
- The most common causes of concern are in toeing, bowlegs (genu varus), knock-knees (genu valgus) and flat foot (planovalgus).
- The role of the physiotherapist in these conditions is to rule out anything more sinister and then monitor the child's development and functional abilities whilst reassuring the parents that they are likely to resolve as the child grows.

Abnormalities of the hip

Developmental dysplasia of the hip

- This term describes the spectrum of hip instability ranging from a shallow (dysplastic) acetabulum to the irreducibly dislocated hip.

- In the infant DDH may present as instability, in a toddler as a limp, and in an adolescent as exercise-induced pain.

- Conservative treatment is likely to be successful only if the diagnosis is made early.

- However, normal hips may be unstable at birth because of ligamentous laxity and stabilise within the first couple of weeks of life so require no treatment.

- The principles of treatment are the same at any age and, put simply are: 'Get it down, Get it in, Keep it in, Monitor'.

- Hips that remain unstable or are dislocated are treated with harnesses or splints which aim to hold the hip in its reduced position of abduction and flexion.

- The most commonly used splint is the Pavlik harness, which allows controlled movement.

- Often it is the role of the physiotherapist to apply the splint and, essentially, to monitor the baby closely whilst in the harness.

- The harness will need frequent adjustment as the child grows to reduce the risk of avascular necrosis and the parents will need to be advised to ensure their baby keeps kicking as failure to do so may indicate femoral nerve palsy.

- In infants over the age of 4–6 months, closed reduction is usually required and the hip held in a hip spica cast for some months.

- The older the child becomes, the less likely it is that reduction by closed methods will succeed and open reduction, together with bony realignment and hip spica application, is necessary.

- Open reduction becomes more difficult and less successful in the older child and so surgery is often not undertaken over the age of 6–8 years in bilateral cases and over 8–10 years in unilateral.

- Physiotherapy involvement in these children will include advising the parents on manual handling and positioning the child in the spica and providing information on suitable buggies/chairs/car seats.

- On spica removal, physiotherapy will be targeted at regaining range of movement and muscle strength and, depending on the age of the child, re-education of gait.

- Passive movement of the knee should be avoided due to the risk of supracondylar fracture but the child should be encouraged to move as normally as possible.

Legg–Calve–Perthes disease

This condition is characterised by the development of AVN of the proximal femoral epiphysis and, once established, follows a relatively well-defined path lasting 3–4 years. This entails collapse and fragmentation of the ossific nucleus of the femoral head followed by healing with revascularisation and regeneration of the bony epiphysis. Prognosis is generally good, particularly of young children and those with partial femoral head involvement. However, during the collapse and fragmentation stages, femoral head deformity occurs.

If a child between the ages of 4 and 8 years complains of aching or pain at the hip or knee, walks with a limp and shows reduced range of hip movement, Perthes disease should be suspected and X-rays requested to confirm this diagnosis.

The primary aim of physiotherapy in these children is to maintain range of movement (particularly hip abduction and extension) through stretches, active exercise and positioning. This will encourage sphericity of the femoral head and hence reduce the likelihood of secondary acetabular dysplasia. Sporting activity may be reduced, particularly those that stress the joint such as trampolining or contact sports, but the use of crutches and/or wheelchairs should be avoided because they promote the adducted and flexed posture that you are trying to avoid. Hydrotherapy is an excellent medium to increase range of movement without placing undue stress on the joint.

The role of operative treatment is controversial. Some surgeons prefer to perform surgery early to prevent deformity secondary to femoral head collapse whilst others advocate later intervention to correct deformity. Postoperatively, physiotherapy will be needed to mobilise and strengthen the limb and re-educate gait.

Slipped upper/capital femoral epiphysis (SUFE)

As this is a fracture through the physis it can be missed on X-ray until it allows the epiphysis to displace on the femoral neck. If a prepubertal child (more commonly boys) complains of hip or knee pain with reduced range of hip movement on assessment and a leg which rests in an externally rotated and shortened position, X-rays should be requested (including lateral views) to rule out SUFE. Most slips are pinned in situ and the role of the physiotherapist is to regain range of movement, strength and re-educate gait postoperatively.

Abnormalities of the knee

Knee pain

Pain or aching around the knee is a relatively common complaint amongst children, particularly those who engage in sport or during rapid periods of growth when traction injuries may occur. As mentioned, referral of pain from the hip, particularly SUFE, should be excluded. Swelling and pain in the knee can also be caused by juvenile rheumatoid arthritis, infections in the knee joint (septic arthritis), and certain types of bone cancer, including osteogenic sarcoma.

Osteochondritis dissecans

The child will complain of localised tenderness and locking of the joint if a loose body occurs. The prognosis is better in children than adults. Management is initially rest, ice and isometric exercises followed by a progressive exercise programme to regain range of movement and muscle strength and to encourage a gradual return to full activities.

Osgood–Schlatter's disease (traction apophysitis of the patella tendon insertion)

The child will complain of pain, swelling and localised tenderness over the tibial tubercle. Initial management is again rest and analgesia. This is a self-limiting condition but ice, taping to reduce the pull of the quadriceps and hamstring stretches can be helpful in managing the symptoms.

Patellofemoral pain (often due to patello maltracking)

As in adults, taping and quadriceps strengthening (particularly VMO) can be very effective.

Abnormalities of the foot and ankle

CTEV

This is commonly known as club foot, and is a deformity of unknown aetiology, in which the foot is in an equinovarus position. Physiotherapy input will depend on whether this deformity is postural or structural.

Postural/positional

Bony anatomy of foot is normal, but foot has been held in an abnormal position in utero.

The foot will usually correct spontaneously but the carer can be shown appropriate passive stretches.

Structural/rigid

- Bony anatomy of foot is abnormal.
- Triplanar deformity with hindfoot equinus and varus, midfoot cavus and forefoot adduction and supination.
- This may be idiopathic, neuromuscular (e.g. spina bifida) or syndromic (e.g. arthrogryposis).
- There are various scoring systems, but the Pirani scoring system is reliable, quick, and easy to use, and provides a good forecast about the likely treatment for an individual foot. It records deformity on a scale of 0 (full correction) to 6 (severe deformity) (Dyer & Davis 2006).

Management consists of serial casting to correct the various components of the deformity. This is commonly carried out by a physiotherapist and commenced as early as reasonable after birth. The most universally recognised method of doing this is the Ponseti method (specific manipulation and casting technique, followed by early Achilles tendon tenotomy and the use of boots and bar to maintain the corrected position up to the age of 4 years). Compliance with treatment may be more difficult as the child gets older but failure to do so is associated with a higher relapse rate. This method is successful in 95% of feet, avoiding formal surgical release, although percutaneous tenotomy is usually required. Tibialis anterior transfer can be used to correct dynamic supination in toddlers.

Congenital vertical talus (CVT)

CVT presents as a 'rocker bottom' foot as the navicular dislocates dorsally on the talus and the head of talus can be felt in the sole of the foot. These feet can also be managed with casting and early results of reverse Ponseti plastering, followed by wire fixation, are promising (Dobbs et al 2007).

Tarsal coalition

Presents as a stiff, painful flat foot and the child may have difficulties walking and running. Physiotherapy will not improve these children but the bar can be resected. In these instances, physiotherapy may be needed to regain range of movement and re-educate gait postoperatively.

Severs disease

Presents as heel pain related to activity. Calf muscle stretches are the mainstay of treatment.

Upper limb abnormalities

Function must be the most important consideration when managing abnormalities of the upper limb. Children cope very well with disability and adapt quickly.

Radial club hand

Commonly associated with other congenital anomalies (e.g. VACTERL syndrome). Physiotherapy management is serial plastering as club foot and splinting.

Radioulnar synostosis

Usually presents some time after birth with fixed forearm rotation. Physiotherapy will not increase the range of movement but input is usually required to assess which position is most functional for the child as osteotomy can change the fixed position but not restore range of movement.

Limb length discrepancy

Limb length discrepancies may be caused by congenital deficiencies or occur secondary to infection, vascular injury, trauma, neurological problems, resection of tumours or conditions such as Ollier's disease.

Management will depend on the amount of shortening predicted at skeletal maturity, the stability of adjacent joints and the wishes of the parents and child.

- A limb length discrepancy of under 2 cm does not require intervention unless the child is complaining of symptoms. In this case, a 1 cm raise can be accommodated within the shoe.
- For a discrepancy of up to 5 cm the family has two choices:
- A shoe raise: in general, the raise should not be the same as the measured discrepancy, as this will result in problems with foot clearance, nor anything over 5 cm as this becomes too heavy to be functional.
- Epiphysiodesis or plates to ablate/slow the growth of the longer leg so that the legs are equal by the time the child reaches skeletal maturity.
- For a discrepancy over 5 cm the options are:
- Limb lengthening with an external fixator
- Combination of limb lengthening and epiphysiodesis
- Extension prosthesis
- Amputation and prosthesis.

Physiotherapy plays an important role in the management of children undergoing any of these procedures. Whilst the intensity and methods may vary, the aims for each are:

- Preoperative planning:
- To ensure realistic expectations of the child and family
- Liaison with school and relevant local services
- Provision of wheelchair and any equipment required.
- Postoperative management:
- Maintain joint range of movement
a Use of splints for joints above and below
b Active and passive exercises
- Encourage functional activity
- Weight bearing as indicated in postoperative notes
a This is usually full weight bearing as axial loading is important for osteogenesis
b Children with congenital causes of limb length discrepancy frequently have upper limb abnormalities and so crutches/walking frames may need adapting
- Transfer practice including bed to chair, on/off floor, stairs
- Independence in activities of daily living.

Spinal abnormalities

Obstetrical brachial plexus palsy (OBPP)

A birth injury due to a tearing force on the cervical nerve roots caused by extreme traction of the head from the shoulder girdle during delivery, resulting in a flail upper limb. The most common type is Erb's palsy (paralysis of nerve fibres from C5–C6). Risk factors include overweight babies (particularly those requiring forceps or ventouse extraction), small babies with breech presentation, prolonged second stage of labour or a previous child with OBPP.

All limbs should be examined to exclude quadriplegia, although bilateral OBPP has been reported. A full assessment with muscle testing can then be undertaken 48 hours after delivery to differentiate the patterns of paresis and determine the nerve roots damaged. Most children achieve full recovery (Eng et al 1996).

Physiotherapy management will consist of:

- Regular assessment of range of movement and muscle power.

- Passive stretches to prevent muscle and joint contractures (hand, wrist, forearm and elbow from birth and shoulder around the age of 5 days). Stretches are very specific and so, whilst the family can be taught them, it is advisable that regular contact is maintained by the physiotherapist (APCP 2001).

- Tactile stimulation.

- Weight-bearing exercises through the affected limb when indicated.

- Referral on to a specialist centre for consideration of surgery if return is not noted by the time the child is 3 months old.

- Advice to encourage awareness and use of the affected limb after 6 months of age.

Congenital muscular torticollis

Torticollis is a descriptive term of abnormal posture in which the head and neck are held in side flexion towards the affected side with rotation of the head to the opposite side. There have been more than 80 causes postulated for torticollis. An algorithm for differential diagnoses was developed by Ballock and Song (Ballock and Song 1996).

Physiotherapy management entails:

- Positioning to improve head position and muscle length and skull shape

- Encouraging active movement to address the muscle imbalance

- Strengthening overstretched muscles through use of postural reactions as the baby gains head control (e.g. head-righting reflex)

- Educating parents on handling, playing and positioning of child's equipment to encourage the desired movements.

Torticollis usually resolves without long-term effects but surgical release may be necessary if restriction of movement persists at the age of 1 year. Following surgical release of the sternomastoid muscle, passive movements may be started by the physiotherapist from 24 hours postoperatively. These should be carried out with the child supine, the shoulder girdle stabilised and gentle traction applied. The parents can be taught these preoperatively and take over from the physiotherapist when able. A child may also be given a collar for support and comfort in the first few weeks postoperatively. Active exercises are also important to redress the muscle imbalance and the child will need verbal and visual prompts to correct their head position. There may be some short-term visual disturbance until the eyes have accommodated to the improved head position.

Positional plagiocephaly

This occurs when a baby spends prolonged periods resting in one position. The child may present with an apparent torticollis and an asymmetrical posture but this will be due to difficulties moving off the flattened skull rather than restriction in passive movement. As movement becomes more difficult it increases the flattening and perpetuates the cycle. Physiotherapy is therefore aimed at restoring active movement by encouraging the baby to turn its head using toys and mobiles and ensuring frequent position changes, including supervised 'tummy time' in the first few months of life. It is also important to encourage the baby's general motor development (Hutchison et al 2004).

There is increasing interest amongst parents in the use of helmets to reshape their baby's heads. Their use remains controversial as the majority of heads recover their shape as babies become more active. However, they may have a place in the more severe or resistant cases.

Scoliosis

- Deformity is multiplanar and includes a rotational component.
- Aetiology may be congenital (underlying bony malformation), neuromuscular, syndromic or idiopathic.
- Back pain associated with scoliosis may be associated with an acquired cause such as infection or tumour.
- Treatment depends on the severity and curve progression – it varies from observation, through bracing, to surgery.
- Physiotherapy management for the idiopathic scoliosis may include exercises (controversial) and postural advice.
- Physiotherapy for the neuromuscular scoliosis will include positioning equipment for lying, sitting and standing.

Motor disorders

This section explores the medical and surgical management of the altered tone found in motor disorders covering focal and more generalised management including reversible and nonreversible changes that can be brought about through treatment (Figure 1.4).

Physiotherapy intervention is covered in Chapter 5 in this volume.

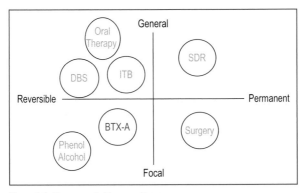

Figure 1.4 Management of increased tone.

Oral medication

Spasticity management

Baclofen

Baclofen works by binding to GABA B receptor sites to inhibit the release of excitatory neurotransmitters at the spinal cord level. It is the drug most commonly used in paediatrics for spasticity management. Side effects can hinder increase in dose to an effective level, e.g. drowsiness, difficulty concentrating at school, increased dribbling, decreased truncal tone and therefore reduced stability.

Benzodiazepines

Diazepam is the most commonly used and works by creating an inhibitory response at the reflex arc. It is particularly helpful in reducing painful spasms that may produce insomnia.

Dantrolene

Dantrolene works at the muscle level and inhibits the release of calcium ions from the sarcoplasmic reticulum, which reduces the force of the muscle contraction. Its greatest effect is on fast twitch muscles. Dantrolene is metabolised by the liver creating a risk of hepatotoxicity. Regular monitoring of liver enzymes is recommended when using this drug.

Alpha-2 adrenergic agonists

Tizanidine is the most commonly used alpha-2 adrenergic agonist, which acts at the level of the brain and spinal cord. It also carries the risk of hepatotoxicity and so regular monitoring of liver enzymes is recommended (Gage et al 2009).

Dystonia management

Trihexyphenidyl is an anticholinergic on the CNS, i.e. it blocks the effect of acetylcholine, therefore re-establishing a balance between excitatory acetylcholine, and inhibitory dopamine. Many side effects are associated with this drug, which again influences the ability to increase the dose. Side effects include urinary retention, constipation, blurred vision, and dry mouth (which may be beneficial if there's a lot of drooling) – they may need to reduce use of hyocine patches if being used.

Intrathecal baclofen (ITB)

Baclofen is delivered to the intrathecal space in the spine via an implanted drug pump surgically inserted into the abdomen. The pump is programmable so dose and timing can be preset. Before an ITB pump is inserted, the child is assessed by the multidisciplinary team and clear functional goals are set.

ITB is usually considered for children of GMFCS levels IV–V with generalised spasticity, dystonia or mixed picture, for pain relief, caregiver satisfaction and ease of care. However, in some centres ITB has been successfully used in ambulant patients (GMFCS LEVEL III).

A test dose tends to be given in most centres to determine whether the child will respond positively.

Although more invasive, the advantage of ITB in comparison to oral baclofen is that lower doses of baclofen can be administered directly via the catheter resulting in reduced side effects for the child.

Deep brain stimulation

Deep brain stimulation (BP-DBS) is a surgical procedure in which electrodes are implanted to stimulate parts of the brain to reduce involuntary movements and tremors.

It has been shown to be an effective treatment for primary generalised dystonia. However, the effect of this treatment on secondary dyskinesias such as dystonia–choreoathetosis as seen in cerebral palsy is not as clear. The deep brain stimulators consist of electrodes placed in the basal ganglia. The leads are connected by wire to the main implant near the collar bone or abdomen. A generator inside the implant sends electrical pulses through the leads into the brain.

Outcome is usually measured using a dystonia scale and quality of life measure.

Selective dorsal rhizotomy

SDR tends to be performed at L1–S2. The roots are divided into sensory and motor divisions. The sensory roots are stimulated with electrodes and those roots associated with an abnormal response are divided to reduce the sensitivity of the muscle spindle.

Centres often have strict criteria to ensure correct patient selection.

These include:

- Neuroimaging consistent with periventricular leukomalacia
- Spastic tone rather than dystonic
- Evidence of fair selective muscle control and muscle strength
- Ability to co-operate and follow through with long-term therapy programme post-operatively
- Walking is prime method of mobility.

Focal management of spasticity/dystonia

Botulinum toxin

Botulinum Toxin A is indicated for the treatment of focal spasticity (Delgado et al 2010). There are two preparations available commercially for use in paediatrics (Dysport and Botox).

Botulinum Toxin A is injected into the muscle usually under sedation or whilst using Entonox in the paediatric population. The effects can be seen 12–72 hours postinjection, but are usually maximal around 2–3 weeks postinjection.

The toxin is injected as close as possible to the motor end plate, and internalised into the nerve ending, which inhibits the release of acetylcholine, causing temporary denervation, resulting in reduction of muscle tone in the injected muscle.

Injection of the toxin is recommended to be carried out with the guidance of US or EMG. The child is usually sedated and in some cases injections take place in theatres under a general anaesthetic.

The dose available to use is limited based on patient weight, so it is important to prioritise the muscles that are interfering the most with function. Setting functional goals with the family and members of the local team is essential to ensure optimal choice of muscles.

Phenol injections

Phenol can be injected directly onto the nerve with electrical stimulation to aid guidance. The phenol causes a neurolysis, which causes denervation with a reduction in afferent and efferent impulses. The phenol neurolysis can take 10–60 minutes to occur and can be painful, and is therefore carried out under general anaesthetic (GA). Phenol blocks generally last 3–12 months and are done on superficial nerves, e.g. obturator nerve.

Alcohol injections

Alcohol can be injected into the muscle to cause denervation. They can be painful and are done under GA, and are usually done for larger muscles.

Orthopaedic surgery

This can be either single or multilevel depending on the needs of the child. Surgery can involve soft tissue lengthening, muscle transfer or bony surgery to correct lever arm dysfunction.

Cardiorespiratory management

Background

- The main goal of physiotherapy is to maximise cardiorespiratory function in children by treating or preventing cardiorespiratory problems.
- This is usually achieved by assisting with the removal of tracheobronchial secretions, removing airway obstruction, re-expanding areas of collapsed lung, reducing airway resistance, optimising gas exchange and reducing the effort of breathing in children with respiratory distress (Wallis and Prasad 1999).

Non-intubated children

- Treating sick children can be very challenging at times.
- It may be necessary to use persuasion and distraction with things like games, songs, storybooks and rewards to build rapport and engage the child.
- It may also be appropriate to involve and direct play specialists to help with physiotherapy treatment, if they work on the ward.
- A non-intubated child could be referred to cardiorespiratory physiotherapy for a number of reasons, including:
- Post-surgery: this may range from seemingly simple procedures in patients with or without underlying chronic respiratory disease to major surgery that might also involve the respiratory muscles themselves.
- Acute lung infections in otherwise healthy children or those with underlying chronic respiratory or neurological disease.
- Parapneumonic effusions that require drainage and re-expansion of the resulting collapsed lung.
- Generally, the main problems identified during assessment relate to retention of sputum, loss of lung volume and increased effort of breathing with visible signs of respiratory distress.
- Physiotherapy treatment techniques used to address these problems are similar to those used in adults, but will need to be modified to be effective in children.
- It is important to remember that the diaphragm is the main muscle of respiration in babies and small children and that it has less fatigue-resistant muscle fibres (Type 1) compared with adults (Keens and Lanuzzo 1979).
- In the sicker non-intubated child with respiratory distress, care should be taken to preserve the function of the diaphragm in order to avoid further deterioration and possible intubation.

Breathing exercises

- Deep breaths help to re-expand collapsed areas of lung and assist with secretion clearance by getting air behind sputum.
- As with adults, mobilisation should be used where possible, especially in the low-risk patient (Bourn and Jenkins 1988).

- In older children, this could be achieved by sitting over the edge of the bed, sitting out of bed or going for a walk.
- If mobility is restricted (usually for surgical reasons) things like incentive spirometers could be considered.
- In younger children, active play, depending on age, ability and postoperative restrictions, should be encouraged.
- Alternatively, blowing games with the child sitting upright could be used, e.g.
- Blowing bubbles
- Blowing into cups of liquid (not soapy!) with straws to make bubbles
- Blowing paint around paper with a straw
- Singing songs and getting them to join in
- Reading stories and getting them to join in, particularly stories with huffing and puffing like the well-known story about the 3 little pigs.

Huffing and coughing

- Forced expiration techniques or huffing assists with sputum clearance by moving sputum from the peripheral to the more central airways where it can be cleared with a cough.
- Huffing from mid to low lung volume can be taught to children as young as 3 years of age and is a very effective airway clearance technique (Pryor and Webber 1979, van der Schans, C. P. 1997).
- Some children may have difficulty maintaining an open glottis, if this is the case, a tube like a cardboard peak flow tube may be used.
- It is important to note that young children are unable to cough to command effectively.
- Children are often unable to expectorate and usually swallow their secretions.
- Getting children to laugh is a good way to encourage coughing and can often be achieved by playing games or tickling the child.
- In babies, changing position, like putting them over your shoulder and patting their back or bouncing them up and down on your lap might encourage them to cough.
- If they are able to sit unsupported then playing games and getting them to move about might work.

Manual techniques

- In sicker, less mobile children positioning with percussion, which is rhythmic clapping to the affected areas of lung, is a widely used and well-tolerated technique (Tudehope and Bagley 1980).
- It is often used clinically in non-intubated children.
- The aim of percussion is to loosen bronchial secretions, encouraging the child to cough spontaneously.
- Contraindications to the use of percussion are the same as in adults.
- There are various ways of performing this technique depending on the age of the child.
- In small babies, the smaller Palm Cups® percussors or three fingers with the middle finger raised to overlap the first and third fingers (tenting) can be used.
- In bigger children, the bigger Palm Cups® percussors or a single cupped hand can be used.

- It is advisable to use a thin layer of clothing, towel or blanket to protect the child's skin.

Suction

- In non-intubated children, suction should only be used when secretions cannot be cleared by any other means and when they are clearly detrimental to the child's condition, e.g. obvious signs of respiratory distress, decreased saturations and increasing oxygen requirement.
- Nasopharyngeal suction in side lying with the child restrained is usually the treatment of choice to minimise the risk of vomiting and aspiration.
- If suction is used then it should be performed quickly with the smallest catheter required to be effective and the lowest suction pressure possible.
- Both the child and the parents will need to be given lots of reassurance.
- It is advisable to have supplemental oxygen and resuscitation equipment on hand.
- Remember that it takes time to build up trust with the family and the child, therefore, where possible, continuity of care is important for all involved.

The paediatric intensive care unit (PICU)

- On average, there are nearly 16 500 admissions to PICU in the UK each year.
- Of these, nearly half are children less than 1 year of age.
- About 60% require mechanical ventilation.
- Most children stay in PICU for 2 days or less.
- The main reasons for admission are cardiovascular, respiratory or neurological problems (PICANet 2010).
- The PICU environment can be hugely overwhelming and stressful for those who have not experienced it before.
- There are lots of factors contributing to this (Box 1.1).
- It is important to appreciate that acutely ill children can change very quickly.
- Not only do they have the potential to deteriorate very rapidly, but they also have a tendency to improve rapidly.
- This makes PICU a very challenging and rewarding environment in which to work where excellent clinical reasoning and problem-solving skills are essential.

Box 1.1 Some of the stressful factors associated with PICU

- Stressful environment, lots of flashing lights and noise
- Presence of parents
- Often immediate intervention is required
- PICU is an emotional area
- There are many people involved in the MDT
- It can seem scary
- There is a lot of equipment for a very small child
- The problems are complex
- Decisions have to be made about whether to treat or not

Intubation and ventilation

- Although they can be intubated orally, children often have nasal endotracheal tubes, which are uncuffed.
- Unlike adults, the narrowest part of the upper airway in babies and children is the circular cricoid ring, so a good seal is possible without a cuff.
- Although uncuffed tubes are thought to be less damaging to the tracheal mucosa, if they don't fit well, there is the potential for substantial endotracheal tube leak.
- This can affect accuracy of ventilation delivery, monitoring of the patient (Main et al 2001) and can also complicate physiotherapy, particularly when trying to interpret sounds during auscultation.
- Intubated and ventilated children and infants are particularly vulnerable to respiratory complications.
- They are also frequently pharmacologically sedated and paralysed, which means that they have no cough reflex.
- Secretion clearance can be a problem in these children and regular physiotherapy assessment and treatment is very important.
- Depending on assessment findings, physiotherapy treatments may consist of positioning, manual hyperinflations, saline instillation, chest wall vibrations and suction.
- Contraindications and precautions for the use of these treatment components in children are generally the same as in adults.

Positioning

- There are many reasons for using positioning as part of physiotherapy treatment.
- In terms of respiratory function, the supine position has been shown to have the least advantages (Dean and Ross 1992).
- Prone positioning is thought to have the most advantages (Pryor and Prasad 2008).
- Due to the association of prone positioning with sudden infant death syndrome, it should only be used when the child is being monitored (Southall and Samuels 1992).

Ventilation and perfusion

- In adults, both ventilation and perfusion are preferentially distributed to the dependent lung.
- In order to achieve optimal oxygenation the diseased lung is placed uppermost.
- Children and infants are different in that they ventilate best in the uppermost, non-dependent regions of the lungs (Davies et al 1985), but perfuse the dependent areas of the lungs best, creating a mismatch in ventilation and perfusion (Bhuyan et al 1989).
- To achieve optimal oxygenation, the good lung should be placed uppermost (Heaf et al 1983).
- However, if the physiotherapy goal is to improve ventilation and facilitate secretion clearance of the diseased lung using positioning and postural drainage, the child should spend a proportion of time with the diseased lung uppermost.

- It is important to note that this position may not be tolerated well and oxygen and ventilation settings may need to be adjusted to achieve this goal.
- There is also the risk of rapid deterioration of the child's respiratory status.
- As with all practice, the physiotherapist would have to clinically reason their decision based on the stability, tolerance and therapeutic goals for the individual patient in conjunction with the multidisciplinary team.

Manual hyperinflation (bagging)

- This technique is performed using an open-ended 500 mL bag in infants and smaller children or 1 L bags in older children.
- It usually involves giving a long inspiration with an inspiratory pause followed by rapid release of the bag.
- This is thought to recruit collapsed lung units and increase expiratory flow moving secretions from the peripheral to the more central airways (Maxwell and Ellis 2003).
- Inflation pressures should be monitored using a manometer in the circuit and should not exceed 10 cmH$_2$O above the peak ventilator pressure.

Chest wall vibrations

- Chest wall vibrations are rapid compressions applied to the chest wall at the start of expiration with a continued oscillatory pressure until expiration is complete.
- In intubated infants and children they are usually performed in conjunction with manual hyperinflation.
- Current research in this area has shown that chest wall vibrations have the potential to augment expiratory flow in order to move secretions from the peripheral to the more central airways where they can be cleared by suction (Gregson et al 2007).
- It has been shown that each physiotherapist has their own unique way of performing chest wall vibrations which is highly repeatable within treatments.
- However, there is huge variation between therapists in magnitude and duration of the chest wall vibrations as well as in the amplitude, number and frequency of oscillations within them (Shannon et al 2009).
- In order to be maximally effective and safe, timing between the chest wall vibrations and the manually delivered breaths should be optimal (Shannon et al 2010).

Saline instillation

- Instilling saline into the endotracheal tube of ventilated patients aims to loosen thick or sticky secretions and assist with their removal using suction (Schreuder and Jones 2004).
- Evidence supporting or refuting this practice is variable and conflicting.
- However, many experienced physiotherapists believe saline instillation to be well tolerated and regularly use saline in their treatment of infants and children.
- The reasons for doing this are to assist with secretion clearance and to avoid narrow endotracheal tubes and suction catheters blocking off.

PICU summary

- As with all physiotherapy practice, it is important to remember that constant reassessment and evaluation is necessary throughout physiotherapy treatment of children and infants in intensive care.
- For more detailed information regarding paediatric assessment and treatment, please refer to Pryor and Prasad (2008, chapter 10).

The references for this chapter can be found on www.expertconsult.com.

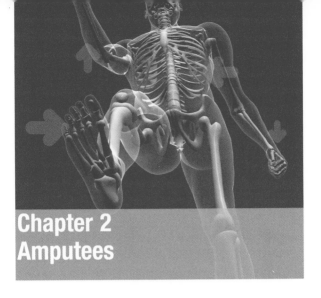

Chapter 2
Amputees

Introduction

- The student or novice physiotherapist may treat the 'primary' and/or the 'established' amputee.

- Where there is no on-site specialist physiotherapist available for supervision and guidance it is important that the therapist knows when, where to seek specialist support, e.g. via a regional prosthetic centre or specialist physiotherapist in the acute setting.

- This volume covers the treatment of the adult amputee with acquired lower limb amputation, with some reference to the adult upper limb amputee.

- Advice on the treatment of the child with acquired amputation or congenital absence should be sought from regional specialist centres.

- Treatment planning requires a holistic, integrated, multidisciplinary approach, enabling effective exchange of information with all involved in the treatment of the patient.

- To encourage patient adherence to rehabilitation, SMART goals for treatment must be agreed initially, between the patient and the team members involved in the patient's management.

- Ongoing evaluation by the physiotherapist (and other team members) of the amputee's ability to achieve treatment goals during the early treatment stage will assist in determining the amputee's suitability for prosthetic referral.

- Physiotherapy treatment is defined by assessment findings. Physical, personal, social and environmental factors will influence the plan and determine how attainable rehabilitation goals will be.

- The amputee and physiotherapist should consider goal setting as something to be done in partnership and the plan should include short and long-term goals.

- The International Classification of Functioning, Disability and Health (WHO 2001) model can assist the evaluation of the assessment findings (Geertzen 2008).
- It is recommended that the 'SOAP' format is used for recording treatment.
- Appendices 2.1 and 2.2 provide additional material for students.

Physiotherapy treatment goals

▲ denotes specific treatment rationale for UL physiotherapy treatment.

The prevention of postoperative complications

- This follows the same principles used for any postsurgical patient and applies to all age groups and causes of amputation.
- The amputee will be an inpatient from 1 week to several weeks, depending on the amputee's health, the service and setting and their home environment circumstances.
- The early postoperative stage is normally within the first week postsurgery.
- The aim within this week is for the patient to progress to attending the therapy gym.
- Routine postoperative chest physiotherapy for all patient groups must be performed, irrespective of anaesthetic procedure
- Bed mobility, e.g. lie to sit, transfers to and from a wheelchair, will facilitate and encourage full lung expansion and prevent the retention of secretions
- Circulation exercises are encouraged to prevent problems such as deep vein thrombosis.
- ▲ Walking as balance allows.

Pain management

Early management

- Pain after amputation is common and to be expected.
- Communication and co-ordination of treatment with other members of the MDT is essential and the timing of physiotherapy treatment must coincide with pain control.
- The physiotherapist should have an understanding of prescribed pain medication and side effects (BNF 2010).
- The amputee experiencing significant postoperative pain will find it difficult to co-operate and engage with physiotherapy treatment, therefore the physiotherapist should provide reassurance and explanation of underlying postoperative pain in the residuum (RLP).
- The patient should be alerted to the possible presence of phantom limb sensation (PLS) which may include phantom limb pain (PLP) (Broomhead et al 2006).
- Information about PLS should be provided by health professionals with appropriate knowledge and training (Mortimer et al 2002).
- It should be explained to the patient that PLS is a normal response and consequence of amputation surgery, which handling, exercise and medication will help to reduce.
- This is important for the safety of the amputee who may sense their amputated limb as being present and could unconsciously attempt to weight bear through it, resulting in a fall.

- Handling the residuum helps to desensitise nerve endings, helps the remodelling of the homunculus and contributes to the amputee's adjustment to their new body image (Ramachandran and Hirstein 1998).

- 'Stump handling' enables the amputee to apply early individual control over the management of their pain and it is important to reassure the amputee that gentle handling will not harm the wound.

- Stump handling along with daily observation is important at all stages of rehabilitation and must become part of normal daily routine for the amputee post discharge to check for skin changes resulting from pathology, prosthetic fit or positioning.

Tip!

Encourage the amputee to look at and handle their residuum as soon as possible post amputation surgery, e.g. first day postoperatively.
Handling takes place over wound dressings.

- Active exercises will encourage resolution of postoperative oedema, which can cause pain.

- Appropriate positioning of the residuum to avoid prolonged and excessive flexion must be emphasised – the patient will instinctively want to flex their residuum if it is painful, therefore maintaining full range and a good resting position is essential and must be reinforced.

Tip!

The physiotherapist must ensure nursing colleagues reinforce effective positioning and handling. A pillow should not be placed under the residuum. The transtibial amputee must use a stump board when in a wheelchair (Figure 2.1).

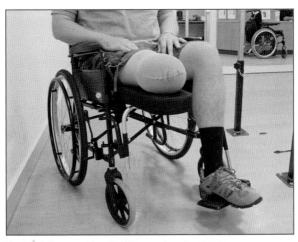

Figure 2.1 Correct position of residuum on stump board.

- Wound healing must be monitored daily by a team member; the physiotherapist should take the opportunity to observe the wound.

Ongoing management

- The amputee may continue to experience either RLP or PLP, or both.
- Where RLP or PLP persists, investigations should be made to identify the cause, e.g. infection, vascular insufficiency, soft tissue injury, referred pain, including joint pain, or breakdown in the myodesis.
- If pain is related to wound breakdown, physiotherapy should be carried out with caution. Exercising may provide some distraction from the pain.
- Where wound healing is compromised and contributing to pain, the use of laser therapy has been reported to be effective (Baxter 1999).
- The physiotherapist must be vigilant in monitoring and evaluating the amputee's pain and communicating this with relevant colleagues, irrespective of the stage of rehabilitation.
- Assessment findings may indicate interventions including:
- Consolidation of residuum handling and desensitisation by the patient, e.g. massaging over stump end or painful area, tapping/percussion, contact with different materials
- Review of medication, e.g. use of tricyclics, antidepressants and anticonvulsants
- Use of graded motor imagery (Butler and Moseley 2003)
- Investigations for referred pain
- Other modalities, e.g. TENS, acupuncture.
- Reference to a 'pain pathway' can facilitate clinical reasoning and support the decision-making processes for a team approach to pain management (Appendix 2.3).
- Progressing with a general exercise programme and use of an early walking aid (EWA) will assist in the management of an amputee's phantom sensation and/or pain (Barnett et al 2009).

Improve functional mobility and balance

Early management

- Where practical, and with MDT collaboration, treatment should be on a daily basis.
- All amputees irrespective of level, age or pathology, should be suitably dressed to participate with physiotherapy, i.e. in day clothes, ideally loose-fitting skirts and trousers with elastic tops, a comfortable and good-fitting sock and shoe with non-slip sole for the single amputee when ready to transfer from bed to wheelchair.

> **Tip!**
>
> Amputees with poor memory or cognitive impairment may respond well to written guidance and/or diagrams for functional activities and exercise, e.g. wheelchair transfers.

- Lie to sit practise will routinely form part of chest treatment and will aid all ADLs.

- Rolling, same rationale as for lie to sit. Incentives for basic functional movements are comfort, preparation for transfers and engaging in active exercises.
- Dynamic sitting balance is essential for transfers, dressing, toileting and ultimately walking, irrespective of level, UL or LL.

Routine balance exercises
- Challenging the amputee to reach outside base of support.
- Rhythmic stabilisations in sitting.
- Rhythmic stabilisations in sitting over the side of the bed/plinth with the remaining foot on the floor. Progress to removing contact with the floor.
- Use of sit-fit cushion, e.g. throwing/catching of ball.
- Core stability exercises.
- ▲ The UL amputee finds dressing difficult and clothes without buttons or zips make this easier.
- ▲ If the UL amputee has had an amputation of their dominant hand functional activities such as dressing, toileting, eating and writing will need to be practised with the remaining limb.
- ▲ Where possible the residual limb should participate in these normal functional activities and a range of devices can assist this, e.g. non-slip mats and a simple gauntlet.
- ▲ The bilateral UL amputee will need specific assistive tools to assist ADLs.
- ▲ A high level or bilateral amputation can affect balance. Balance exercises in sitting, standing and walking should be practised (Figure 2.2).

Wheelchair provision
- Occupational therapists traditionally provide wheelchairs and cushions, in some situations it can be the physiotherapist's responsibility.
- The amputee and/or carer will need to be instructed how to use the wheelchair, including use of brakes and footplates (Broomhead et al 2006).
- All LL amputees, irrespective of age, should be provided with a loan wheelchair on the first day postoperatively.
- A standard 8 L wheelchair (17 inches × 17 inches (43 cms × 43 cms) seat size) is suitable for most adult amputees.
- In some cases a bariatric (heavy-weight) wheelchair is required for the larger amputee.
- Two- to three-inch cushions are standard.

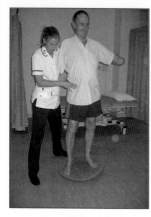

Figure 2.2 Balance exercise for UL amputee.

- Where amputees are at high risk of developing pressure areas a pressure-relieving cushion is necessary.
- Bilateral and bariatric amputees need special assessment and provision.

Transfers

- This is an essential requirement for independence and meeting criteria for prosthetic rehabilitation.
- In some instances amputees will not be able to initiate independent transfers; they may be apprehensive, in discomfort or unable to follow appropriate instructions.
- A manual handling risk assessment should be carried out to identify appropriate assistive devices, e.g. sliding boards, hoists.
- All amputees need to be supervised until assessed as safe to transfer independently.

Tip!

The recommended transfer procedure for a single amputee is the standing pivot:

- Suitable foot wear
- Chair positioned at 90° to the side of the bed/plinth and to the side of remaining leg, brakes applied, footplates positioned away
- Side of wheelchair removed to ease procedure initially and assess amputee's ability
- Amputee places hand flat on seat cushion and transfers partway across
- Amputee then places hand on the side of the wheelchair to enable completion of transfer
- To return, carry out the reverse procedure
- The procedure can be progressed to a transfer without removal of side of wheelchair
- In some instances the amputee may require the use of a sliding board.

> **Tip!**
>
> Some examples of physiotherapy techniques to enable the amputee to transfer include increasing UL strength, e.g. use of push up blocks, balance exercises, core stability and rhythmic stabilisations in sitting.

> **Tip!**
>
> All bilateral amputees should be taught 'sideways' and 'forwards backwards' transfers.
>
> Sideways transfer from bed to wheelchair is often the preferred method of transfer for bilateral transtibial amputees. Procedure:
>
> - Wheelchair is positioned at 90° to the bed
> - Arm rest is removed
> - Sliding board is positioned to facilitate transfer
> - Amputee places hand flat on cushion and transfers across
> - Amputee moves hand across to other wheelchair side to enable completion of transfer
> - To return, carry out the reverse procedure
> - A therapist may be required to stand in front of the wheelchair to offer support and confidence.
>
> 'Forwards backwards' transfer from bed to wheelchair is often the preferred method of transfer for bilateral transfemoral amputees:
>
> - The chair is positioned face on to the bed/plinth, brakes applied
> - The amputee bottom shuffles backwards onto the wheelchair using the arm rests to assist
> - To return, carry out the reverse procedure
> - A therapist may be required to stand behind the wheelchair to provide confidence to the amputee (Figures 2.3 and 2.4).

- All transfer procedures can be applied and progressed in relation to setting, e.g. toilet, car.

> **Tip!**
>
> The younger amputee may express frustration with mobilising in a wheelchair and will want to hop with or without crutches. The physiotherapist must explain the importance of minimising hopping, as this will impact on the resolution of oedema and could increase the risk of falls.

Ongoing functional ability and balance

Core exercises

- Core exercises have an important role in the treatment of all amputees, UL and LL, whether they progress to rehabilitating with a prosthesis or remain as an independent wheelchair user.
- Despite limited research into the benefits of 'core stability' exercises in amputee rehabilitation, it is felt that core stability is essential when using a prosthesis or wheelchair.

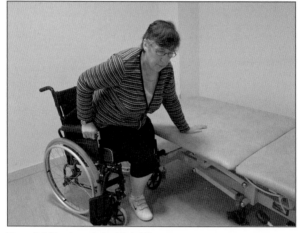

Figure 2.3 Transfemoral wheelchair drill.

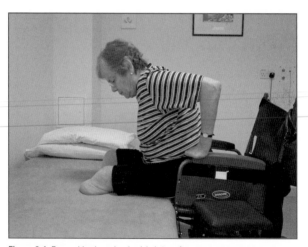

Figure 2.4 Forward backwards wheelchair transfer.

- Progression with these exercises will be dependent on the amputee's cognition, exercise tolerance and ultimate level of activity.
- The independent wheelchair user will benefit from simple mobilising and strengthening exercises (PIRPAG 2005).
- Working closely with OT colleagues, treatment should focus around achieving good dynamic sitting balance to enable independent ADLs and transfers.

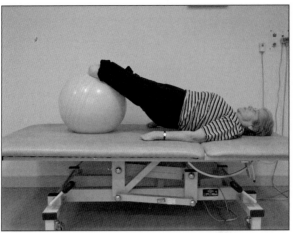

Figure 2.5 Gym ball exercise.

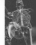

- To progress this, more challenging balance exercises can include:
- Use of the gym ball (Figure 2.5)
- Group games to encourage more dynamic balance reactions, e.g. badminton, indoor bowls
- Use of Nintendo Wii Fit sport, sitting in wheelchair.
- The prospective limb wearer will benefit from all the above and should be further progressed to incorporate treatments that challenge their balance in an ever-decreasing base of support.
- Progression can include:
- 4-point kneeling
- 2-point kneeling
- Rhythmic stabilisations
- Progression with Gym ball
- Use of Nintendo Wii Fit.

Maintain and increase joint range

Early management

- When the amputee is ready to attend the therapy gym, provided it is practical and safe to do so, he/she should be encouraged to make their own way in their wheelchair.

Tip!

Using a wheelchair is an excellent way for the amputee to mobilise and strengthen their arms.

- Active exercises for the remaining and residual limb maintain joint range, improve circulation and wound healing, reduce residual oedema and prevent postoperative complications, e.g. deep vein thrombosis.
- It is important for the amputee to appreciate that the responsibility for practising exercises is theirs for achieving and maintaining functional mobility and independence.
- Frequent exercise practice should be encouraged, i.e. daily exercise sheets designed specifically for the patient can facilitate commitment to exercise.
- The same principles of exercise apply to the UL amputee:
- ▲ Active exercises for the UL amputee should concentrate on all movements of the shoulder joint and shoulder girdle, i.e. elevation, depression, protraction and retraction, as these are important to enable the amputee to operate a prosthesis
- ▲ The bilateral UL amputee may have to use their lower limbs, chin, neck and trunk to perform some ADLs and therefore maximising active ROM of all these joints is essential.
- Use of EWAs is another way to maintain joint mobility.

Tip!

For examples of standardised exercises for lower limb amputees refer to Physiotherapy Inter Regional Prosthetic Audit Group exercises (PIRPAG 2005).

Prevention of contractures

- The promotion of active stretching through positioning and the adaptation of certain exercises will assist in preventing contractures (Figure 2.6).
- Encourage the transfemoral amputee to lie supine each day, to prevent hip flexion and abduction contracture following prolonged sitting or as a consequence of pain.

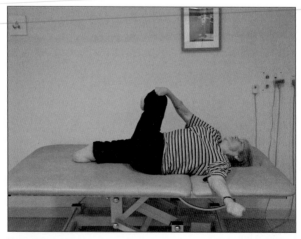

Figure 2.6 Stretches.

- For transtibial amputees the use of a 'stump board' on the wheelchair will help prevent a knee flexion contracture.
- ▲ There is a tendency for the UL amputee to acquire a posture of internal rotation of the glenohumeral joint, cervical lordosis and side flexion to the affected side; trunk side flexion to the affected side with minimal arm swing (of the residuum); and trunk rotation in walking.
- ▲ Encouraging early attention to posture in sitting, standing and walking will help prevent loss of range and contractures.

> **Tip!**
>
> Encourage the UL amputee to regularly move their neck, trunk and both shoulders through available ranges on a daily basis.

Maintenance and increase in muscle strength

- Considerations for progressing exercise will include the level and cause of amputation, PMH, age and goals.
- Exercises should be designed and graded to achieve progression, incorporating strengthening, joint mobility and endurance.
- The amputee needs to have good endurance of both muscles and cardiovascular system in preparation for prosthetic mobility (Waters and Mulroy 2004).
- The older amputee will require an exercise programme of a more repetitive nature, whereas the younger amputee will require greater variation, challenge and resistance training (Velzen et al 2006).

> **Tip!**
>
> Cardiovascular demand will depend on the level of amputation. The physiotherapist must be mindful of the associated risk of resisted exercises with cardiac compromised amputees.

- Techniques and equipment include:
- Manual resistance e.g. PNF, rhythmic stabilisations
- Resistive equipment, e.g. pulley systems, weights, variable resistance equipment such as motomed and Thera-Band (Figure 2.7)
- Progression of resistance to include power and endurance training.

> **Tip!**
>
> The physiotherapist must be aware of the risk of overuse injuries when setting treatment plans.

> **Tip!**
>
> Consider the anatomy of the residuum and the potential for muscle imbalance in relation to surgical technique, e.g. the predisposition for flexion contracture in the knee disarticulation and trans-femoral amputee.
> The hip flexors iliopsoas are not affected surgically.

Mobilisation with early walking aid to prepare for prosthetic mobility

EWAs

- EWAs are examples of specialist equipment and guidelines recommend that therapists should be familiar with their use (BACPAR 2008).

- The use of EWAs as a form of mobility can be indicated as early as 5 to 7 days post-amputation.

- This will enable a LL amputee to stand and mobilise partial weight bearing as part of the assessment and in preparation for prosthetic mobility.

- The physiotherapist introduces sit to stand practice, followed by weight transference in standing, progressing to mobilising.

- Endurance is developed in terms of cardiovascular conditioning and residuum tolerance to weight bearing and pressure.

- In addition to enabling the amputee to prepare for prosthetic mobility, EWAs can provide a psychological boost allowing the amputee to recognise that walking is possible again.

- Early walking is not an activity performed in isolation; it must be combined with other aspects of physiotherapy, e.g. PIRPAG exercises, balance and core work.

- The period of mobilisation using an EWA can be from 1 week post amputation up to an average of 3–4 weeks.

- In some situations this may be prolonged while awaiting referral to the prosthetic centre or while residual oedema slowly resolves and the residuum heals.

The Pneumatic Post Amputation Mobility Aid (PPAM Aid)

- The PPAM Aid is a popular low-cost tool to assist single leg early transtibial, knee disarticulation and transfemoral amputee pre-prosthetic mobility (Figure 2.8).

- It consists of a metal frame (available in four different sizes and heights), an outer and inner pneumatic sleeve/bag.

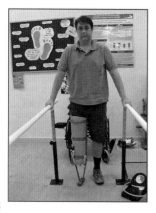

Figure 2.8 PPAM aid.

- There are two outer bags, one for the transtibial and knee disarticulation levels, the other for the transfemoral.
- The stump is suspended through inflation of the bags within the metal frame.
- Inflation must be through a calibrated pump with the outer sleeve being inflated to 40 mmHg to allow partial weight bearing.
- As the amputee walks in the PPAM Aid the pressure increases and decreases alternately, stimulating circulation and oedema resolution.
- Initially amputees may only tolerate sitting in the PPAM Aid for the first session, they should be progressed to daily mobilisation for periods of up to an hour or more at a time.
- It must be remembered the PPAM Aid is a partial weight-bearing device for indoor use and requires the amputee to be supervised as their mobility progresses from the parallel bars to using crutches (Dawson et al 2007).
- There is recent evidence illustrating that mobilising with a PPAM Aid promotes healing in a wound that would otherwise require further surgery, leading to successful prosthetic rehabilitation (Van Ross et al 2009).
- As a matter of course, wounds and residuums should be inspected before and after using the PPAM Aid.
- If soiled during use it must be cleaned after each application and again thoroughly once the amputee starts prosthetic mobility.

Tip!

Cautions with using of the PPAM Aid include:
- Ischaemic wound
- Pain
- Grossly infected wound
- Hip and knee flexion contracture
- Bilateral transfemoral amputee with or without a prosthesis
- Cognitive impairment
- Short transfemoral residuum which prohibits suspension.

- The manufacturer of the PPAM Aid provides additional useful information on their website (www.ortho-europe.com).

The Femurett

- This is an alternative EWA for the transfemoral amputee. It consists of three sized sockets, a thigh component with simple uniaxial knee, a shin tube and a foot (Figure 2.9a, b).
- The lengths of the components and the size of the sockets can be adjusted to suit individuals.
- This is a partial weight-bearing tool for use within a physiotherapy department under supervision only.
- The same principles of progression, wound and residuum care, and equipment management as for the PPAM Aid, apply.
- The manufacturers of the Femurett provide additional useful information on their website (www.ossur.co.uk).

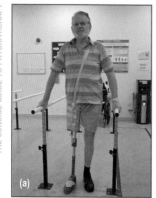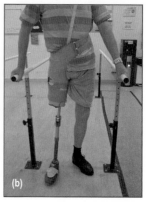

Figure 2.9 (a) Femurett. (b) Femurett with additional suspension from a Tesbelt.

Tip!

Indications for mobilising with the Femurett:

- Used for transfemoral amputees.
- A short and/or flexed transfemoral residuum unable to tolerate the PPAM Aid.
- If an amputee is considered to be 'borderline' with respect to potential for prosthetic mobility, the Femurett can be a useful assessment tool as the construction in terms of weight and socket design bears greater similarities to a basic transfemoral prosthesis than the PPAM Aid.

Tip!

Considerations for the bilateral amputee using an EWA:

- An EWA should not be used for a bilateral primary amputee, unless the amputee was previously a prosthetic user as a single amputee and uses a prosthesis in conjunction with the EWA.
- In the case of a bilateral transfemoral amputee, advice should be sought from a specialist centre with respect to the appropriate use of EWAs.
- To reduce energy expenditure, ease sit to stand and improve balance, it is recommended that the existing prostheses are reduced in height.

Prosthetic referral

- Within the first few weeks post surgery it will become apparent if an amputee is suitable for prosthetic referral.
- Fundamental criteria need to be considered in the decision-making process of whether an amputee will be able to use a prosthesis functionally and safely:
- The residual limb wound must be healing – an unhealed wound may compromise prosthetic prescription
- The amputee must be able to understand and remember instructions – this is an issue of safety

- The amputee must demonstrate independent transfers to and from a wheelchair – reflecting safety and the ability to function independently
- Independent wheelchair mobility indoors – as above
- The amputee must be able to push up from sitting to standing independently within parallel bars and remain standing, using the bars demonstrating strength, endurance and balance
- Wound healing permitting, the patient should be able to mobilise with an EWA – this challenges strength, balance, co-ordination and cardiovascular tolerance.

The non-prosthetic user

- The decision to refer an amputee for prosthetic referral should be made by the MDT in agreement with the amputee.
- The physiotherapist's evaluation of the amputee's ability to achieve treatment goals will influence this decision.
- The decision not to use a prosthesis may be the amputee's own choice, or failure to meet the criteria.
- Not all amputees will proceed to prosthetic rehabilitation, e.g. prosthetic outcomes for older dysvascular amputees are poor (Callaghan and Condie 2004; Cumming et al 2006; Davies and Datta 2003).
- In situations where an amputee does not fully meet the centre's required criteria, but is motivated to walk, a review appointment may be made to reassess potential.
- This agreement should be known to all relevant members of the team and the physiotherapist in the referring team should plan and co-ordinate treatment accordingly.
- For patients not proceeding to prosthetic rehabilitation there must be collaboration with OT colleagues to ensure they become safe and independent wheelchair users within their home setting or identified discharge destination.
- Physiotherapy should include an exercise maintenance programme, e.g. the future potential for a transtibial amputee to achieve prosthetic mobility will be compromised if a knee flexion contracture develops through insufficient rehabilitation; additionally there is the potential for a flexed residiuum of a non-ambulant transtibial amputee to break down due to excessive distal pressure applied via the stump board or bed.
- Discharge planning involves appropriate MDT input during home visits with referral to social services or intermediate care services (ICT) to provide ongoing support as required.
- ▲ The upper limb amputee is likely to be discharged earlier, i.e. within the first week.
- ▲ Referral to the prosthetic centre for assessment must be made in good time.
- ▲ A visit to the centre may or may not include specialist physiotherapist advice about posture management, normal movement and prevention of problems, e.g. overuse of remaining arm, reduced trunk rotation and arm swing, symptoms related to poor body image, lack of confidence and pain.
- ▲ This advice should be provided prior to discharge from the acute setting.
- ▲ Prosthetic rehabilitation focuses on function and cosmetic use involving working between the OT and the physiotherapist to prevent and manage physical limitations.

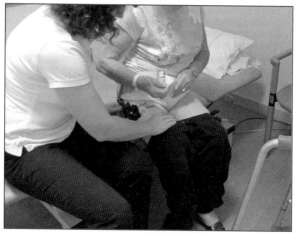

Figure 2.10 Teaching a patient how to donn a prosthesis.

- Modifications to prosthetic suspension should be explored as necessary to aid donning and doffing, e.g. the use of velcro to replace buckles.
- The physiotherapist must explain the correct procedure for donning and doffing, supervising this to ensure the amputee understands how the prosthetic socket and liner fits and when alterations are required to maintain correct fit (Figure 2.10).
- With the exception of the transpelvic and some transfemoral levels, most sockets require a liner of some kind.
- Poor prosthetic fit and/or a poor donning/doffing technique can result in a damaged residuum.
- The amputee must regularly inspect the skin of their residuum.
- To achieve a comfortable and effective prosthetic fit, appropriate use of 'stump socks' is crucial.
- The amputee is given a supply of cotton socks at fitting. These come in varying lengths, widths and thicknesses to suit the individual amputee.
- Amputees must learn to alter the number and/or thickness of socks to ensure the correct prosthetic fit.

Sit to stand, transfers and standing balance

- Physiotherapy concentrates on:
- Upper and lower limb strength
- Balance (Velzen et al 2006)
- Weight transference with manual facilitation and stepping practice (Gailey and Clark 2004).

Walking

- Gait re-education commences within parallel bars progressing to appropriate walking aids, in- and outdoors as relevant.

- The natural progression is through sit to stand, transference of weight through step practice, to walking.
- The physiotherapist should use the skills of close handling, facilitation of weight shift, verbal prompting and biofeedback, e.g. full-length mirror.
- Once the amputee is confident and safe to walk independently within the parallel bars the physiotherapist can begin to observe and analyse the gait pattern to identify existing or potential gait deviations.

Gait analysis

- The physiotherapist uses their skills of observation to identify the cause of any presenting gait deviation. The use of video or access to the facilities of a gait laboratory can assist this.

Potential causes of gait deviation include

The amputee, e.g. physical limitations in strength, joint range of movement, pain.

- Physiotherapy treatment of 'amputee' causes include:
- Strengthening exercises for identified weak muscle groups
- Stretching of flexion contractures
- Exercises to increase joint range of movement
- Balance exercises
- Pain management
- Improving confidence.
- Physiotherapy treatment modalities may include (Gailey et al 2004):
- PNF
- Resisted walking, manually and with use of theraband (Figure 2.11)
- Rhythmic stabilisations
- Weight shifting in all planes

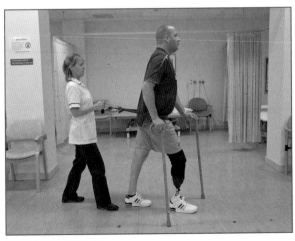

Figure 2.11 Resisted walking.

– Step ups

– Trunk work.

Prosthetic cause of gait deviation

- Accurately assessing a prosthetic cause is a specialist skill; however, there are some broad areas to consider and identify in the overall judgement of the cause of a gait deviation; and this information must be relayed back to the specialist rehabilitation centre for review.

- Potential prosthetic causes may include (Appendices 2.4 and 2.5 for 'prosthetic checkout' procedures):

– Uncomfortable socket fit

– Length discrepancy

– Amputee changes shoes, i.e. heel height impacts alignment

– Incorrect prosthetic alignment

– Poor suspension.

A combination of amputee and prosthetic, e.g. flexion contracture and long prosthesis

- The amputee's past habitual walking pattern, e.g. stooped, toe walkers.

– This is a question to ask of the amputee or a relative, as this is infrequently observed preamputation. Recognition of any habitual gait deviation should be accommodated within both the prosthetic prescription and physiotherapy treatment.

- Uneven timing and/or step length, i.e. commonly a longer prosthetic stride.

– This is the most common gait deviation.

- Circumduction/abducted gait.

– Commonly caused by pain in groin area (transfemoral), a length discrepancy between prosthesis and remaining leg/prostheses, or the transfemoral amputee's inability to hip hitch effectively with a locked knee prosthesis.

- Lateral trunk bend.

– Commonly triggered by removing walking aids too soon in the younger amputee.

- Reduced trunk rotation and arm swing.

- Vaulting.

– Raising of the heel on the contralateral foot, common in transpelvic levels.

- As the amputee gains in confidence and ability through practice within the parallel bars they can progress to the use of walking aids, firstly within the bars and then beyond.

- The support of parallel bars can mask gait deviations and progression to walking aids may demonstrate gait deviations not previously observed. Addressing these will follow the same treatment approach.

Functional walking and activities

- The ultimate goal for the amputee, physiotherapist and OT is using a prosthesis for functional tasks with the prospect of participating in ADLs, social activities, work, hobbies, sport and leisure.

Steps, stairs and kerbs

- Initially for all levels, the amputee will be taught to ascend leading with their non-prosthetic leg and to descend leading with their prosthesis, ascending and descending one step at a time.

Tips!

Some transtibial amputees will eventually manage stairs reciprocally, i.e. leg over leg.

Some transfemoral amputees, if their prosthesis has a yielding prosthetic knee, can be taught to descend reciprocally.

Advice should be sought from specialist centres.

Slopes

- Similar to steps and stairs in that the non-prosthetic leg leads the ascent and vice versa for descent.
- However, some transfemoral amputees will prefer to do this facing sideways, in the same manner as described with non-prosthetic leg leading the ascent etc.

Different surfaces, e.g. carpet, grass, rough ground

- Amputees need to be exposed to different terrains in- and outdoors, incorporating this into treatment sessions.
- Walking outdoors allows the amputee to experience many other factors such as weather conditions, e.g. wind, noise, traffic, crowds.

Cars, public transport, out and about

- Practising transfers in and out of a car, getting on and off a bus, an escalator and a train will be advanced skills but necessary for some amputees.

Home and work environment

- Treatment should include opportunities to walk and perform everyday functional tasks as relevant, e.g. making a meal in the kitchen, working at a desk, gardening.
- The physiotherapist needs to work closely with OT colleagues within the hospital setting or social services and/or ICT.
- The physiotherapist may need to refer to an employment re-ablement officer directly or via OT if the amputee is returning to previous work which is assessed as physically problematic.

Management of falls

- The likelihood of the amputee falling during rehab and at home is high. Studies describe the incidence of amputees falling as 20–53% (BACPAR 2008).
- Many health care organisations have a falls policy and/or advisor who can assist the physiotherapist in assessing and monitoring risk factors.
- Physiotherapy interventions addressing strength, balance, endurance, proprioception, pain and the provision of appropriate walking aids are key in falls prevention. The physiotherapist should also be aware of the influence of medical management, e.g. effects of medications and environmental modifications on falls.

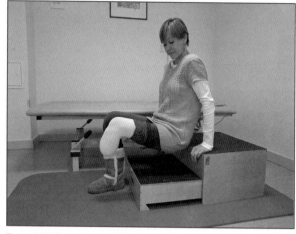

Figure 2.12 Forward and backward chaining.

Teaching the amputee to get on and off the floor safely

- This procedure should be incorporated into treatment sessions.

Forward backward chaining

- Using available equipment the amputee is taught to lower themselves gently from the plinth to a lower surface and then the floor (Figure 2.12).
- To return to the plinth the reverse procedure must be practised.
- This skill can be used by the amputee who needs to ascend and descend stairs at home without a prosthesis.

Kneeling

- Having reached the floor using the chaining method the amputee is shown how to kneel with their prosthesis (transtibials and knee disarticulation amputees can kneel without a prosthesis) followed by positioning themselves in front of a secure surface, e.g. plinth.
- Whilst kneeling through their amputated side they can use their remaining leg to push up and rise from the floor (Figure 2.13).

> **Tip!**
>
> This is the opportunity to discuss with the amputee how this can be managed at home.

Provision of patient information

- The physiotherapist must ensure the amputee understands the reason for their treatment at all stages.

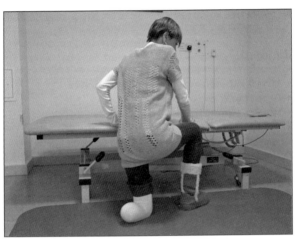

Figure 2.13 Getting up from the floor.

- Some amputees will benefit from written material, e.g. transfer procedure, falls guidance. Relevant information will reassure, encourage understanding and compliance and promote realistic goals.
- Provide information gradually; beware of information overload and raising unrealistic expectations.

Tip!

Many amputees will seek 'information' from the web.
Some information may be misguided and physiotherapists should encourage the amputee to discuss their individual needs when attending their specialist centre.

- Regional prosthetic centres will have written information for the amputee, e.g. introducing the centre, stages of rehabilitation, benefits and entitlements, user support groups (Appendix 2.6), advice on driving.

Roles and responsibilities of the MDT

Medical

- Physiotherapy assessment can help inform medical colleagues with regard to level selection and potential prosthetic outcome.
- There should be communication with the vascular/orthopaedic surgeon regards referral to prosthetic centre, wound healing and commencing EWAs.

Prosthetist

- In prosthetic centres the physiotherapy liaises closely with the prosthetic department around prosthetic fit and comfort, alignment and gait.

- Suggestions for management are:
- Step practice
- Use of mirror/video feedback
- Gradual progression of tolerance to the prosthesis through time, wearing and walking practice to avoid soreness and tissue breakdown
- Resist relinquishing walking aids too early.

The knee disarticulation amputee

- Appropriate for the nonprosthetic user (single or bilateral). Benefits include a whole lap to rest things on in sitting and a weight-bearing residuum which can assist the single amputee with transfers.
- This level is favoured over a transfemoral level in children as the retained epiphyseal plate allows the residuum to continue growing and results in a residumm of good length when the child reaches physical maturity.
- The appearance of a knee disarticulation prosthesis can be poor cosmetically with a longer 'thigh' than the remaining limb and consequently a shorter shin when sitting where the foot may not reach the ground.
- However, as prosthetic componentry advances, appearance and gait outcomes are improving.
- This level retains intact muscle balance, thereby providing a strong lever.
- The ability to prosthetically end bear depends on full hip extension and exercise programmes should reflect this.
- The length and strength of the residuum impacts on gait re-education, i.e prosthetic stride length must be modified to facilitate step through of remaining limb.
- Suggestions for managment:
- Preprosthetically, preparation for loading can start with four- and two-point kneeling and loading through a stool in the parallel bars with decreasing amounts of support
- Attention to stride length
- Biofeedback.

The transfemoral amputee

- A common level for the elderly dysvascular amputee:
- Weak hip extensors and short residuum impact on gait re-education and require the physiotherapist to maximise range of movement and muscle strength
- Energy consumption at this level is high, and therefore exercise tolerance and gaining endurance takes time
- Upper limb strength, hand strength and dexterity influences ability to donn and doff, and sit to stand.
- Prosthetic prescription will influence gait re-education.
- The locked knee gait requires the amputee to control stride length and to learn to hip hitch to avoid circumduction.
- Suggestions for managment:
- PIRPAG hip-hitching exercises in lying and sitting and in standing with facilitation and manual resistance over iliac crest (PIRPAG 2005)
- Biofeedback.

'Free' knee amputee

- The physiotherapist must have a sound understanding of the mechanics of the relevent components, e.g. swing phase is control by alignment, pneumatics or hydraulics (Divers and Scott 2005).
- The inexperienced physiotherapist should liaise directly with the amputee's prosthetic centre.

Transpelvic amputees

- An uncommon level of amputation, with the commonest cause being sarcoma. Consequently prognosis, simultaneous treatment, e.g. chemotherapy/radiotherapy may influence physiotherapy goals.
- The prosthesis for amputees at this level is bulky with three prosthetic joints and no residuum to act as a lever to aid propulsion, momentum and mobility.
- Energy expenditure is high; cadence is slow with vaulting of the remaining leg a common deviation, often unavoidable in the hemipelvectomy amputee.
- Amputees often choose to combine prosthetic mobility with wheelchair and crutches.
- In the early stages of rehabilitation the physiotherapist must liaise closely with the OT around the provision of suitable wheelchair seating.
- Suggestions for management (prosthetic and/or wheelchair user):
- Strength of back extensors and remaining leg
- Core stability
- Pelvic tilting
- Balance
- Strengthening remaining limb
- Sit to stand ability
- Increase endurance.

The bilateral and multiple limb loss amputee

- The main consideration for all levels of bilateral lower limb amputees is to facilitate balance and reduce energy expenditure by lowering their centre of gravity, i.e their height (Uellendahl 2004).
- Physiotherapy must include balance and core exercises with and without the prostheses (Figure 2.15).
- The likelihood of a bilateral amputee reducing from using two walking aids when walking to one is reduced and therefore the abilty for upper limb function will be restricted.
- It is important to consider the level of mobility and function achieved as a single amputee previously, since this will influence goal setting and prosthetic prescription.

The bilateral transtibial amputee

- For the amputee who has both amputations at the same time, the use of EWAs needs to be carefully considered.
- The following recommendations state:
- Application of one PPAM Aid and one prosthesis is an acceptable combination for gait re-education for the bilateral amputee
- A minimum of two staff should be involved with bilateral PPAM Aid use

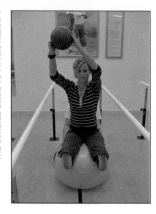

Figure 2.15 Balance exercises for the multiple amputee.

– Standing only with two PPAM Aids should take place in parallel bars (Dawson et al 2007).

The mixed bilateral, e.g. transtibial and transfemoral, amputee

- If the amputee had originally been a single amputee, the use of an existing prosthesis will contribute to gait re-education.
- Ideally the prosthesis should be shortened to facilitate early mobility with the EWA.

The bilateral transfemoral/knee disarticulation amputee

- Short Rocker Pylons or 'stubbies' are used for the bilateral amputee as a method of EWA to assess ability and prosthetic potential.
- The shortened height lowers the centre of gravity assisting stability.
- These are valuable in physically preparing the amputee for articulated prostheses.

Multiple limb loss including upper limb loss

- Priority for rehabilitation may well be the achievement of ADLs and upper limb functional use, with or without an upper limb prosthesis.
- Upper limb ability will assist gait re-education, when this stage is reached.
- Adaptations to walking aids may be required and advice and provision can be sought from the specialist prosthetic centre.

Outcome measures

- Outcome measures can illustrate an amputee's progression towards personal goals.
- There are a growing number of outcome measures and it is often difficult to select which ones to use.
- For the amputee there are validated measures including (Condie et al 2006):
- Activities-specific Balance Confidence Scale – UK (ABC-UK)
- Amputee Mobility Predictor with a prosthesis (AMPPRO) (Gailey et al 2002)

- Houghton Scale of prosthetic use in people with lower-extremity amputations (Devlin et al 2004)
- Locomotor Capabilities Index 5 (LCI-5) (Franchignoni et al 2004)
- The Trinity Amputation and Prosthesis Experience Scales (TAPES) (Gallagher and MacLachan 2004)
- Timed Up and Go test (TUG) (BACPAR 2010).

- There are challenges in measuring outcomes in the acute setting and for the non-prosthetic user. Suggested measures would include COPM (2005) and GAS (Rushton and Miller 2002).

Referral and review of the prosthetic user

- Once initial prosthetic rehabilitation is complete decisions need to be made regarding appropriate onward referral and review.
- The amputee may require further rehabilitation within their home, school environment or work setting.
- Information in the form of a discharge report outlining rehabilitation progress and outcomes must be forwarded to the relevant professionals, e.g. community services, school staff, GP.
- Prosthetic centres arrange routine follow-up appointments where progress, prosthetic mobility, function and outcomes are reviewed.

Support for physiotherapists working in amputee rehabilitation

- Members of the Chartered Society of Physiotherapy (CSP) may join the British Association of Chartered Physiotherapists in Amputee Rehabilitation (BACPAR).
- BACPAR can provide contacts and advice for those working with amputees and aims to promote best practice in the field of amputee and prosthetic rehabilitation for the benefit of patients and the profession.
- It supports the promotion of evidence-based practice and research, is committed to education and providing a network for the dissemination of best practice in pursuit of excellence (www.bacpar.org.uk).
- The network for amputee rehabilitation is hosted on the CSP interactive site (www.interactivecsp.org.uk).

The references for this chapter can be found on www.expertconsult.com.

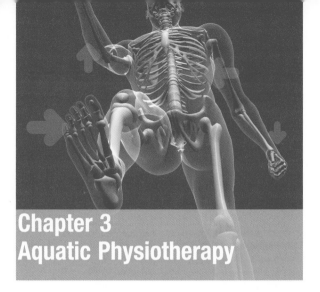

Chapter 3
Aquatic Physiotherapy

Treatment methods

- The physical properties of water covered in the assessment chapter facilitate the application of treatment techniques that can be used to provide therapeutic benefits for patients managed in a pool. Methods of utilising these physical properties of water are as follows.

Uses of buoyancy

- To progressively strengthen concentric muscle actions (assisted – neutral – resisted)
- To resist eccentric muscle actions
- To resist isometric muscle actions
- To assist joint movement
- To assist prolonged muscle stretches
- To provide weight relief
- To assist relaxation
- To assist in the application of the metacentric effect.

Uses of turbulence

- To assist movement.
- To resist isometric muscle action.
- To resist isotonic muscle action.
- To maintain balance.
- To displace balance.
- To restore balance.

- To assist walking.
- To resist walking.

The grading of muscle actions in water

- Muscle strength is graded on land according to the Oxford or Muscle Test Rating scales. In water these scales are modified so that muscle strength can be finely graded utilising hydrodynamic principles. As on land this scale is subjective, especially when there is no 'normal' limb to compare against.

Muscle strength grading in water

Grade 0	No contraction
Grade 1	Assisted by buoyancy
Grade 2−	Buoyancy counterbalanced
Grade 2	Buoyancy counterbalanced with speed
Grade 2+	Against buoyancy
Grade 3	Against buoyancy with small float or with speed
Grade 3+	Against buoyancy with larger float
Grade 4	Against buoyancy unstreamlined
Grade 4+	Against buoyancy with large float with speed
Grade 5	Against buoyancy unstreamlined with maximum speed or with largest float able to be moved

Muscle actions during immersion

Concentric

When considering the effect of buoyancy (alone), on movements at slow speed, the effect is as follows:

Buoyancy assisted   Moving a limb or body part towards the water surface

Buoyancy counterbalanced   Any movement of a limb or body parallel to the water surface

Buoyancy resisted   Movement of a limb or body part downwards against the upward thrust. This resistance can be increased by the use of additional flotation aids, or by lengthening the lever arm.

Eccentric

- These contractions can only be achieved by moving a limb towards the surface at a slower rate than the upthrust effect is trying to produce. Extra flotation aids will be required for effective muscle work due to the close relative density of water and the limb.

Isometric

This type of muscle action can be achieved by:

- Buoyancy   Maintaining the position of a limb or body part against the upthrust forces.
- Metacentre   Holding an adopted position with altered body shape against the rotational forces caused by an imbalance between the forces of buoyancy and gravity.

- Turbulence   Holding the position of a limb or body part against the drag created by an area of turbulence (low pressure water) created by the physiotherapist.
- Drag effect   Holding a posture against the drag effect created when the therapist moves a patient through the water.

The latter two effects can equally be used to promote concentric dynamic muscle action.

Muscle strengthening: using buoyancy, turbulence and the metacentric effect

Buoyancy

Resisted concentric

- The body part is moved away from the water surface – limbs will need a flotation aid due to their higher relative density, e.g. to strengthen the left shoulder adductors a float is held in the left hand. The patient stands, leaning over to their left side with the shoulder immersed. The left arm is pulled down from the surface through the water to come to the patient's side.
- These techniques are generally written as 'buoyancy resisted'.

Resisted eccentric

- The patient has a hand float attached around an ankle and the ankle is allowed to be taken towards the surface, passively flexing the knee. The patient controls the rate of movement of the ankle, so that it rises to the surface at a slower rate than the float is trying to take it. For example, an eccentric quadriceps exercise requires the patient to stand at the pool side with a float round their ankle. They let the knee flex slowly so that the float gradually moves towards the surface.
- These techniques are generally written as 'buoyancy resisted'.

Assisted

- The body part is moved towards the water surface using the assistance from a float (usually a very small one). The speed must be slightly greater than that created by upthrust alone.
- These techniques are generally written as 'buoyancy assisted'.

Counterbalanced

- The body part is moved parallel to the water surface.
- These techniques are generally written as 'buoyancy counterbalanced'.

Utilising turbulence

Therapist created

- The therapist creates an area of fast-moving water to create drag on a body part. The patient resists movement towards this area of low pressure, e.g. to create resistance for the biceps. The patients arm is supported on a float at water surface. The therapist then creates turbulence over the posterior forearm and outwards.
- These techniques are generally written as 'turbulence resisted'.

Patient created

- The patient moves a body part through the water, thus creating an area of low pressure behind the moving part, e.g. to create a strengthening exercise for the shoulder flexors and extensors the patient moves their arm briskly backwards and forwards through the water.
- These techniques are generally written as 'speed resisted'.

Via the 'drag' effect

- The patient is moved through the water while they hold a position against the drag of the water. For example, to strengthen the trunk side flexors the patient is supported supine on floats. The therapist holds the patient either at the ankles or the shoulders and swings them sideways through the water while the patient tries to prevent side flexion.
- These techniques are generally written as 'drag resisted'.

Utilising the metacentric effect

- The patient holds a position against the turning forces created, e.g. patient in supine lying, works against the following movements to prevent the tendency for the body to rotate along its longitudinal axis:
- – Turning the head
- – Taking an arm or leg out to the side
- – Lifting an arm out of the water.
- Patient in standing or in the 'box position' (squatting in the water as if sitting on a chair), supine lying, works against the following movements to prevent the tendency for the body to rotate around its transverse axis:
- – Taking the head forward, backward, or to the side
- – Taking the arms forward or backward
- These techniques are generally written as 'metacentre resisted'.

Physiological considerations

- Comparing oxygen consumption and heart rate responses during exercises performed on land and in the water, both heart rate and oxygen uptake are greater during exercises in water.
- Evidence indicates that viscosity and turbulence provide a greater load during exercise than the resistance of gravity during land exercises.
- Oxygen consumption increases by about ten times over resting values in the water for male subjects performing leg exercises and about seven times for women.
- Arm exercises performed in water require less energy than leg exercises in water.
- However arm exercises require significantly more oxygen when performed in water than the same exercises performed on land (Johnson et al 1977).

Improving range of movement (ROM)

Utilising buoyancy

Buoyancy assisted

- The body part is moved towards the water surface, assisted by a float. This can be done as a contract/relax technique or as a prolonged stretch (Figures 3.1–3.17).
- These techniques are generally written as 'buoyancy assisted'.
- Therapist created turbulence can be added to assist the effect.

The lower limb stretches

- Keep trunk upright allow float to take leg up towards surface of pool (Figure 3.1).

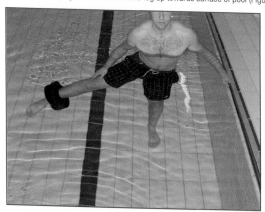

Figure 3.1 Stretch for hip abductors (right illustrated).

- Trunk braced against poolside, patient instructed to hold a lordosis, allow float to take leg up towards surface of the pool (Figure 3.2).

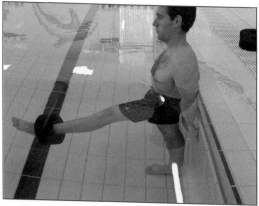

Figure 3.2 Stretch for hamstrings (left illustrated).

- Patient holding onto side of pool (elbows flexed to help keep body upright). Patient flexes left knee and hip to eliminate lumbar hyperextension (Figure 3.3). Allow float to take leg towards surface of pool, patient instructed to keep knee in extension.

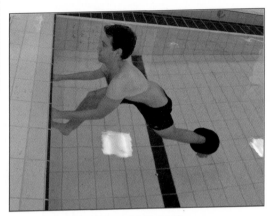

Figure 3.3 Stretch for hip flexors (left illustrated).

- Patient holding side of pool with elbows extended. With left hip and knee flexed, allow float to bring the flexed leg towards pool surface (Figure 3.4).

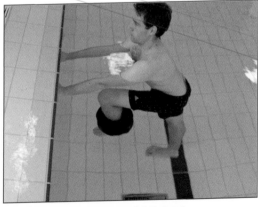

Figure 3.4 Stretch for hip extensors (left illustrated).

- Patient with trunk braced against pool side, right hip flexed to 90°, right hand to fix knee to enable rotation around axis of femur to occur. Allow float to bring the foot up (Figure 3.5).

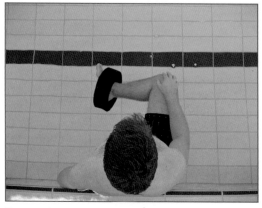

Figure 3.5 Stretch for hip rotators (right lateral rotators illustrated).

- As per stretch for lateral rotators, but with opposite rotation of femur (Figure 3.6).

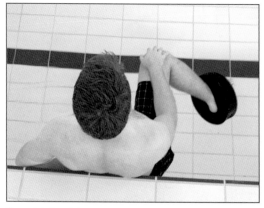

Figure 3.6 Stretch for hip rotators (right medial rotators illustrated).

- Patient holds side of pool to keep trunk upright and thigh in neutral position. Allow float to bring foot up towards pool surface (Figure 3.7).

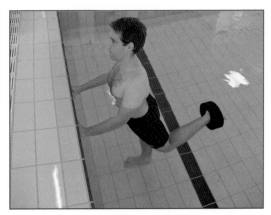

Figure 3.7 Stretch for knee extensors (left illustrated).

- Patient facing pool side with both forearms on rail. Tread on inside of inner surface of ring. Twist knees to R and flex both up the wall to the R so that L thigh is against wall. Both feet and float remain under the knees (Figure 3.8).

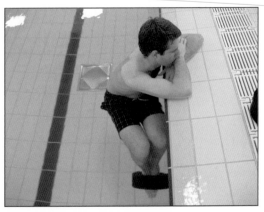

Figure 3.8 Stretch for hip extensors and spinal rotators.

- Patient in standing or sitting on stool, flex hip to 90°. Patient to fix thigh position and allow float to bring foot up to surface of pool (Figure 3.9).

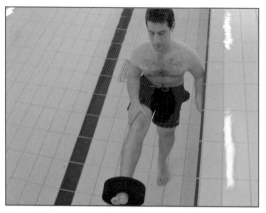

Figure 3.9 Stretch for knee flexors (right illustrated).

- Patient with trunk horizontal to water surface, left hip in 90° flexion, allow float to take foot up to surface of pool (Figure 3.10).

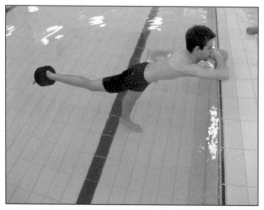

Figure 3.10 Stretch for hip flexors and quadriceps (right illustrated).

The upper limb stretches

- Patient supported by floats in right side lying, facing side of pool. Keeping elbow extended allow wrist float to bring the arm through abduction to surface of pool (Figure 3.11).

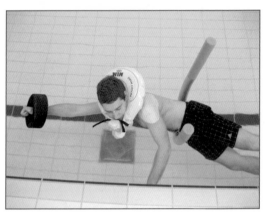

Figure 3.11 Stretch for shoulder adductors (right illustrated).

- Patient with trunk parallel to pool surface with waist float. Keep elbow in extension allow float to bring hand to surface of pool (Figure 3.12).

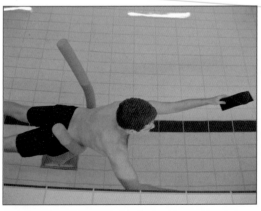

Figure 3.12 Stretch for shoulder to increase flexion (left illustrated).

Trunk stretches
- Patient prone, keeping knees extended allow float to bring legs to surface of pool, producing spine extension (Figure 3.13).

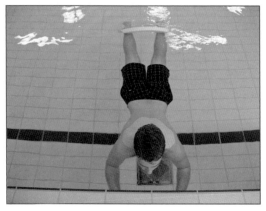

Figure 3.13 Stretch for abdominals.

- Patient to grasp side of pool, keeping shoulders level and thighs against pool side, allow float to bring the legs up towards pool surface (Figure 3.14).

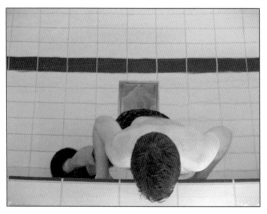

Figure 3.14 Trunk side flexors (left illustrated).

Specific stretches using drag

Muscle group	Starting position
Trunk side flexors	Supine lie
Trunk rotators	Supine lie, therapist adds rotation as the body moves through an arc
Trunk flexors/extensors	Side lie
Hip adductors	Supine lie
Shoulder adductors	Supine lie
Shoulder extensors	Prone or side lie
Pectorals	Standing – walking forwards holding bats in both hands – walking in a circle holding a bat in the hand of the arm to be stretched
Elbow flexors	Standing – walking forwards holding bats in both hands – walking in a circle holding a bat in the hand of the arm to be stretched

Therapeutic methods developed to utilise the properties of water

Other treatment techniques that rely on the use of the physical properties of water include the Bad Ragaz Ring Method, and the Halliwick Concept.

The Bad Ragaz Ring Method (BRRM)

- Bad Ragaz, spa town, Switzerland (BR).
- Ring Method (rings = floats).

Bad Ragaz, background

- In the 1930s, land exercises were applied in water without attention to the properties of water, Dr Knupfer from Germany developed exercises where the physiotherapist acts as a fixed point for movement and the patient is supported in supine lying with pelvic and neck floats.

- During the 1940s and 1950s the polio epidemic in the USA led to the development of the proprioceptive neuromuscular facilitation (PNF) techniques by Knott and Voss in the USA during the 1960s (Voss et al 1985).

- Bad Ragaz techniques were developed through a combination of the earlier German techniques and the PNF techniques in Bad Ragaz, Switzerland, which gives the method its name.

- The most significant developments of the Bad Ragaz Ring Method (BRRM) took place between the early 1960s and 1990. Initially these techniques were developed by Dr Zinn and Nele Ipsen and later by Bridget Davies and Beatrice Egger who published articles outlining the therapeutic processes and the benefits to be gained from this form of therapy (Davies 1967, Zinn 1975, Egger and Zinn 1990).

Features of BRRM

- The method utilises the properties of water of turbulence and streamlining, with buoyancy being used as a support and not as a means of resistance during exercise.
- Turbulence provides resistance due partly to negative pressure behind the moving body i.e. 'negative drag,' resulting from the formation of eddy currents, which impede forward movement.
- Turbulent drag is directly proportional to the speed of movement through water, therefore the faster the patient moves, the greater the resistance. This is controlled by the patient and therefore the method is 'self regulating'.
- It restores anatomical, biomechanical, physiological movements of joints and muscles in functional patterns.
- The therapist is one to one with a patient in the water.

PNF and BRRM

- There are some similarities and some important differences between PNF techniques and BRRM.
- The similarities to PNF are:
- Functional patterns of movement
- Commands are short with as few words being used as possible
- Weak muscles are recruited in patterns by overflow from stronger muscles
- Patterns may be unilateral or bilateral
- Maximal resistance is used.
- Sensory stimulation is maximised.
- Traction and approximation may be applied, but due to the instability of the body in the water this is more difficult than on land.
- The differences to PNF are:
- Resistance is provided principally by the movement of the body through the water causing turbulence together with the directing manual force applied by the physiotherapist.
- Stretch stimulus is not generally possible for facilitation of a muscle contraction because the patient is free floating.
- In BRRM the patient controls the resistance applied by controlling the speed of movement during isotonic patterns. In PNF the therapist applies the resistance according to the patient's ability.
- Generally PNF is open chain and BRRM is closed chain.
- In BRRM the therapist provides the fixed point during isotonic patterns. In PNF the therapist moves with the working part of the patient's body.

Principles of the technique

- The patient's starting position may be supine lying, side lying or prone lying and is varied according to the aim of the exercise and by the position of the limbs.
- Usually the patient floats with a neck collar or floatation helmet and a large body ring or float around the pelvis.
- Smaller floats are attached to the legs and arms as necessary.
- The density of all the floats is varied according to the size and weight of the patient.
- The floats provide support and correct positioning of the patient.

- In order to have control of the patient and to be able to grade the strength of a movement and the resistance given, the physiotherapist must be stable in the water with the patient on a one-to-one basis.

- The therapist must be in walk or stride standing with feet at least shoulder width apart and hips and knees slightly flexed.

- The therapist transfers body weight from one foot to another according to the direction of movement and the specific exercise.

- The water level should be between the waist and axilla of the physiotherapist who may wear special non-slip shoes to provide more friction. The floor of the pool must be even, with non-slip tiles. This enables the physiotherapist to maintain control of the movements.

- The position of physiotherapist hands on the patient influences the stability and direction of movement of the patient and the amount of isotonic or isometric work required.

- If the patient is severely disabled, anxious or afraid of water or has extensive muscle weakness proximal supports are used to increase patient confidence and therapist control.

- Distal supports at the end of a limb or trunk allow for greater range of joint movement and stronger muscle action due to lengthening of the lever.

Aims of treatment with BRRM

- Increase joint range of movement.
- Increase mobility of neural and myofascial tissues.
- Improve muscle function.
- Relieve pain.
- Improve stability of trunk and proximal stability of the limbs.
- Preparation of lower limbs for weight bearing.
- Restoration of normal patterns of movement including co-ordination in upper and lower limbs.
- Restoration of patient's confidence.

Indications for BRRM

- Orthopaedic and rheumatology conditions, e.g. rheumatoid arthritis, spondylosis, osteoarthritis, including pre- and postsurgery, fibromyalgia, ankylosing spondylitis.
- Post fracture, e.g. spine, pelvis and lower limb.
- Soft tissue injuries.
- Thoracic or breast surgery.
- Neurological conditions, e.g. cerebrovascular accident, spinal injury, Parkinson's disease, head injury. Patients exhibiting hypertonicity should be treated by experienced practitioners in order to avoid exacerbating any increase in tone. Rapid and fatiguing activities should be avoided for the same reason.
- Problems associated with learning disabilities.
- Children, particularly those with juvenile idiopathic arthritis.

Contraindications and precautions

- Patients are screened for all contraindications to aquatic physiotherapy.

- Programmes must be planned to avoid fatigue of patients (the freedom of the water may encourage too much activity).
- Patients receive a large amount of vestibular stimulation during treatment (avoid giddiness).
- Caution during treatment for those patients with acute conditions of spine or extremities, due to the possibility of over stretching painful, swollen or hypermobile joints.
- Patients with neurological conditions where active or resisted exercises increase spasticity in the trunk or limbs, or in the presence of hypertonicity.

Application of BRRM techniques

- Teach or show the patient the movement pattern passively on the affected limb to ensure correct movement components or teach on the unaffected stronger limb first.
- Bilateral patterns may be used initially if the patient's balance in water is poor.
- Where there is limited joint range of motion, muscle weakness and pain.
- Limbs, begin with trunk patterns. This is on the basis that the trunk muscles are strong and this utilises the use of overflow into weaker muscle groups or induces movement in areas that may be painful.
- Start with limbs patterns, in order to treat trunk problems, e.g. low back pain.
- Muscle weakness (lower motor neuron pathology), use overflow from stronger muscles.
- Pain, start with isometric patterns. Control range to pain free movement only.
- PNF techniques such as slow reversals (reciprocal patterns), repeated contractions and rhythmical stabilisations may be applied.
- Initially BRRM techniques may form only 5 to 10 minutes of the aquatic physiotherapy session, progressing to 10 to 20 minutes of the total. This will be dependent on the nature of the patient's condition, age and ability to learn and perform the patterns.

Patterns of movement

- The patterns of movement can be divided into lower limb, upper limb and trunk patterns.
- The limb patterns can be unilateral or bilateral.
- They can also be classified as isometric and isotonic in relation to the type of muscle work performed by the target muscle group.
- In isometric movements the patient holds the limbs or trunk in a set pattern while being pushed through the water by the physiotherapist.
- In isotonic movements the patient moves towards or away from the physiotherapist who acts as a fixed point.

Examples of patterns: isotonic muscle work

- Bilateral hip abduction and adduction patterns:
- The patient lies supine with neck and pelvic floats.
- The physiotherapist stands at the patient's feet and places the hands on the lateral side of the feet, particularly the heels.

- The patient abducts both legs and moves through the water towards the physiotherapist, who stands steady and provides the force, against which the patient pushes into abduction. The therapist guides the movement.
- The patient then relaxes, the physiotherapist steps backwards and passively adducts the patient's legs and the movement is repeated.
- Hip extension and medial rotation movements can be added to the abduction movement.
- The pattern is reversed for adduction, with the physiotherapist's hands being placed medially over the patient's heels.
- The patient adducts the legs and moves away from the physiotherapist, who has to step forward and move the patient's legs passively into abduction. The movement is then repeated.
- Hip flexion and lateral rotation movements can be added to the adduction pattern.
- The patterns can be repeated one after the other without a break (PNF slow reversals).
- The physiotherapist remains in one place and transfers body weight from back foot to front foot (abduction pattern) and from front foot to back foot (adduction pattern).

Examples of patterns: isometric muscle work

- Arm abduction patterns
- Bilateral pattern
- The patient abducts both arms in a pain free range and maintains this position as the physiotherapist holds the feet and at the same time pushes the patient through the water, head first.
- Unilateral pattern
- The patient is instructed to hold one arm in abduction and the physiotherapist's hands are placed on the trunk. The patient is moved by the physiotherapist walking in a clockwise direction so that the right arm is working isometrically against the turbulence of the water (Voss et al 1985).

Adaptations of patterns

- Patterns may be adapted by the physiotherapist using therapeutic principles, e.g. one limb can provide stability working isometrically whilst the other limb works isotonically. For example, extension, abduction and medial rotation of one leg working isometrically and flexion, adduction and lateral rotation of the opposite leg working isotonically or upper and lower limbs working simultaneously, one side isometrically and the opposite side isotonically.

Adaptation of patterns to patients

- As a patient improves resistance can be increased by:
- Increasing the speed of the body moving through the water
- Making the body less streamlined e.g. add floats or change the shape of the body
- Moving the physiotherapist's hand position distally i.e. increasing the lever arm
- Using larger and quicker movements
- Using quick reversal and reciprocal patterns, i.e. working into and out of the negative drag effect and cumulative increased turbulent drag

- Changing direction of movement, with the point of fixation being moved in the direction of the movement
- Increasing the repetitions.
- If the patient becomes weaker demand for muscle work can be decreased by:
- Decreasing the speed of the body through the water - less turbulence and therefore less resistance
- Making the body more streamlined
- Moving the manual hold proximally thereby decreasing the leverage
- Movement of the point of fixation in the opposite direction to the movement
- Using slower smaller range movements
- Working in one direction only – so that the there is a work/rest ratio of activity for the patient.

The Halliwick concept

Halliwick background

- The Halliwick concept is an approach to teaching people water activities, with particular focus on those with special needs, to enable them to become safe and independent in water and in some cases swim independently.
- Water happiness is the key to the success of the concept.
- The Halliwick concept was developed by James McMillan in the 1940s at the Halliwick School for Girls with Disabilities in London.
- The concept is now managed by the Halliwick Association of Swimming Therapy (Halliwick AST) (http://www.halliwick.org.uk/).
- The concept has developed internationally and in 1994 the International Halliwick Association (IHA) was formed.
- There is strong emphasis on ability, rather than disability and on the application of the effects of water on the human body.
- The concept uses the term 'swimmer' for the person who is learning and 'instructor' for the helper or teacher.
- There is a one to one ratio of instructor to swimmer until the swimmer has reached a stage of proficiency, e.g. safe independence in water.
- No flotation aids are used, so that the swimmer learns to use the support of the water and the instructor, rather than floats, to facilitate their activities.

Ten Point Programme (TPP)

The concept is based on the application of the TPP.

Mental adjustment

- This is a continuous process from the start of a programme.
- The Swimmer learns to adjust to the effects of turbulence and buoyancy, so that they gain good body control and become safe and water confident.
- The Instructor teaches breathing control, which is essential for safety and progression and this is the first skill that is taught:
- The swimmer is encouraged to breathe out every time the mouth comes into contact with the water.

– First, with the face out of the water, the swimmer blows on to the surface of the water or on a floating object.

– This is repeated with the mouth at water level.

– Then with the mouth under the water (oral breathing, blowing bubbles).

– Followed by the nose submerged (nasal breathing blow bubbles from the nose or hum).

– Progression is made by maintaining rhythmical breathing and controlled bubble blowing when the face is in the water, while performing different activities in different positions.

– Breath holding and over ventilation is avoided at all times.

• Different activities and movements are introduced in order that the swimmer experiences the various ways in which the water affects balance and control of the body. Good mental adjustment results in a happy, relaxed swimmer.

Disengagement

• This is a continuous process.

• A swimmer is encouraged to reduce the reliance on the instructor and become independent in the water.

• At the start, the instructor judges and applies the amount of manual support required for the safety and confidence of the swimmer and this is gradually reduced as the swimmer progresses.

• The process involves turning from facing the instructor, to having the back to the instructor thereby reducing eye to eye contact.

• Instructors can be changed so that the swimmer is moving from parents to others.

• Further progression can be gained by: moving away from the side of the pool, changing from feet on floor to lying back, reducing verbal instructions, independent entry to the pool, introducing basic swimming strokes, changing groups and further social integration.

• Disengagement is necessary as each new skill is learnt. The swimmer begins with full support and this is gradually reduced until, where possible, it is reduced altogether and the swimmer is independent of the instructor.

Transversal rotational control

• This involves movement in the sagittal plane around a transverse axis, e.g. regaining the upright position from the horizontal position and the horizontal position from the upright position. The most advanced form of this is somersaulting.

• Due to the long radius, movement in this plane is difficult to initiate, alter and to stop.

• Changing from supine to the upright position requires flexion of the cervical spine, flexion of the trunk, hips and knees and balance of the head over the body to regain and maintain the vertical position. Swimmers with hydrocephalus and spina bifida have particular difficulties achieving this.

• Changing from the upright to supine requires some extension of the cervical spine, trunk, hips and knees.

Sagittal rotational control

• This involves movement in the transverse plane around a sagittal axis, i.e. any activity which involves trunk side flexion such as side stepping.

- It may be the upper trunk or the lower limbs moving side to side and can be performed in the upright or horizontal positions.
- The whole body may move, e.g. the instructor moves the swimmer side to side at the waist. These movements are helpful in gaining relaxation, which in turn promotes confidence and mental adjustment.
- Application to functional activities occurs when the swimmer is in a wheelchair for example, retrieving objects from the floor.
- The rotation is a useful activity for releasing tightness on one side of the trunk and also for actively working trunk side flexors.

Longitudinal rotational control

- This involves movement round a longitudinal axis, i.e. any activity that involves rolling over.
- It may occur in two positions, when the patient is standing movement can occur around a vertical axis and when they are lying a movement can occur around a horizontal axis.
- Due to the short radius it is easy to initiate and difficult to control.
- The swimmer may initiate this movement by turning the head or by positioning the arm or leg across the body in the direction of movement.
- As the body is asymmetrical rotation may occur naturally.
- Asymmetry may occur due to alteration of body density or shape, e.g. following stroke or head injury.
- Importantly the swimmer must learn to control this rotation in order to become confident balancing in the water when it becomes 'choppy' due to the turbulence created by other people moving around.
- The radius can be increased, e.g. by spreading the arms sideways, to increase the stability around the axis in early stages.
- As a progression the swimmer should be able to control the rotation with a short radius.
- This rotation works the rotator muscles of the trunk, upper and lower limbs and is useful for trunk mobilising with patients with Parkinson's disease.

Combined rotational control

- This is the ability to produce or control any combination of rotations executed in one movement.
- This is necessary for the patient to be able to achieve the upright position from the horizontal prone position and from an independent entry to a pool so that they can achieve a safe breathing position.
- On reaching the side of the pool in a supine position the swimmer reaches over to grasp the pool rail, turns to the vertical and is safe.
- If a swimmer falls forward in trying to get the feet off the floor then turning the head to look at the Instructor facilitates this control and ensures safety.
- Mastery of this rotation means that the swimmer can control their position and is therefore safe in water.
- Inhibition of unwanted rotational movements may be necessary to remain in a safe breathing position.

Upthrust

- This involves developing the swimmer's awareness of the effects of buoyancy and in learning that the water always pushes upwards.

- It may be introduced by demonstrating that when a low density ball is pushed under the water and then released it bobs up to the surface.
- The swimmer can appreciate the force when attempting to crawl on the pool floor. A few people are natural sinkers and must learn to push up from the floor of the pool.
- Advanced level of breathing control is necessary, it is essential that bubbles can be seen leaving a swimmer's mouth and nose during submersion.
- As the swimmer progresses, particularly with breathing control, submersion activities facilitate an understanding of upthrust and assist the swimmer to overcome the fear of water.
- The activity is useful for swimmers requiring improved respiratory control.

Balance in stillness

- This involves teaching the swimmer to maintain a relaxed body position while floating e.g. lying on the back while the water is moving and tending to turn the body.
- By experimenting with different body shapes the swimmer learns to float in a position that is stable and is a safe breathing position.
- This requires the swimmer to make constant controlled adjustments to keep the body balanced.
- Everybody has a balanced position in water in which the body can float, but this is not necessarily horizontal.
- The swimmer may start to learn this by 'sitting in a chair' (chair position) and the Instructor creates turbulence at the front, sides, and back. Ideally the swimmer starts in still water and progresses to turbulent water.

Turbulent gliding

- This teaches the swimmer to control the body position in lying while being moved through the water by the instructor.
- The instructor creates turbulence under the swimmer's shoulders and the swimmer's body is pulled along by the turbulence as the instructor walks backwards.
- There is no touch contact between the swimmer and instructor.
- The swimmer is not involved in the creation of movement through the water, but must control any tendency to roll.
- This is likened to ducklings floating along in the turbulence created by the mother.

Simple progression, basic swimming stroke

- This is the beginning of the progression to moving independently through the water.
- The first simple propulsive movements made by the swimmer are usually elementary movements of the hands close to the body in supine at the centre of balance, sculling actions or side clapping movements. If the hands do not produce the propulsion then leg or shoulder movements may be used.
- When balance and co-ordination have developed this should enable the swimmer to combine both arm and leg movements.
- Further progression is to try swimming strokes, often modified arm backstroke.
- In this stroke both arms are taken low and wide over the water (if too high the body sinks) to enter at '10 to 2' in relation to the head at being at '12 o'clock'.

- The hands are then pulled slowly through the water to the side of the body.
- During the resultant gliding action arm movements are stopped.
- Leg action can be added if appropriate; however, only 73% of swimmers with physical disability can use only the arms.
- Bilateral movements avoid lateral instability and the supine position allows easy breathing.
- This stroke is useful for many swimmers, but any stroke that can be adapted to suit individual needs is suitable.
- The ten point programme takes the swimmer to a basic stroke only and is the starting point for other swimming strokes.
- The programme gives a logical order for teaching and all points must be mastered to produce a safe and independent swimmer

Summary of benefits of the use of the Halliwick concept

- The concept enables people with disabilities to acquire the skills of the ten point programme by working with one instructor at a time.
- Some swimmers go on to be entirely independent in the water; however, others need instructor support all of the time.
- In clubs the Halliwick philosophy is to encourage siblings who may be able bodied to join in the activities and for parents to act as instructors. This encourages family activity and social interaction.
- In addition to the benefits from the activities outlined the Halliwick concept swimmers experience the general effects of water immersion and exercise such as increased function of the cardiovascular, respiratory, renal and immune systems. Mobility, muscle strength, stretching, pain relief and gait activities, e.g. walking across the width of the pool while blowing a sponge or ball combines gait and breathing control.

Group work in aquatic physiotherapy

- Aquatic physiotherapy provides the physiotherapist with a variety of ways in which they can treat patients.
- Patients can be treated individually in a pool on a one to one basis, while others may enter the pool as part of a group.
- Patients may be treated as a group even with different conditions and individual treatment programmes.
- Where patients have the same condition it is possible to include them in a group class, where they will have the opportunity to share their individual experiences with other patients who can be sympathetic and tend to have a high degree of empathy.
- Group work can engender comradeship, which can be used in a positive way to motivate patients to work hard at their exercises.
- Groups may interact socially and sometimes appropriate levels of competition can be introduced to assist them to achieve their rehabilitation goals.

An example of group interaction

Total knee arthroplasty class

- Each patient would be referred into the pool because they are struggling with some aspect of rehabilitation.
- There are identified problems of achieving either desired knee flexion or extension.

- The patients have been given a programme of exercises to increase the range of motion, strength, core strength and exercise tolerance.
- Each patient will have their range of motion measured and they will tend to compare the amount of improvement with other group members.
- The patients will tend to be motivated to work harder by each other (external motivation), whereas patients that have individual programmes have to motivate themselves (internal motivation) to achieve progress through exercising.

Clinical examples of the application of aquatic physiotherapy

- The following case studies show how physiotherapists can use a range of treatment techniques that can be tailored to a variety of patient presentations.
- These case studies are based around 'real life' reports by experienced aquatic physiotherapists based in different units around the UK .

Case study: acute back pain

- Background
- The patient was 3 weeks postpartum and had suffered from severe right sacroiliac joint (SIJ) pain in the final weeks of her pregnancy.
- She was still experiencing severe levels of pain (VAS 10/10) and could only walk with crutches.
- The patient had been referred for outpatient physiotherapy; however, the therapist had been unable to palpate her spine due to the intensity of her pain.
- SIJ disruption was diagnosed by an extended scope physiotherapist (ESP).
- Electrotherapy modalities (Interferential therapy, TENS, acupuncture) were tried to reduce pain, with no benefit being gained.
- The ESP felt that Maitland's joint mobilisations were indicated, but not possible at present.
- The benefits of trying aquatic physiotherapy were discussed by the ESP and the pool therapist and it was agreed to try this as a means of mobilising the SIJ.
- Treatment outline
- Session 1
a The patient was placed in supine floating for 20 minutes to facilitate general relaxation and to allow gentle movement of the spine via the movement of water.
b 'Sea weeding' (dragging through the water while keeping a steady side to side movement) from shoulders was used by the physiotherapist to encourage movement with minimal pain.
- Session 2
a Supine floating (10 minutes) was repeated, in addition to sea-weeding from both legs and sea-weeding from the right leg only to enable mobilisation of the right SIJ.
b Standing in deep water with gentle leg swings (alternate legs) was used to encourage active movement, with minimal weight bearing.
c Supine floating with active alternate and bilateral leg abductions was also included into treatment during the session.

- Session 3

a The patient reported an improvement in pain levels (VAS 7/10). Treatment was repeated as per session 2 with the addition of a passive left rotation stretch being performed by the physiotherapist to the point of discomfort. Following this the patient was found to be sufficiently relaxed to enable joint mobilisation to be performed in the water.

b Buoyancy-assisted rotations to the left were taught and the patient was passed back to the outpatient therapist to be taught stabilising exercises and self mobilisations.

- Postscript

a The patient called 2 days later and reported that her pain was much better (VAS 1/10).

b She reported that she no longer needed the support of the crutches and she was continuing the exercises as these were continuing to help.

c The patient also said that she was convinced that without the aquatic physiotherapy she would have been suffering her symptoms for a much longer period.

Case study: cerebral palsy

- Background

- 'Jason' a 17-year-old boy with cerebral palsy, who can walk unaided for short distances.

- His condition has resulted in him having a spine that is side flexed to the left all the time, and he walks with flexed knees with hardly any hip movement.

- On his initial assessment it was agreed with his parents that aquatic physiotherapy would provide the best options for improving Jason's flexibility and strength.

- Jason liked the water, and it was agreed that Jason would attend with either his parents or a carer, so that the physiotherapists could work with them to take over his treatment in the longer term.

- Treatment outline

- Early sessions

a Early treatment concentrated on stretching out the tight left side.

b Using the warmth of the water made this goal easier to achieve as it facilitates a lowering of high muscle tone and in addition enables patients to relax.

c The physiotherapist used sweeping, taking Jason through the water to stretch the left side using the resistance of the water.

d Buoyancy was used with Jason being placed in left side lying the movement of his lower body and legs towards the surface producing a stretch in the tight left side.

e The stretching proved helpful, and similar techniques and stretches also helped to improve mobility in his hips and tight hamstrings.

- Later sessions

a Once Jason was more flexible the physiotherapists concentrated on improving his balance by getting him to stay still while the water was swept around him.

b   To improve his muscle tone techniques such as rolling and correcting his
    position, tipping side to side and stopping the movement part way through
    were incorporated into his treatment.

–   Postscript

a   Jason regularly goes swimming with his parents or carers.

b   They and Jason all report that he is much more flexible and has much
    improved balance. He has also noted improvements in his walking abilities and
    his levels of stamina have markedly improved.

Case study: pain management

•   Background

–   A 29-year-old female police officer was referred for physiotherapy following an
    injury sustained during a violent arrest.

–   She initially complained of neck pain, back pain and right hip pain.

–   She was referred for aquatic physiotherapy after an initial assessment in
    outpatients.

–   The aims of aquatic physiotherapy were to decrease her pain, increase her
    range of movement in her lumbar spine, thoracic spine, cervical spine and
    right hip as well as regaining strength in her core and lower limbs.

–   'Sally' was very low in mood when she started aquatic physiotherapy as she
    was keen to get better quickly and return to work.

–   She had been carrying out the advice she had been given on dry land, but had
    completed her programme vigorously in the belief she would get better quicker
    and had made her symptoms worse.

•   Treatment outline

–   Early sessions

a   Sally was introduced to the pool and a gentle range of motion programme was
    commenced with an element of relaxation carried out by floating her supine in
    the pool.

b   She responded well to the graded movement programme, initially regaining
    confidence in trying to move her right hip.

c   This was carried out over a 3-week period.

d   After gaining confidence in the pool, strength work for the trunk and lower
    limbs was introduced. This consisted of using buoyancy-resisted exercises and
    drag to increase strength.

e   Trunk flexion and extension was maintained by carrying out movements holding
    onto the rail at the pool side.

f   At this time Sally complained of a particular tender spot around her right
    scapula, therefore as part of the holistic approach to her treatment she
    received trigger point acupuncture on dry land to release the tight muscles
    identified around her shoulder girdle. This treatment enabled Sally to continue
    with the exercises in the pool.

g   She continued to improve her lower limb strength and core stability over a
    period of 7 weeks.

–   Later sessions

a   She completed an initial course of aquatic physiotherapy and asked
    for a review on dry land in order to gain advice about returning
    to work.

b Sally was still struggling to manage pain so she was referred to a pain management group. She commenced a pain management programme in the aquatic physiotherapy pool while completing a course of acupuncture.

c Gua Sha and cupping on dry land was introduced to help relieve tight trigger points and promote some relaxation and well being.

d The aquatic physiotherapy programme ran for 10 weeks, consisting of a graded programme of exercises aimed at maintaining range of movement, building strength, promoting the ability of the patients to relax and improve their well being.

e The programme commenced with trunk movements of flexion, extension, trunk side flexion and rotation. Lower limb hip flexion and abduction movements were included and calf raises and squats were included to promote range of movement and the muscle activity associated with the movements. The exercises were commenced with 6 repetitions initially, increasing to 12.

f All movements were performed without pain and as soon as the patients could complete 12 repetitions comfortably buoyancy aids were introduced to make each task a little harder.

g Side flexion was carried out with blocks in hands to facilitate stretching. Hip flexion and abduction was carried out using either an arm band or a woggle.

h Core strengthening was introduced by pushing and pulling a kick board back and forth or cycling in the corner of the pool.

i The patient practised gait exercises in the pool walking tall initially, then walking and pushing buoyancy aids in front to provide resistance.

– Post Script

a Sally was able to complete the programme and has managed to return to work on a phased return programme.

b She is currently working on her strength and endurance in order to return to beat duties. Her pain is controlled; she feels more positive in her attitude and is planning to apply for specialist training that could lead to promotion in the coming year.

Case study: ankylosing spondylitis

• Background

– 'John', a 19-year-old boy with AS, was diagnosed two years ago and had been attending the local National Ankylosing Spondylitis Society (NASS) group on a weekly basis.

– He is a builder by trade.

– He was experiencing an acute flare-up of the condition in his left hip, which caused him severe pain and had consequently forced him to take time off work. This he did reluctantly as he works as a self-employed builder.

– When he woke up in the mornings he was experiencing prolonged stiffness, finding it difficult to move.

– It was taking him half an hour to get ready in the morning and he could walk only with the assistance of two elbow crutches.

– He felt mornings were made easier by having a hot shower and doing some gentle exercises.

- Due to the enforced inactivity, other joints started to stiffen up as well and his posture began to take on an increasing stoop.

- He was sleeping badly at night, on average for 2 hours and tended to doze off during the day, lying slouched on a settee, watching television.

- On his initial assessment the Bath Ankylosing Spondylitis Metrology Index score was 4/10, where previously it had been between 1 and 2 (Jenkinson et al 1994).

- Treatment outline

- Early sessions

a During the first aquatic physiotherapy session John carried out walking, moving up and down the pool in the deep end up and down in the deep end of the pool.

b Subsequently his whole body was immersed in water, which helped to ease the pain and to relax his muscles. The physiotherapist also carried out some 'sea weeding' and in addition whilst John was floating on his back, supported by floats, the physiotherapist walked backwards and moved John's body gently from side to side through the water, using the drag effect.

c This resulted in a gentle stretch of his trunk side flexors and generally aided his relaxation. That night he slept a lot better and undisturbed for 6 hours.

d In the next few sessions, John also did some gentle buoyancy-assisted stretches for his hamstrings and quads, using a small float on his foot.

e He also performed some hip abduction and adduction, with neutral buoyancy whilst floating supported by floats in supine.

f John had progressed from using crutches to walking with one stick held in the opposite hand to his symptomatic hip.

- Later sessions

a As he started to feel better, he was able to introduce some water aerobics, i.e.: jogging and jumping in the deep end, with the full support of the water, so that it didn't aggravate his joints. Whilst jumping he moved his legs apart and together, gradually increasing the mobility of his hip abduction.

b On his last session he used larger floats for the stretches, added a stretch for the hip adductors and also did some buoyancy-resisted exercises.

c While he was lying on his back, he pushed a ring (around his ankle) down against the buoyancy of the water, working the hip extensors concentrically down into the pool and eccentrically as the leg raised up from the bottom of the pool with buoyancy. He performed this exercise with his trunk in an extended position in order to counteract the stooping posture.

d By that time he was quite comfortable doing his walking in the shallow end and he was able to do this in a backward and sideways direction as well.

- Postscript

a When he was measured again, his BASMI showed improvement at 2.5, not quite back to where it used to be.

b Pain was greatly reduced and he had given up the use of walking aids as he no longer felt the need for the support.

c He was planning to return to work in the short term and had rejoined the local NASS group. Initially taking part in the aquatic physiotherapy class, then after another month he joined in with the dry land sessions as well.

The references for this chapter can be found on www.expertconsult.com.

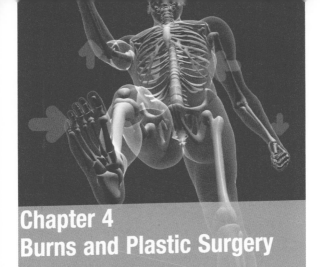

Chapter 4
Burns and Plastic Surgery

Introduction

- Early intervention of therapy is imperative for a successful outcome in burns management.
- From admission, splinting, positioning and exercises all become part of the patient's daily routine.
- The patient and team commitment to treatment and restoration of function is vital in order to achieve good outcomes.
- Careful consideration of the care, rehabilitation and management of multiple problems in this group is needed by a multidisciplinary team.
- A clear insight into the reasoning processes that enable treatment progression and decision making is vital.
- The ultimate goal is to assist the patient to return to their preinjury status, or as near as possible, physically, psychologically and functionally to this.

The burns team

- The team consists of a number of dedicated professionals, who have a variety of roles in the management of a burns patient (Table 4.1).
- The roles of the team will overlap and merge in units around the country; they have been listed above to provide an indication of the variety and diversity of skills needed by each professional.
- For the purposes of this volume, treatment has been divided into pre- and post-healing stages.

Table 4.1 The burns management team

Surgeons	Psychologist
Burn resuscitation Wound care Debridement and grafting Nutrition Prescription of medication	Psychological support
Nurses	**Physiotherapist**
Wound care and dressings Administering of medication Fluid monitoring Emotional support	Respiratory treatment Maintain joint range Prevent contractures Increase muscle power and function Mobility
Dietician	**Occupational therapist**
Nutrition Swallow assessments	Scar management Prevent contractures Emotional support Discharge planning Functional restoration
Social worker	
Discharge planning Psychosocial needs Assistance with financial claims	

Pre-healing stage

Acute medical management

- This will include pain management encompassing sedation if necessary, giving humidified oxygen, maybe via continuous positive airways pressure (CPAP) or intermittent positive pressure ventilation (IPPV) to maintain gas exchange, fluid resuscitation, feeding (possibly via nasogastric (NG) tube), dressings, excision and grafting.

Respiratory physiotherapy treatment

- Standard respiratory physiotherapy assessment and treatment techniques apply, but there will be a few key differences.
- The effect of smoke inhalation and thermal injury has been covered in Volume 1 of this book.
- Inhaled smoke will affect the respiratory function of patients.
- They may not initially present with any signs of underlying respiratory damage; however, they can deteriorate rapidly and may need admitting to an Intensive Care Unit at short notice.
- The therapist must be mindful of the patient's pain levels and especially of the location of the burns when performing manual treatments.
- Graft sites must not be disturbed for at least 5 days postoperatively, to avoid shearing, although respiratory problems will take precedence over the burns as they are more likely to become life-threatening.

Aims of physiotherapy treatment

- Maintenance of the airway.
- Removal of secretions.
- Improvement of gaseous exchange.
- Prevention of atelectasis.
- Maintenance of thoracic expansion and general mobility (Keilty 1993).

Intubation

- This may be necessary, especially if the patient is suffering from facial or neck burns, with accompanying oedema, or poor blood gases.
- Intubation can be by endotracheal tube, or tracheostomy, and can allow mechanical ventilation to be used.
- IPPV is required in patients with respiratory failure, with this being indicated by:
- Hypoxaemia (paO_2 less than 8 kPa with an inspired oxygen concentration of 50%)
- CO_2 above 7.5 kPa and rising
- Falling pH
- Increasing respiratory rate
- Increasing pulse
- Cyanosis
- Exhaustion of the patient, and an inability to cough effectively
- The patient is sedated
- Pulmonary oedema.
- It is not the aim of this book to cover all respiratory treatments; however, the following treatments may be encountered in addition to ventilation:
- The use of intermittent positive pressure breathing (IPPB) or CPAP may be sufficient, although facial burns would preclude the use of a face mask
- Oxygen should be humidified and saline nebulisers may also be needed to improve dehydration in the airways, and assist secretion removal (Keilty 1993)
- Postural drainage is contraindicated in the presence of facial oedema so treatment may need to be modified to positioning patients on their side and regular turning carried out
- Suction must be gentle and minimal, and preferably only on intubated patients due to the damage to the nasal mucosa
- Manual hyperinflation may be necessary if the patient is ventilated (Harvey-Kemble and Lamb 1987)
- Vibrations and shaking are contraindicated if there are graft sites on or near the chest wall, due to the risk of shearing
- Patients will need regular monitoring of the blood gases, for signs of respiratory and metabolic acidosis, i.e. 'burns shock'
- Constant monitoring of the respiratory system is necessary especially during treatment sessions, as these patients tend to be very unstable due to the major fluid changes they are experiencing
- For example, the cardiac output can fall quickly during position changes, so must also be monitored closely

- The burns patient is also at risk of developing adult respiratory distress syndrome (ARDS), with reduced lung compliance and associated raised airway pressures
- This is caused by persistent pulmonary oedema, the formation of hyaline membrane and ultimately interstitial pulmonary fibrosis
- Regular chest X-rays and blood gases will help the team identify any developing complications
- Treatment will need to be applied little and often, to avoid fatigue
- Burns patients can deteriorate quickly, particularly during the first week, and after recurrent surgical interventions
- Even if there do not appear to be any chest complications the patient will need daily reassessment by a respiratory or burns physiotherapist.

Flaps and grafts

- Early excision and grafting is preferable for a number of reasons:
- Increased rate of healing
- Decreased mortality
- Prevention of ischaemic compression
- Decreased risk of wound infection
- Decreased energy demand for healing
- Decreased length of hospital stay.
- Skin grafts are used to facilitate healing in deep dermal or full-thickness burns.
- The most commonly used graft is a split-thickness graft (SSG), which contains a variable portion of the dermis.
- Burns are first debrided to a viable capillary bed; the donor skin is harvested and moved to cover burnt areas.
- The donor site will heal in 10–14 days; however, this can be very painful initially.
- A skin graft may be meshed to provide coverage of a greater surface area at the recipient site. The spaces between the meshing allow bacteria and fluid to drain.
- The appearance of the mesh will remain long term, which may influence the choice of graft used in cosmetically sensitive areas.
- Different types of split skin grafts:
- Autograft, uses the patient's own skin to provide permanent skin cover. Skin, however, may be limited in large burns and re-harvesting of donor skin may be necessary.
- Allografts or homografts use donor skin from another person. These grafts will not take in the long term. They are used to provide a temporary cover for 2–3 weeks to reduce pain, fluid loss and infection.
- Xenografts or heterografts involve the use of pig skin and can be used as a temporary dressing.
- Cultured skin and synthetic skin is a growing area of development. New grafts include cultured epithelial autograft (CEA), which uses skin cells from the burns patient to grow new cells in the laboratory. Other products include Integra that contains animal products with silicone to provide a permanent dermal substitute.

- A skin flap composed of skin and subcutaneous tissue with its own blood supply, may be required to cover exposed bone, tendon or joints, as a skin graft would not take, due to the poor underlying blood supply.
- Grafts and flaps over joints need to be immobilised with dressings and splints until the doctors are happy the skin graft has taken.
- At this point therapy can begin to manage the joint range.

Positioning

- This is fundamental for successful burns rehabilitation, in order to minimise chest complications and pressure areas, to enable wound care and healing, to decrease oedema and maintain tissues in an elongated state to prevent contractures.
- The areas of the body most likely to contract are the neck, axillas, elbows, thumb and finger web spaces, knees, ankles.
- If possible the patient should be turned regularly in the bed, and nursed on a pressure care mattress.
- Once they are out of the acute phase, they should be encouraged to sit out of bed for periods during the day.
- Patients with burns to the anterior neck should be nursed without pillows to prevent early contractures developing.
- Oedema will develop within a few hours of the burn injury and peaks at approximately 36 hours; therefore, consider elevation of the extremities, using foam slings, wedges or pillows.
- Positioning may be maintained with suitable splints, e.g. resting splints for the hands in a POSI, or foot-drop splints for the feet, which can be applied between treatments, or overnight only.

Positioning of the upper limbs

- Axilla burns, anterior chest, and lateral posterior trunk burns are prone to developing contractures preventing shoulder abduction and flexion (elevation), therefore the shoulders must be positioned and stretched into these positions.
- Burns to the antecubital fossa lead to elbow contractures, especially as a flexed elbow tends to be a position of comfort for the patient to rest in.
- Elbow extension splints may be required at night, including the positioning of the forearm into supination.
- Elevation of the hands in Bradford slings designed to assist swelling control. If the shoulders do not permit this, then the hands should at least be elevated on pillows.

Positioning of the lower limbs

- Hips need to be positioned in neutral rotation and slight abduction using foam wedges, towel rolls or sandbags.
- Prone lying is an excellent position to stretch tight hip flexors, if the burns permit it and the patient can tolerate it for short periods.
- Knees should be positioned in extension when the patient is in the bed, avoiding use of a pillow under the knees, which would encourage flexion contractures.

- Plantar flexion contractures of the foot are the most common encountered, so the ankle should be placed in a neutral position, unless the burn is isolated across the anterior surface of the ankle and foot.
- This can be achieved with the use of splints, pillows, or foam.

Musculoskeletal treatment

- The aim is to maintain range of movement, especially over joints in the hands, which will contract quickly, if not stretched regularly.
- If the patient is conscious, it is important to encourage active movements.
- If the patient is not conscious then passive stretches will be necessary.
- It is essential to avoid being too aggressive or vigorous as this can rupture fine muscle fibres and vessels surrounding the joint, producing a haematoma within the joint space, which may eventually lead to fibrosis or heterotopic calcification (Richard and Staley 1994).
- Passive movements should be slow, gentle and controlled, aiming to achieve full range of movement.
- Donor sites can be moved and they will feel sore, but there are no restrictions to movement of this area.
- However, joints in close proximity to newly grafted sites must not be moved until the surgeon has agreed the graft has taken.
- This will be approximately 5 or more days post graft application.
- If a surgeon feels the graft has not 'taken' they may instruct the therapist to move the joint, until further surgical management can take place.
- Care is needed to avoid stressing areas of deep tissue damage, such as exposed tendons or joints.
- Respect the patient's wishes and their tolerance of pain, although ultimately it is essential to treat in order to avoid long-term contractures.
- Patients tire easily during treatment, partly due to the increased energy expenditure that accompanies the loss of the skin barrier.
- They may lose up to 10% of their body weight during the post-injury period, despite careful monitoring of their calorie intake and nutrition.
- Therefore, careful consideration of the frequency and timing of treatments is important and liaison with the nursing and medical staff is essential to avoid clashes of treatment.
- Individual hospital policy or staffing may dictate whether the patient receives 5, 6 or 7 days of treatment in a week.
- Treatment may be carried out whilst the patient's dressings are in situ, although it is vital to view the burns during their healing phase, in order to facilitate good handling by the therapist and to predict areas of possible contractures.
- Assisting the nurses during dressing changes can be helpful, although once the dressings are in place they can help to cushion the therapist's hands and spread the pressure applied during the manual treatment.
- There is a high risk of infection due to the loss of the skin barrier, so use of infection control techniques is even more fundamental in the burns patient than usual.
- Liaising with the patient's relatives/carers is crucial, and they may be keen to be involved in their relative's rehabilitation, perhaps performing correctly taught passive movements between therapy sessions.

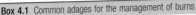

> **Box 4.1** Common adages for the management of burns
>
> - 'Mornings are always the worst due to stiffness from inactivity during the night'
> - 'ROM first'
> - 'Burn scar contracture is a lack of tissue to go around'
> - 'Stretch opposite the burn, e.g. elbow extension if the burn is in the antecubital fossa'
> - 'The sum of the parts does not always equal the whole' (i.e. may need to stretch multiple joints at a time)
> - 'If it's white, it's tight and needs to be stretched'
> - 'Pinching pain (to be avoided) or stretching pain (to be expected)'

Richard and Staley, 1994.

- The family should be educated regarding the aims and all other aspects of the therapy programme, including the benefits of treatment and the risks of non-compliance (Leveridge 1991).
- The advice may include some of the common adages relating to burns (Box 4.1).

Mobility

- As soon as the patient is medically stable and coming out of the acute phase, consideration of their mobility must be of prime importance.
- Transferring out of bed into a chair or wheelchair, followed by gait assessment and re-education can be carried out by the therapy team. This will include the provision of appropriate aids, seating and advice.
- If the patient has been in bed for a prolonged period of time, they may need to be treated on a tilt table initially to enable them to be brought gradually up into an upright posture.
- Likewise the gradual introduction of lower limb dependence ('dangling') may be required before the patient can tolerate weight-bearing on their legs.
- In the presence of grafts on the legs, the dressings must be covered with double Tubigrip when mobilising.
- If they have stairs at home, they must ascend and descend a flight of stairs prior to their discharge to ensure safety and independence.

Hand burns

- Initial elevation in a Bradford sling is vital to assist the reduction of oedema.
- The hand may be dressed, or may be enclosed in a Flamazine bag, which will be changed daily.
- The most common posture of an untreated burnt hand is with the MCP joints in extension, the IP joints of the fingers in flexion, and the thumb in adduction.
- This can be corrected with the use of thermoplastic splinting in the 'intrinsic plus' position, or position of safe immobilisation (POSI) between therapy

89

treatments (wrist at 30–40°, MCPJs at 45–70°, IPJs in neutral and the thumb abducted), to maintain the length of the collateral ligaments and volar plates).

- The splint can be fabricated over the Flamazine bag or dressings, and adjusted regularly as required to ensure a good fit and therefore effective positioning of the joints.

- Active exercises can begin from day 1 post-admission if the patient is conscious and able to comply.

- If not, or if the amount of active movement is poor, passive movements are essential to maintain joint range and muscle length, as well as preventing contractures.

- The exercises are best carried out soon after analgesia has been administered, and preferably without the dressings in situ.

- Passive flexion should be avoided if there is damage to the extensor apparatus of the fingers, otherwise exercises should consist of taking all affected joints through their full range of movement, or as near as the patient can tolerate if they are in pain.

Burns dressings

- The qualities of a good dressing are that they have high humidity but allow removal of excess exudate, they are impermeable to bacteria, are comfortable and last long enough to avoid frequent changing (Appendix 4.1).

Post-healing stage

- Once the patient is discharged from hospital they will need to continue their care as an outpatient.

- This will probably take the form of hospital outpatient visits, in which they will be seen by a number of team members.

- Dressings will generally be managed by the nursing team.

- Monitoring of healing will be carried out regularly by the surgeons, with the planning of future surgery, if necessary for any further grafting on unhealed areas, scar revision or contracture release.

- The patient will need provision of a tailored home exercise and stretching programme and this will need regular reviews and the addition of appropriate progression.

- Range of movement should be recorded at each therapy session using a goniometer.

- Graded muscle-strengthening exercises involving exercise bands, weights and springs can increase muscle strength, whilst aerobic exercise, such as using an exercise bike, will improve endurance and stamina.

- The patient should be setting goals in conjunction with the therapist, in order to keep motivation levels high, and to ensure that there is tangible progress to measure.

- The community team may be able to help with nursing or therapy provision for those patients who are unable to travel back to the burns unit on a regular basis.

- These health professionals will need to liaise closely with the hospital team, especially if additional information or technical skills are required.
- Aids or adaptations may be required in order to promote self-care activities once the patient has been discharged.
- Splints for positioning and stretching are likely to be an ongoing necessity, so regular appointments will be required to ensure correct fit and continuing effectiveness.
- Family members are often keen to offer support, so it may be useful to compile a list of activities the patient can manage independently and those with which he or she requires assistance.
- Patients may need assistance from members of the therapy team with tasks such as filling in disability claim forms or advice about driving and the questionnaires associated with this.

Scars and healing

- Often a scar settles within 2–6 months, to become white and appears as a fine line. However, scars can become keloid or hypertrophic.
- Keloid scarring is scar tissue which goes beyond the original parameters of the wound, and expands into the surrounding tissue.
- It is often bulky and can be shiny, or red and painful to the touch.
- The type of scar formed after a burn will depend on the depth, type and location of the burn on the body.
- It is very difficult to predict, unless the patient has previous scars which have become keloid, although it is most common in people with Afro-Caribbean heritage.
- Certain areas will be more prone to hypertrophic scarring, e.g. over the sternum, deltoid and the ear (O'Brien 2008).
- Generally it seems that if the burn is healed within 3 weeks the scarring will be minimal, but if this takes longer than 3 weeks the scar is likely to be significant and will probably require some form of treatment.
- Hypertrophic scars are raised, itchy, lumpy, red and painful, and typically develop a few months after the burn, once the site has epithelialised.
- Scars can be seen to get worse within the first 3–6 months before they improve, which needs to be communicated to the patient, so they are forewarned and do not become dispirited by what seems to be a deterioration of their situation.
- Keloid scars extend beyond the original site of the injury and can stay active for several years.
- Contributing factors to hypertrophic scarring include: age, location of the scar, depth of the burn, skin tension and race.
- These types of scars are prevalent in 70–80% of all scars following burns.
- The aims of scar management are to prevent or reduce functional limitation, reduce pain and irritation and to gain an optimal appearance.

Scar management

- The approach to scar management includes the following:
- Creams
- Scar massage

- Stretching and exercise
- Silicone gels and elastomers
- Pressure garments, to help make the scar softer, flatter and paler in colour
- Steroid injection – if unresolved scar in an obvious place.

Creams

Grafted skin tends to dehydrate and requires regular moisturising with aqueous creams, to avoid blistering, cracking and overgranulation of the skin (Richard and Staley 1994).

Scar massage

The aim of massage is to break down collagen that has been produced in response to the burns, or other soft tissue injury and thus relieve underlying tethering, as well as assisting desensitisation. Care must be taken on newly healed skin grafts, to prevent shearing or blistering of the fragile skin (Richard and Staley 1994). Once healing has been established, deep tissue massage and frictions break down the excess collagen formation and encourage the matrix to form along the most functional lines (Hunter 1998).

Stretching and exercise

Regular stretches and exercises are required from the time the burns and skin grafts are healed, to prevent the development of contractures and assist in the elongation of the scar tissue, especially that which extends over one or more joints (Richard and Staley 1994). Scarred areas in soft tissue mimic the tissue they replace but it is difficult for them to replace it completely. The application of movement and forces across the healing tissues encourages the collagen matrix to form with the most suitable tensile strength to encourage it to replicate the damaged tissue as closely as possible (Hunter 1998).

Silicone gels and elastomers

It is not fully understood just how these work and there is very little evidence to support their clinical use. However, anecdotally they have been found to be very beneficial. Current research theorises that the gel promotes hydration of the scar, by means of the reduction of water vapour loss reducing capillary activity and therefore reducing collagen deposition (Sepehrmanesh 2006).

Pressure garments

The physiological effects of pressure garments are also not fully understood. There are two theories that are referred to in the literature: the first is that the pressure applied causes increased stasis, leading to a reduction in the fibroblastic activity and therefore the production of collagen. This would account for the decrease in the mass of hypertrophic tissue to promote faster maturation of healing tissue (Edwards 2003). The second theory is that the pressure garments reduce the blood flow to the covered area, and the levels of gamma globulins which would otherwise inhibit the scar remodeling process (Williams et al 1998).

- Pressure garments are deemed unnecessary if the grafts have taken early or are healed within 2–3 weeks.
- A scar must be fully healed for a pressure garment to be fitted.
- There are advantages and disadvantages to using pressure garments (Table 4.2).
- Pressure garments may need changing every 6–12 weeks, depending on the patient's activity levels, and change in their weight or muscle bulk after discharge from hospital.

Table 4.2 Advantages and disadvantages of pressure garments

Advantages	Disadvantages
Custom made, therefore fit well and can be adjusted	They need to be worn 23 hours per day
The patient can function fully within them	Patients can find them hot and rather cumbersome
Improvements can be noted relatively quickly	The garments are expensive
	They are labour-intensive to make, and require specialist skills

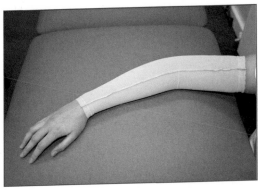

Figure 4.1 Pressure garment.

- The garments are likely to be needed for as long as the scars are active, i.e. approximately 12 months or longer (Figure 4.1).
- Ultimately the scar should flatten and fade to a paler colour.
- In addition to the disadvantages of wearing pressure garments there are a number of complications associated with wearing them, e.g. swelling, blistering and scar breakdown.
- Scars can be monitored for varying factors using tools such as the Vancouver scar scale (Table 4.3).

Protection from the sun

- Education on protecting the scar from exposure to sunlight is essential. Risk of sunburn is increased due to the newly healed skin having none of the protective pigment normally found in skin and therefore being highly sensitive to ultraviolet rays the patient is particularly vulnerable to the adverse effects of sunlight.
- Patients are instructed to avoid sun exposure for at least 1 year after a burn and to use a high-factor sunscreen on areas of skin which cannot be covered up.
- Cosmetic camouflage has been developed to diminish the distress of facial and hand scarring, in order to improve the patient's self-esteem.
- The correct application of the waterproof opaque creams can cleverly disguise disfiguring scars and these usually contain a sunscreen.

Table 4.3 Vancouver scar scale

Pliability	0	Normal
	1	Supple
	2	Yielding
	3	Firm
	4	Adherent
Height	0	Normal
	1	1–2 mm
	2	3–4 mm
	3	5–6 mm
	4	6+ mm
Vascularity	0	Normal
	1	Pink
	2	Red
	3	Purple
Pigmentation	0	Normal
	1	Slightly
	2	Moderately
	3	Severely

Baryza and Baryza (1995).

Psychological aspects of burns

- The psychological effects of burn injuries cannot be underestimated, although for most patients they are temporary.

- Psychosocial care is essential following a burn, and this may be carried out at different times by all members of the team, e.g. nursing staff, OTs, physiotherapists, social workers, psychologists and medical staff.

- Common complaints in the early post-burn period are anxiety, sleep disturbance, confusion and delirium.

- The focus in the initial management of a burn patient tends to be on immediate survival and physical problems. The team should follow the patient's lead and only confront the long-term implications of the injury if this is directly requested by the patient.

- Family members should be encouraged to avoid showing their own anxiety in front of the patient. They should be encouraged to appear calm, hopeful and supportive.

- Once out of the ITU setting patients will often begin to experience more negative emotions, such as depression, post-traumatic stress disorder, nightmares and anxiety.

- The majority of patients learn suitable coping mechanisms to deal with their situation, but sometimes stronger behavioural problems such as direct hostility, regression or dependence can manifest themselves.

- At this stage it is extremely helpful if an experienced burns psychologist or psychiatrist can become involved in the patient's care, and give guidance to other team members and the family on how to react and handle these behaviours.

- Some departments have clinics where the patient can be assessed by the doctor and then given advice by the therapist outlining what they should expect from the surgery and the postoperative intervention and treatment.
- Some departments provide patients with comprehensive leaflets which cover the same information.

Ward-based treatment

Respiratory management

- If a patient stays overnight on the ward, the minimum intervention would involve the patient receiving a day one chest check.
- This usually entails a check of the SaO_2 levels, the respiratory rate and auscultation of the patient's chest.
- If a patient is having difficulty taking deep breaths due to pain, physiotherapists are ideally placed to inform the doctors or nursing staff of this and to ensure the patient has adequate pain relief in order to ensure that the optimum conditions are available for the patient to expand their airways and prevent chest complications.
- Head and neck patients who have had a radical neck dissection or those undergoing an ENT procedure may have a tracheostomy in situ.
- Some patients may have spent a period of time on ITU following their surgery and they will have their own unique respiratory requirements due to an element of ITU deconditioning with or without tracheostomies in situ or following major head and neck reconstruction. This can include flaps inside the mouth and palate.
- Patients who have spent time on ITU may need encouragement to take deep breaths, and will require gentle and gradual activity pacing and progression so they do not become fatigued.
- This can occur after any time spent on ITU. Patients who require ITU input tend to be those with more extensive surgery and those who can be more unwell prior to surgery or less mobile, e.g. flaps related to gynaecological cancers follow a slower rehabilitation stream.

Mobility

- Early intervention from the physiotherapist providing a mobility assessment either pre- or post-operatively can provide the information that enables the team to discuss the plans for treatment relating to the mobility and function required by the patient.
- This also identifies any blocks or hurdles there may be to achieving a timely discharge home for a patient from the ward.
- There need to be good communication channels between all the support services and the medics, to ensure the patient is discharged to the appropriate place, whether this is to a community hospital, intermediate care bed or to the patient's home.

Bedrest

- Some patients may be on a period of enforced bed rest whilst in hospital, e.g. some departments may not allow patients to mobilise on day one following the establishment of a muscle flap.

- They may require a period of 'dangling' while the congestion of the flap is assessed over a period of 4–5 days with gradually increasing timescales from 30 seconds up to a period of five minutes.

- There should always be an awareness of the needs of the patient as a whole to ensure full range of movement (ROM) is being maintained in all non-affected joints, particularly in elderly patients and those with polytrauma where immobility may lead to increased joint and soft tissue stiffness.

- Bed exercises should be provided to maintain strength of muscles in the unaffected limbs. This will ensure that the patient will have sufficient power to enable them to mobilise safely with walking aids.

- Bed exercises will also have an effect on maintaining the flow of the circulation, preventing complications such as deep vein thrombosis and encouraging deep breathing as an exercise can help prevent chest infections or other complications as a result of the reduced airway expansion from enforced bed rest.

- Some departments encourage transfers into a chair before dangling commences, and it is important that the patient and nursing staff know how to do this safely and in a protected manner.

- Teaching the patient how to use a banana board or a rotation plate can facilitate early sitting out.

- How a patient mobilises will depend on the surgery undergone and other co-morbidities.

- Some equipment which you will be familiar with are pulpit frames, gutter frames, Zimmer frames, crutches, sticks and standing hoists.

- Any and all of these may be used on plastic surgery wards and the physiotherapist should familiarise themselves with each piece of equipment in order that the patient can be shown all the relevant health and safety checks relating to the equipment and its use.

Outpatients

Dressings

- Often the nursing staff will carry out wound dressings on the ward, and may take them down in clinic prior to you seeing a patient.

- Sometimes, however, the physiotherapist will be required to do the dressings.

- Be familiar with the departments' infection control protocol.

- Dressings should only be changed using an aseptic technique.

- Depending on what requires dressing, e.g. with hand surgery (tendon repairs and similar) the lighter the dressing is, the more likely it is that the patient will begin moving early and easily.

- If a dressing is very bulky, the patient will find it difficult to do their exercises and may well not bother. There are various factors to consider when deciding which dressings to apply (Table 4.4).

Splinting

- Following the application of dressings, the tendon repair or fracture should be protected to provide a safe environment for exercise and rehabilitation.

- There are many different splints which can be provided for patients. These can be pre-formed or made specifically for the patient.

Table 4.4 Type of wound and choice of dressing

Type of wound	Dressing to use
Dry and clean. Suture in place	Non-stick Use something like 'Jelonet' covered with gauze or plaster
Oozing wound, but not open	Non-stick May need more gauze, held in place with bandage or tubinette
Open and oozing	Antiseptic dressing, like Inadine or a Betadine spray Covered with gauze and bandage to secure it

- Splints are most commonly made out of thermoplastic for rigid splints, or neoprene for those which need to be less rigid, or which need to be less hard.
- Thermoplastic materials have a variety of different properties.
- Some can be very hard and rigid, but may also be quite bulky.
- Some are lightweight, but also can be very strong.
- Some are very easy to work with and they can be formed easily, but they may have a very short working time.
- Some thermoplastic can be so malleable that it can feel like a piece of chewing gum. Having a very malleable material can be difficult to form into the shape required, but it often drapes well to give a better conformity.
- Depending on what the splint is required to do will dictate which type of material is used for its construction.
- Every department has slightly different protocols relating to splinting, the length of time patients should wear them, and what types of exercises can be carried out whilst the patient is wearing the splint.
- Figures 4.3–4.6 illustrate examples of some of the more commonly used splints for protecting tendon repairs.
- The splints illustrated in Figures 4.3–4.6 have been made out of Ezeform thermoplastic and are fastened with Velcro straps.
- Splints are not always the rigid, static structures that are used to prevent movement as illustrated in Figures 4.3–4.6.
- They can be made with a hinge incorporated into the slab, or with elastic structures that facilitate movement and are generally known as dynamic splints (Figures 4.7 and 4.8).
- Dynamic splints are used to help with digit and wrist extension, e.g. following a radial nerve palsy.
- A dynamic splint may improve a patient's functional ability, i.e. if a patient is able to flex the digits, but is unable to use the hand functionally due to their inability to extend the wrist and extend their fingers, then a dynamic splint can assist the wrist and fingers to be moved into extension to enable the patient to be able to grip objects with the finger flexors.
- A dynamic splint is used primarily to restore function to the patient, although they do have to have a fairly high level of compliance in order to wear the splint and achieve meaningful function.

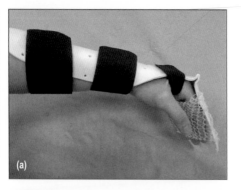

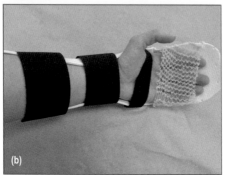

Figure 4.3 (a and b) Flexor hood for tendon treatment.

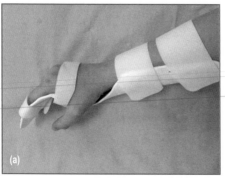

Figure 4.4 (a and b) Splint used for extensor tendon repair of the digits.

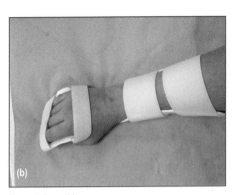

Figure 4.4, cont'd.

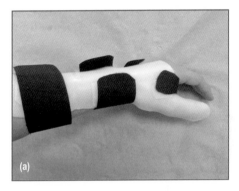

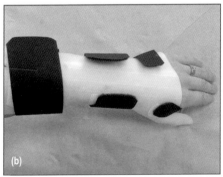

Figure 4.5 (a and b) Splint used for flexor tendon repairs of the thumb.

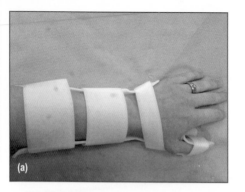

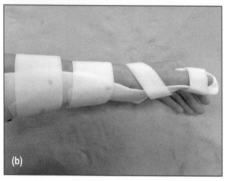

Figure 4.6 (a and b) Splint used to protect extensor tendon repairs of the thumb.

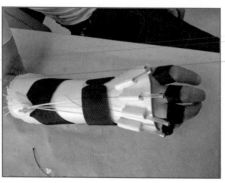

Figure 4.7 Dynamic splint.

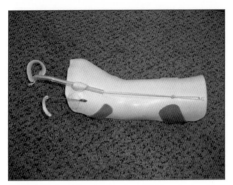

Figure 4.8 Dynamic splint.

- The patient may need a splint to restrict movement in one area in order to facilitate another joint to increase its functional range.
- Sometimes a joint needs to be supported if it is hypermobile, for example. This will encourage muscles to work more effectively, within an optimum range and length to increase the stability of the joint.

Scarring

- Whenever there is a wound to the skin or soft tissue structures, there will always be the deposition of scar tissue. The treatment of this has been covered in detail in the burns section.

Heightened sensitivity/decreased sensation

- A scar can become sensitive during the course of remodeling.
- If a nerve has been damaged this can lead to sensitivity of the area or altered sensation in the part of the limb supplied by that nerve.
- When this sensation is increased it is called peripheral sensitisation.
- Central sensitisation can be experienced by people with complex regional pain syndrome.

Touch

- A variety of different textures and different pressures are required to stimulate nerve recovery.
- If there is heightened sensation the patient can start with exposure of the area to a texture or level of pressure which is uncomfortable, but not painful.
- After a short period of approximately 1–2 minutes, they progress to a texture or level of pressure which is comfortable.
- After a further 2–3 minutes they return to the original texture or pressure.
- The patient should find that the discomfort has eased and they should be able to tolerate the texture or pressure more easily.
- This reduction in sensitivity is due to there being a reduction in the nerve firing threshold and in the number of signals being sent to the brain.

- The brain does not continue to process the signals as pain and the discomfort level is simultaneously reduced.

- If the patient is encouraged to look at the painful area as they are touching it, this helps to stimulate visual input into the somatosensory cortex.

- This reduces cortical reorganisation and encourages neural regeneration (Svens & Rosén 2009).

- Touch through massage over an area of altered sensation or a painful scar can stimulate blood flow, which in turn improves the interstitial fluid balance. This has the effect of removing any potentially harmful inflammation away from the tissues and from around nerve endings.

- If the inflammation is left it can become a source of peripheral sensitisation as it will become a stimulus for nociceptive fibres which can lead to the perception of pain.

Tapping

- Tapping is a form of touch, which is a more specific way to stimulate the deep pressure and vibration sensory nerve fibres found in the dermis, e.g. Merkel receptors and Pacinian corpuscles.

- The vibration sense is often the first area of 'nerve feeling' to return.

Visualisation

- This involves hiding the hand or affected area and imagining the movement as if it is actually being performed. This is a strategy during the later stages of nerve recovery (Butler & Moseley 2003).

- Mirror therapy is another useful technique.

Oedema

- Along with altered sensation oedema may be present.

- The pressure caused by oedema can alter nerve conduction, which leads to an alteration in the blood flow to the affected area, which in turn can increase the interstitial fluid.

- Other causes of inflammation and oedema could be infection, CRPS, overuse or underuse of the affected area.

- In the first stages of wound healing and inflammation, oedema is required as a necessary part of the healing process.

- However, if this state continues for longer than 2–3 weeks, it can become problematic.

- Long-term oedema can lead to stiffness in the hand and contractures of the soft tissues.

- It can prevent free gliding of the tendons and nerves through their interfaces and it can affect circulation, which subsequently has an impact on nerve healing and on skin condition.

- Oedema can be managed by using pressure garments, similar in design to those used in burns management which can be either made-to-measure or of-the-shelf garments.

- As with burns they ideally need to be worn for 23/24 hours a day to gain the most benefit.
- Massage can be used to help to improve circulation and to help to move the swelling out of the affected areas and into the lymph system.
- Warming an oedematous area both prior to and after massage can improve the circulation further.
- Using a piece of equipment called a 'chip-bag' can assist in moving stubborn oedema, particularly from the dorsum of the hand or arm.
- This consists of lots of small pieces of foam or neoprene chips inside a cloth bag. This is placed over the affected area and held into place with a bandage to create compression.
- It should be removed and repositioned periodically when it is worn to ensure the 'chips' create different areas of pressure over the oedematous part of the body.

Loss of range of movement
- Swelling or oedema can lead to a loss of range of motion.
- Other causes include fractures, altered tissue length leading to contractures around joints, a lag in movement where the soft tissues are too 'baggy' to contract fully and nerve damage resulting in reduced motor nerve signals getting to the muscles.
- Treatment modalities will be dependent on the cause of the loss of movement.

Fractures
- These could lead to a loss of range of motion due to pain, or because the area feels unstable or vulnerable to movement. Before you can work on soft tissue changes the skeletal system has to be strong enough to support movement. This would commonly be fixed through surgical means if required, but as therapists we can help with splints or braces to support the skeletal system whilst allowing some movement. Movement at a fracture site can help to stimulate bone regrowth so long as the fracture edges are close enough together to promote healing.
- Refer to Chapter 17 for further detail.

Contractures
- These can be caused by tight, stiff tissues restricting the amount of movement available at a joint, or due to scar tissue preventing movement from being retained.
- If the contractures are due to scar tissue, the patient should be encouraged to undergo deep tissue massage of the scar and close surrounding area.
- Splinting of the area, particularly in the hand will allow the tissues to stretch.
- If you apply the physics of tissue lengthening to contractures, tissue creep, where the tissues are placed under a low load for extended periods of time slowly lengthens the tissues without causing pain (Flowers and LaStayo 1994; Jordan et al 2000).
- Ideally the splints should be worn for at least 12 hours of the day/night, but the best results are obtained if the splints can be worn for longer than this (Glasgow et al 2003).

- Making static progressive splints where the tension of the stretch can be increased gradually by the patient allows the elasticity of the tissues to return without a high demand on the therapy services.

- Static progressive splints can be made to improve both flexion (Figure 4.3a) and extension of a digit or digits, but you have to make sure that the patient understands that the splint application should almost feel like nothing is happening to the tissues (i.e. very low load of stretch) as otherwise when worn for extended periods of time it becomes painful.

- The patient is unlikely to comply with the splinting for the time required to achieve a result if it is painful.

Lengthened tissue

- Splinting can also be used to help to shorten tissues where they have lengthened. This can happen after a fracture when the bone has lost height. By splinting the tissues in a shortened position it can help to tighten the structure.

Nerve damage

- The level or type of nerve injury will affect the functional deficit and changes to the ROM (Table 4.5).

- The higher the nerve damage (the more proximal to the spinal cord) the more extensive the functional input. The more damaged the nerve the more likely there will be functional deficit.

- This can be treated through sensory re-education and also the use of splinting to provide a functional position of joints.

- Examples are the foot drop splint, which is used when there has been damage to the common peroneal nerve of the leg, which results in the inability to dorsiflex the foot and toes (Figure 4.9). Another is the dynamic splint as seen earlier in the chapter which can be used for radial nerve injury in the upper limb (Figure 4.10).

- Splinting should also be used for positioning the affected limb to prevent the development of contractures as the nerve recovers.

- Surgery may be required to create a more functional limb; for example muscle transfers or nerve grafting in the longer term after injury.

Table 4.5 Nerve injuries (Seddon 1943)	
Type of nerve injury	Definition
Neuropraxia	Compression, or generalised bruising to a nerve. Segmental demyelinisation
Axonotmesis	Damage to the axonal layer of the nerve. Slow recovery. Wallerian degeneration below level of damage
Neurotmesis	Damage to the internal structure of the nerve. Complete loss of continuity with Wallerian degeneration below the level of the injury. Requires surgery to recover
Avulsion	Complete rupture of the nerve at the root. Often non-salvageable even with surgery

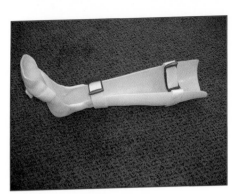

Figure 4.9 Foot drop splint.

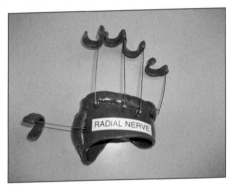

Figure 4.10 Dynamic splint for radial nerve injury.

Pain and complex regional pain syndrome (CRPS)

- Pain is one of the features of complex regional pain syndrome (CRPS) and can be very disruptive for normal movement and for therapists trying to encourage movement or a return to function.
- Movement may stimulate and increase the pain sensation. It is described by the IASP (International Association for the Study of Pain) as being:

  …an unpleasant sensory and emotional experience associated with actual or potential tissue damage, or described in terms of such damage.

- Note that it talks about 'actual or potential' damage to the tissues. If the brain perceives something to be a threat, we as therapists have to educate the patient to understand which pain behaviours are useful for recovery and those which can become ingrained and dysfunctional.
- Nociceptive pain can be treated using regular analgesia, heat or ice therapy, massage, ROM and stretches.

- Neuropathic pain, described as 'burning, hot, deep bone type pain' has elements of peripheral and central sensitisation and should be managed using a multi-modal approach (Svens and Rosén 2009).
- Peripheral sensitisation is common in CRPS presentations and should it become chronic then central changes can occur.
- Other symptoms of CRPS are stiffness, allodynia or hyperaesthesia, changes to hair and nail growth (either increased or decreased), changes to sweating and temperature of the hand, changes to the condition of the skin and altered ROMA patient with CRPS may have all, or only some of these characteristics, and they do not necessarily follow a timeline.
- Sometimes they can occur weeks or months after the initial trauma to the body.
- This therefore makes it very difficult to predict, and the treatment should be designed to fit the current symptoms.

A multimodal approach to treatment

- The sensorimotor cortex of the brain is made up of links to many different parts of the brain which include sight, sound, smell and hearing.
- Treatment of CRPS and pain has to use elements of all of these senses.
- Simple pain relief, such as paracetamol or anti-inflammatories plays a part in the treatment of CRPS.
- When we ask them to give a painful area more attention, it can make the pain worse initially, so we need that 'window of opportunity'.

Analgesia

- Most common medications used are amitriptyline (below 50 mg), which is taken at night. It should be taken regularly and does not work effectively if taken 'as and when'.
- Another form of medication is gabapentin or pregabalin (Lyrica).

Education

- This is the most important aspect of treating CRPS.
- The patient must be reassured that the development of CRPS is not their fault.
- Some people develop it and others do not and we have a limited idea as to why.
- Education around pain behaviours and pain responses will help the patient to see that even though the exercises are painful, it is not causing actual tissue damage.

Desensitisation

- This type of treatment can be used to incorporate the multimodal approach.
- When the patient touches the different textures, you can also use textures which have smell, such as citrus peel; sound, such as crinkly sweet wrappers, or rough Velcro; and vision, by looking at which body part is being touched, when it is being touched.

Hand laterality tasks

- This uses vision to start recognition of the affected limb, whether it is hand, foot or other body part, in different positions.
- Moseley (2005) found that this was useful in reducing pain and disability in his patient group with CRPS of the hand.
- Using flash cards with limbs in different positions over time by patients can help to reduce pain.
- The cards are mixed together and picked out at random and the patient has to state whether they are a right or a left limb.

Graded imagery

- This is related to the visualisation tasks as described in the nerve injury section.
- The patient should first start with the laterality tasks, and then imagine their own hand or leg in the positions on the cards.
- Once this is comfortable and does not cause them pain they should then start to place their own affected hand or limb into the positions seen, using only the cards related to their affected side.

Mirror therapy

- Mirror therapy was described as a useful tool for treating phantom limb pain by Ramachandram and Hirstein (1998), and its use in other areas of pain associated with cortical reorganisation has been steadily gaining ground.
- Due to the homunculus and the brain itself being open to plasticity and change, mirror therapy is a way of harnessing this change for positive recovery.
- The patient is set up with their good limb visible in the mirror, devoid of any distinguishing features such as rings, watches or socks.
- The affected limb is placed behind the mirror screen so the patient looks at the non-affected limb in the mirror.
- By moving the non-affected limb, and seeing the reflection in the mirror, the brain 'recognises' that the affected limb is moving, and pain can reduce as a result.
- Mirror therapy should be used by the patient daily and should be repeated 5–6 times per day for 5–10 minutes each time to get the best result from the treatment modality (Grünert-Plüss et al 2008).
- Ideally it should be done under supervision the first time, to ensure the patient's pain levels do not increase on the affected side. Should this happen the treatment should be stopped, and the patient returned to laterality or graded imagery (Moseley 2005).

The references for this chapter can be found on www.expertconsult.com.

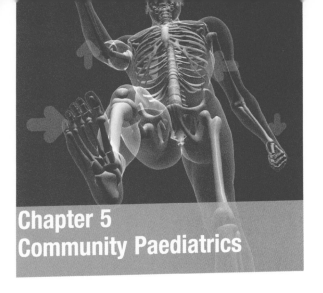

Chapter 5
Community Paediatrics

The development of the child

- A physiotherapist working in paediatrics should have an awareness of the stages that infants and young children progress through during their development.
- The physiotherapist may identify issues associated with motor function or the presence of a visual or hearing impediment.
- The physiotherapist should also be aware of the levels of development achieved by children and what would normally be expected in order to assist the planning of treatment interventions.

Locomotor development development

- The development of a child will include their ability to move independently, use their hands and to be able to interact with their environment through the use of their senses of vision, hearing and cognition.
- Most children follow a regular pathway of development, during which the different stages may be reached at different times.
- The presence of impairments such as vision or hearing or premature birth may lead to delay in or even failure to achieve certain developmental milestones.
- The major milestones for infants involve sitting independently (6–11 months), crawling (6–12 months), independent walking (18 months).
- Some children miss out the crawling stage and move on to standing and walking from sitting, if the walking is achieved later, e.g. 20–24 months, then this may be indicative of a child with low tone or of developmental delay.
- Children begin grasping objects during their first year, initially with both hands and then with one.

- The grasp begins to become more dextrous with sufficient precision being developed to build a column of blocks by the end the first year and hold a pencil by the age of 3.

- Dominance in either hand tends to develop after 2 years.

Speech development

- The earliest signs of communication occur when a child begins to point to objects (9–18 months).

- Between 9 months and 1 year children will begin to show understanding of simple words and sentences.

- During the second year the number of recognisable words increases so that by 3 the child will be able to distinguish between something being in or on something.

- Most children will be able to combine multiple words by the second year.

- Fluency in speech occurs by 4 years although when angry or excited they may stammer during their speech.

Hearing

- Infants react to sound from birth, by turning their eyes in the direction of the sound.

- By 4 months the child will turn towards the sound.

- By 7 months once sitting ability has developed the child will turn directly towards their parent or carer.

- A hearing impairment is often missed unless it is profound and identified by the child's parents.

Vision

- Infants will turn their head towards light and from 1–3 months an infant will fix on a parent's face and follow their own hand movements. By nine months they are able to see and poke small objects such as crumbs. By one year they will watch objects such as birds in a garden or a car passing by.

- The concerns of parents may help to discover impending problems, e.g. inability to fix vision.

- Potential vision issues in small children need to be assessed by an appropriately trained professional (Frost & Sharma 1997).

The management of children with neuromuscular disorders

- Duchenne muscular dystrophy is one of the commonest inherited diseases found in children and as a consequence physiotherapists working in community paediatrics will encounter these children in their practice.

- The role of the community physiotherapist is primarily to monitor those children who are at risk of developing debilitating contractures in the hips and around the ankles when the child is able to walk and then progressively in the remaining limb joints once the child becomes wheelchair-dependent.

- The physiotherapist will be responsible for teaching the parents/carers and school staff how to stretch the tendo-Achilles to maintain range of dorsiflexion and hip flexion in order to maintain range necessary for independent gait to be maintained.
- These will need to be carried out on a daily basis and the presence of contracture monitored carefully.
- Night splints should be provided to maintain the ankle in dorsiflexion at night and these tend to be ankle foot orthoses (AFOs).
- The physiotherapist should encourage regular, moderate amounts of active exercise in order to maintain joint motion, avoiding the use of resisted exercises.
- Aquatic physiotherapy will benefit these children, enabling joint motion to be maintained as the child has fun in the water.
- As the child shows signs of losing the ability to walk the physiotherapist will need to ensure that the child is referred to a specialist centre for the provision of knee ankle foot orthoses (KAFOs) and possible release of tendons such as the Achilles to facilitate joint motion compatible with achieving independent gait.
- The longer the child can remain able to walk the later they will develop the impending spinal scoliosis associated with constant wheelchair use.
- Once the child has been provided with KAFOs the physiotherapist in the community will be monitoring the ability of the child to maintain the ability to walk.
- With the loss of walking ability the child will need to be taught wheelchair skills.
- At this stage skin care will become important and will need to be reinforced with the child, parents/carers and school staff.
- Spinal posture will have an adverse effect on respiratory function and spinal jackets will need to be provided to prevent the deterioration of the spinal posture. At this stage the child will be monitored by the specialist centre for the need to operate to maintain the spinal posture (Eagle 2007).
- The reader is referred to the acute paediatric chapter in this volume for further detail regarding the management of neuromuscular disorders.

The management of children with musculoskeletal disorders

- Children will present with a wide range of musculoskeletal disorders, which may be managed by the physiotherapist in the school or home environment, however, there will be situations where a child may present with a problem or a condition that is beyond the competence of the community physiotherapist.
- In these cases it is important to liaise with musculoskeletal specialists either in the community or in the nearest specialist centre.
- The community physiotherapist should draw on their core knowledge and skills to manage children with musculoskeletal dysfunction.
- The reader is referred to the section covering the management of musculoskeletal disorders in the acute paediatric chapter in this volume for further detailed information on the treatment modalities and approaches that can be used.

The management of children with neurological disorders

- Successful treatment of children with long-term neurological conditions will be dependent on the physiotherapist having an effective working relationship with the child's family and/or relatives or alternative carers.

- Physiotherapy treatment will be ongoing, often for the whole of childhood, but despite the amount of physiotherapy involvement it is the people who are with the child the most who will have the greatest impact on their development.

- A child may be referred for physiotherapy at different stages of the medical pathway, for example a child born prematurely or perhaps into a socially deprived environment where there is a high incidence of morbidity or alternatively where health and social care issues have already been identified, will ideally be referred to a number of community services on discharge from hospital.

- Many children will be referred later, with or without a diagnosis, with parents being aware or potentially unaware of their problems.

- The timing of the referral can impact on the relationship the family have with the physiotherapist. For example, does the family want the input, do they know their child has problems? Are they still in the stage of denial?

- Often the child's problems are not isolated. An initial need for physiotherapy intervention may sooner or later develop into the need for many other professionals and services to become involved in the child's management.

- Children with a disability often have a huge multidisciplinary team around them and reliable inter-professional communication is vital. Physiotherapists need to prioritise their time and establish which meetings or clinical appointments they should attend.

- The purpose of attending a meeting may be to provide or to obtain information, but it needs to be considered that both can be achieved through the provision of reports, emails, letters, and phone calls if necessary.

- The physiotherapist may find themselves the health representative within an educational setting or a child's advocate during a hospital clinic appointment.

The physiotherapist and their relationship with parents/carers

Developing respect and confidence

- The parents or carers are usually the most important people in a child's life, and therefore it is essential that they are able to respect and have confidence in their child's physiotherapist.

- There is a strong possibility that a physiotherapist will be working with a child and his or her family for a number of years, therefore the physiotherapist must strive to ensure that there is a positive working relationship.

- It is not trite to say, that the parents need to like their child's therapist.

- Setting up good early relationships is vital; it helps if the child doesn't cry every time that the physiotherapist pays a visit too!

- Some basic organisational details are crucial to getting off to a good start. Setting appointments at a time that is convenient for the family.

- Arriving for appointments at a previously agreed time.

- Setting up communication channels, whether via email or phone.
- Giving the parents/carers confidence that you are easily contactable and will return calls within a relevant time period are all small details that are key to developing a good effective working relationship with the child's family or carers.
- As with any service there must be access to interpreters and written information sheets or leaflets explaining what physiotherapy intervention entails, and what is to be provided by the therapist, and in turn what is expected of the family and other settings in providing the physiotherapy programme.
- Information must be presented in a way that is appropriate for the recipient and is respectful of the cultural or religious beliefs of the family or carers.

Skills required by the therapist

- Communication:
- The most important of these is communication skills to enable effective working with the child, parent/s and the multidisciplinary team, including education and social services.
- A small infant may be suspicious of anyone and will need to be engaged through their parent or carer, whilst the child is on their lap or playing on a mat with them. Parents can be taught how to carry out movements of the child's limbs or specific activities to encourage their developmental skills.
- Treatment can be delivered through play and using toys, incorporating a game they like to play or a favourite toy.
- Ask the people who know the child, they will tell you what motivates and what worries the child.
- Negotiation may work with older children.
- Non-verbal communication will indicate mood or feelings.
- Be aware of your body language, e.g. sitting slightly turned away from the child with arms folded gives an impression of indifference. Leaning towards someone and mirroring their body language shows interest and empathy.
- Conflict awareness:
- Be aware of the signs that a person is aggressive and angry.
- Conflict awareness training can help develop the therapist's ability to deal with situations that can develop.
- If treatment is likely to be contentious, plan in advance how to manage the situation, e.g. by having another person present, or seeing the family in clinic or at school where it will be easier to maintain control and support is present.
- Parents:
- Be aware of the issues facing parents, e.g. if a child has been newly diagnosed the parents may be grieving for the expectations they had.
- These expectations will need to change, but they need time, understanding and to be managed tactfully.
- Acceptance can be variable, some parents will accept their child is unlikely to walk and act by being proactive, e.g. sourcing equipment to assist their child.
- Others will need considerable support, only coming to terms with a diagnosis after several years.

- Forcing issues around acceptance is likely to lead to them refusing to have you as their therapist.
- Building a relationship with parents and the child takes time, but it is only when they trust you that you will be able to work together for the benefit of the child.
- Listen to their concerns, be realistic but tactful in response.
- A child's problems or disability may become apparent when they become older.
- Children who seem to have many problems early on may improve beyond expectation and do well, unfortunately the reverse can also be true.
- The therapist will need to help the families to maintain a positive outlook and assist them to deal with what can be major issues.
- Admit when you don't know something, offer to go and find out the answer.
- You need to be positive and reliable, if you say you will find out or do something it is important to fulfil the promise.
- Teaching:
- Teaching parents management techniques can be done in a variety of ways:
- Demonstration of exercises with the child.
- Providing a written programme, including diagrams.
- Guiding their hands so they learn kinaesthetically.
- Photograph programmes are a really good way to motivate the child, and to show parents, carers or school staff how to position, use equipment or do an activity.
- It is important to teach others how to effectively carry out therapy to ensure SMART goals are met and to maintain the confidence that parents have in you.
- Manual handling:
- Manual handling and physical activity is a big part of the role of the paediatric physiotherapist.
- The physiotherapist should be aware of the effect that treating children can have on their body.
- Children with disabilities require a handling risk assessment to be carried out which outlines the process of handling required to reduce the risk of injury to anyone handling them.
- Organisations should have their own risk assessment paperwork.
- Any stooping activity should be interspersed with standing or sitting to avoid prolonged stress on the spine and lower limb joints.
- Equipment such as wheeled stools can make things easier when working with a small child.
- In a clinic or school setting there may be a therapy plinth that will enable the height to be adjusted to enable treatment to be carried out at a suitable height for the physiotherapist.

Working with the multidisciplinary team

- Within a paediatric setting, the medical team is extended to include education, parents, carers, social teams.

- Children with disabilities may often require a high number of interventions and support and within the school setting 'Statementing' is in place to enable the child to receive the support required to access and achieve an education.
- The Common Assessment Framework (CAF) and Team Around The Child (TAC) are used by education, health and social teams to assess a child's overall needs.
- CAF and TAC are also used when there are concerns about a child if they are considered to be at risk.
- This system is available to any child whether they have disabilities or not.
- The child and family may require support to deal with many issues, e.g. the family may need some respite care for their child to provide time for them to deal with family life.
- Respite care is often quite limited, but may consist of some hours per week, or a day or overnight stay in hospice or supportive accommodation.
- The therapist may need to liaise with respite care in order to teach a number of people how to carry out the child's physiotherapy or 24-hour positioning programme.
- Physiotherapy reports need to be both succinct and timely as they may provide a paediatrician or orthopaedic consultant with information about how a child is progressing, or not.
- Educational support for children under the age of 5 years can vary.
- Some areas may have a system called Portage, where an LEA (local education authority) employee visits the family at home to help with the child's development.
- Social services (renamed as children and families teams) have systems that oversee a child's safety and support children with disabilities to the extent of recommendations for housing adaptations.

Following the assessment

Goal setting

- When the assessment process has been completed the physiotherapist will formulate a problem list and in conjunction with the child and/or parents/carers set objectives for treatment. This should ensure that all parties understand the issues and the plan for managing these in the short and long term.
- It is critical to achieving a successful outcome that the child and the family have ownership of the objectives and enter freely into a contract with their physiotherapist.
- This should ensure that the child and their family or carers have a good understanding about exactly what their commitment needs to be.
- The physiotherapist will assess the child with a view to this being an ongoing process that evaluates the specific needs and enables the modification of treatment as indicated by the assessment findings. This should ensure that the treatments plan is successful and the goals are achieved.
- Each treatment session should effect a change in the child; if it does not achieve the desired outcome then this indicates that the treatment is not appropriate.

Table 5.1 Regulations relevant to physiotherapists working with children

Common assessment framework (CWDC 2009)	Identifies problems early and offers holistic co-ordinated approach to supporting families Non statutory guidance
National Skills Framework for Child Health and Maternity (DOH 2004)	Programme to improve children's health. Sets standards for Social Services and Health. For latest amendments refer to: DOH: NSF for child health and maternity
Convention on the Rights of the Child 1990 (UN 1990)	International laws protecting a child's civil, cultural, economic, political and social rights Formal agreement between states belonging to the United Nations
Education Act 1996 (UK Gov 1996)	Duties for educating children with special educational needs in mainstream or special schools Statutory regulation
Early Support 2010 (DCSF 2010a)	Supports parents and carers of disabled children aged five and under Covered by the Childrens' Act 2004
Transforming Community Services 2009 (DOH 2009)	Setting the agenda for commissioners and providers of community healthcare Guidance document
Working together to Safeguard children (DCSF 2010b)	The responsibility of all adults working with children Statutory guidance

Standards and treatment guidelines

- Physiotherapists work according to a number of national and international standards and/or guidelines and in addition have to work within mandatory and statutory policies.

- The specialist area of community paediatrics requires physiotherapists to be aware of the additional legislation involved in working with children in the community.

- A physiotherapist working with children must be familiar with all of the regulations and guidance listed in Table 5.1.

- The reader is referred to the assessment volume for community paediatrics for additional working practices particular to working as a physiotherapist with children.

Treatment environment

- Treating children in a hospital setting is relatively straightforward, with purpose-designed treatment rooms, plenty of space, relatively few distractions with equipment on hand to make the task easier to carry out.

- Treating in a hospital environment has many advantages; however, it is difficult to replicate the home in a hospital department.

- If treatment is organised to take place where the child lives, the interventions can be designed to fit realistically into the child's daily life.
- This can be repeated at school or other settings the child attends, so that a broader team is brought into the treatment process.
- The broader team will involve anyone who spends sufficient time with the child, such that they need to be trained in how to contribute to their physiotherapy programme.
- Treatment in school educational settings is obviously vital, but at the different stages in a child's life the emphasis of the interventions will change as the child matures and develops.
- Suitable rooms and privacy can become an issue as the child gets older, for example, while treatment within the classroom might be ideal in primary school, it is not appropriate when the child is attending mainstream secondary education.
- The transition between primary and secondary is often a time where the emphasis of therapy changes, as the pressures of time within a school day intensify.
- Physiotherapy within school may be about hands-on therapy, but it is also important to provide advice for PE staff or for staff to become familiar with the requirements of the child mobilising generally around the school environment.

When to treat

- This requires effective communication with the parents/carers to establish the times of day when maximum benefit can be achieved and also how often treatment sessions need to take place.
- Decisions need to be made about whether treatment takes place after a young child's day time sleep, rather than before or alternatively earlier in a tiring day, rather than later.
- As parents gain confidence in handling their child and develop an increasing understanding of their child's condition they may not feel they need to see the physiotherapist so often.
- At times of change such as transition or orthopaedic intervention the direct physiotherapy input may need to be increased to provide the more specialist input required to manage the changes that may be seen in the child.

Treatment following orthopaedic intervention

- Children often find themselves being seen by staff in both acute and community settings as they attend paediatric community appointments or are reviewed by an orthopaedic team in a hospital.
- The child may have a condition that requires this pattern of input from acute and community staff. An example of this would be any child with bilateral cerebral palsy needing to have a baseline hip X-ray taken by the time they reach 30 months, or perhaps earlier, if there is evidence of problems such as asymmetrical hip abduction, leg length discrepancies, wind-sweeping.
- The child in this situation is introduced at an early age to orthopaedic services, even if initially only for monitoring.
- Effective team working involves an orthopaedic surgeon and physiotherapists working together to consider intervention options and their timing.

- The success of orthopaedic interventions such as orthotics, serial casting, botulinum toxin injections, soft tissue surgery, bony surgery, multilevel surgery are all dependent on the team approach to the child's care.

- Following botulinum toxin injections or surgical intervention are specific times when the frequency and intensity of physiotherapy intervention will need to be increased quite dramatically, to ensure that the child will return to his or her previous levels of functional ability or to have the greatest impact on maximising the benefits of any procedure undergone by the child.

- Whilst tight or spastic muscles are weakened by the effect of botulinum toxin, opposing muscles should be re-educated and strengthened and this will need to be frequent and specific in order to maximise the benefit of the injections.

24-hour management

- A child's objectives can be met by considering their entire daily routine and thinking about how they could incorporate exercises into their everyday life. How a parent transfers, carries or handles a young child will influence the child's alignment.

- If the parent is taught how to handle the child appropriately this can be used as a successful strategy to activate muscles.

- 24-hour postural management is another approach linking physiotherapy into the child's whole day.

- If one considers the amount of time during a 24-hour period that a child spends asleep it is important to manage their posture while they are asleep. Ideally the child should be positioned symmetrically in supine lying with the aim being to achieve the position of a Chailey ability level 3 (Box 5.1).

- There are several sleep systems commercially available or alternatively smaller T-rolls, pillows, cushions or cuddly toys can be used to influence a sleeping position.

- Some children of relatively low ability may also be spending time awake in lying, so their position may need to be controlled in prone, supine or side lying.

Box 5.1 Chailey level 3, supine lying ability

Maintains symmetrical posture

- Loadbearing through head, shoulder girdle, pelvis and feet
- Neutral pelvic tilt and shoulder girdle neutral giving general trunk curvature
- Hips abducted and externally rotated
- Chin tucked but not retracted and head able to turn freely from side to side
- Controlled eye movements possible
- Beginning of unilateral grasp to side of body, takes fist and objects to mouth

---

CHCS 2010.

Seating and standing frames

- Static chairs and wheelchairs will be used to control posture during the time the child spends in sitting (Figure 5.1).

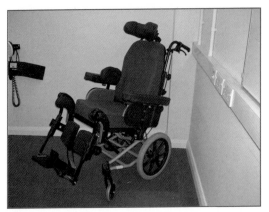

Figure 5.1 Specialised seating is provided to maintain optimum sitting posture.

- From the normal developmental age for standing, the use of standing frames can be included in the child's daily routine.
- In the early stages there are benefits to be gained from having an adult facilitate standing, so that they can be responsive to efforts being made by the child and to make the activity more dynamic.
- As the child grows in size a standing frame is a more realistic way that they can be facilitated to stand for prolonged periods of time.
- In the 'targeted training' therapeutic technique a frame may be used to support lower joints, as the child learns to control their trunk, pelvis and hips.
- Using a standing frame with thoracic support may not teach a child to stand, but it will affect them in a positive way psychologically as well as physically by holding their joints in a weight-bearing alignment.
- The area of seating provision crosses the boundaries between physiotherapy, occupational therapy and specialist wheelchair services in different parts of the UK, with the services having different roles.

Individual or group work?

- Group work cannot completely replace one-to-one therapy sessions, but this can be a very successful way to integrate therapy into different aspects of a child's life.
- Early intervention, where families join in to work together with the physiotherapist and other members of the team can often bring about improved outcomes when compared to the child being treated by one person.
- Working together with other children and families can be very beneficial where both a child and parents have been isolated.
- The group work can provide opportunities for the children and the families to form relationships with others in similar situations.

- This can also ensure that educational as well as therapeutic targets can be integrated into the child's overall management programme by the team that is composed of early years teachers, speech and language therapists, occupational therapists and physiotherapists.

- The older child may become bored of continuing therapy and therefore they may be more compliant if they can meet and work with other children, either after school or during the weekends or holidays.

Treatment modalities (neurology)

- The choice of treatment modalities available is extensive and is predominantly determined by the objectives that are set and a child's underlying condition.

Floor work

Initial preparation

- Floor work and exercises are particularly useful if the child has abnormal tone. One of the initial priorities is to influence that tone, i.e. if tone is raised then it needs to be reduced and if the tone is low it will need to be increased.

- One of the approaches used frequently in the management of children with abnormal tone is the Bobath concept. The Bobath concept is useful as it includes tone influencing patterns as part of the intervention.

- Positioning, movement, facilitation, weight bearing and the use of gravity can all be used to influence tone and are all part of the preparation of the child for treatment.

- Children with neurological conditions may benefit from tone-influencing medication such as baclofen, taken orally or intra thecally with the physiotherapist being in the position of being able to monitor beneficial or detrimental effects of the treatment. There may be a variation through the day as doses are taken, or wear off.

- The reader is referred to the acute paediatric chapter for further information on pharmacological management.

Alignment

- The preparation is then followed by improving alignment in all appropriate positions.

- This may include the alignment of the head on the trunk, the trunk over the centre of gravity and limb alignment.

Muscle activation

- With tone and alignment influenced the child needs to actively move.

- Their muscles need to be activated, especially the muscles important for maintaining appropriate body position and function.

- If a child cannot perform a movement, then facilitation techniques can be used to assist them to achieve the desired movement.

- As the child's own movement improves the therapist withdraws their support more and more.

- It is important to consider the joint range to work in, e.g. if a child lacks full hip extension in standing, then it will be the inner range of the hip extensors that must be targeted.

- Although muscle weakness may not be the primary problem, it is often found as a secondary problem in conjunction with other issues.
- Children with cerebral palsy will be at increased risk of losing function during growth spurts, muscle strengthening has been advocated as a method of improving function without increasing the level of spasticity (Dodd et al 2002).
- These children may not be able to isolate individual movements and their weakness will be in particular muscle groups.
- Functional activities can be used to develop muscle endurance and power, e.g. the child can be asked to assist as they are brought up to a sitting position from lying down.
- Exactly the way in which the task is achieved will influence correct activation of the neck and trunk muscles.
- Often introducing rotation into a gross functional movement will enable specific muscle groups to be worked.
- As a child is able to move into standing this provides an opportunity to introduce dissociation of one lower limb from the other if they perform the manoeuvre through half high kneeling.
- Consider which leg the child prefers to lead with to achieve the desired outcome. The leading leg should take more weight and the extended hip can be encouraged to achieve greater hip extension.
- As a child prepares to stand up, then they can be discouraged from using their hands and this in turn will increase the effort required from the lower limb extensors to achieve standing.

Stretches and passive movements

- There is a lack of consensus amongst paediatric physiotherapists about the effectiveness of stretches and passive movements.
- They are considered by some to be useful for improving muscle flexibility.
- Spastic muscles stiffen when not being used, therefore helping a child move their limbs is thought to improve flexibility and prepare muscles for work.
- Movements can be performed that mirror normal movement to give a child the feeling of normal movement patterns.
- Profoundly disabled children may have little active movement, therefore passive movements of their limbs can provide experience of normal movement.
- It is also thought that contractures may be prevented and muscle spasm inhibited by applying sustained stretches.
- Various techniques are used in practice, e.g. shaking a limb and applying traction whilst moving the limb out of a spastic pattern.
- It has been found that for effective muscle lengthening to occur the stretch should be held for 6–8 hours a day.
- To achieve the prolonged stretches splinting using ankle foot orthoses can maintain a good position at the ankle to lengthen gastrosoleus and increase ankle range of movement (Teplicky et al 2002).
- Sleep systems, standing frames, supportive seating or adaptive wheelchairs can assist in maintaining alignment, symmetry and muscle length.
- Passive stretches alone are unlikely to be effective for increasing range (Pin et al 2006).
- There is evidence suggesting sustained stretches to be superior to manual stretches for the reduction of spasticity and improvement of range.

- Rapid periods of growth (spurts) can affect biomechanics and this can be predicted to a degree as children tend to have growth spurts around age 6–7, again aged 9–10 and finally before and around puberty.
- The pre-pubertal growth spurt is earlier in girls, around age 10–12, and in boys, as late as 14–16 years.
- Rapid growth initially occurs in bones with soft tissue catching up more slowly.
- Activities to maintain flexibility can help reduce problems associated with growth.

Constraint induced movement therapy (CIMT)

- Constraint induced movement therapy (CIMT) is a method used to improve function in the affected limbs of stroke patients and with children presenting with cerebral palsy.
- There is some evidence to support the use of CIMT in rehabilitation of appropriate patient groups (Taub et al 2004; Hoare et al 2009).
- The child is encouraged to use the affected arm whilst some form of restraint is applied to the non-affected arm.
- Various forms of restraint have been tried and for varying lengths of time.
- If this is going to be something the families continue with it has to be manageable from their perspective.
- A group session can be a very successful way to first introduce the treatment. The physiotherapist needs to come up with many imaginative ways to engage the child in new and interesting activities that are geared to making them use their affected arm.
- To ensure success the activities have to be carefully chosen and the less able children need to be assisted through facilitation to succeed.
- Activities can be functional and could include making a sandwich, dressing up games, fun activities such as lucky dips, where the child immerses their hand in sand to search for hidden treasure or drawing pictures on a mirror covered in shaving foam.
- The restraint should be as little as possible, e.g. a child could be provided with a glove to wear on their unaffected hand.
- This helps them and others to identify which hand they should not be using and discourages use of that hand.
- At home the parent would need to identify games that are specifically chosen for the CIMT sessions.
- The sessions should be run for a realistic length of time, e.g. from 30 minutes up to an hour will be a useful length of time to achieve benefit.

Hippotherapy

- Also known as riding for the disabled, hippotherapy may or may not be provided as one of the community services in a child's local area.
- There are numerous benefits claimed for hippotherapy, ranging from improvements in tone, postural mechanisms and functional abilities (Silkwood-Sherer & Warmbier 2007).

- The movement of the horse is transmitted to the rider providing rhythmic three-dimensional movement that is thought to stimulate the sensory and motor systems within the child.

Aquatic physiotherapy

- The physiotherapist faces additional challenges when working in a pool.
- They must familiarise themselves with the operating and emergency procedures and practise the evacuation procedure.
- It is important to feel comfortable and be relaxed in the pool, nervousness or tension is picked up by children.
- The depth of water affects stability, with water at waist depth around 50% of body weight passes through the feet enabling stability to be maintained during the delivery of manual resisted exercises.
- The child should be assessed prior to attending for pool treatment, what this will involve will depend on the child's diagnosis.
- Conditions that can benefit from aquatic physiotherapy and some of the challenges (Figure 5.2):
- Juvenile idiopathic arthritis
- Cerebral palsy, due to increased tone, there will be higher muscle density, which can cause affected limbs to sink
- Hemiplegia, the child has to learn to counteract horizontal rotation in lying when one side sinks in comparison to the other side
- Diplegia, altered balance and possible muscle wasting may entail a child needing support to prevent them from having their head thrust under water.
- The Halliwick concept of teaching swimming to people with disabilities is a method of using the properties of water to enable confidence and some measure of independence to be gained.

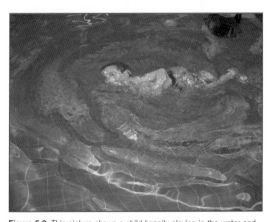

Figure 5.2 This picture shows a child happily playing in the water and independently propelling himself. He has learnt to hold his breath, or to blow bubbles to prevent water entering his mouth and nose. He is unable to swim with his head above water whilst in prone.

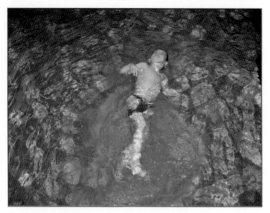

Figure 5.3 Rolling from back to front independently.

- Breathing control and confidence are taught to enable the child to relax and be able to listen to and learn new instruction.
- Games can be used to help motivate and can be individual or carried out in groups. Balance in the water both vertical and horizontal needs to be gained so the child recognises when they are in the correct position, and can correct themselves if they move out of this.
- A child can be encouraged to turn to look at someone to start a movement, following the movement with the arm will assist the child to roll. See Figure 5.3.
- Praise needs to be instantaneous to encourage younger children or those with learning difficulties to try again to achieve a goal.
- A child must learn to float on their back, and this is usually achieved once the child is confident working with an adult, and have become familiar with being in a pool environment.
- Initially this may be achieved by them lying back with their head on the adult's shoulder.
- This is progressed to supported floating, independent floating and learning to propel independently through the water. See Figure 5.4.
- Independence in the pool environment can be started in the changing room. The child can be encouraged to roll, sit, and help to change themselves.
- Child protection must always be considered, and changing should be appropriate. Modesty is important to children and care should be taken to ensure this is respected and that the child has a say in how they are changed and by whom.

Fun

- Children need to enjoy their physiotherapy sessions and the physiotherapist must be prepared to be imaginative and flexible when trying to achieve treatment goals.
- For a session to be successful it is important to know what level of cognitive skill a child can perform to and also their personal interests.

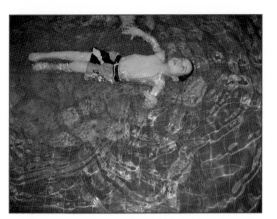

Figure 5.4 This child with quadriplegia has learnt to float independently. The head is tipped back to assist with horizontal position and helps keep the legs and pelvis floating. Arms are spread and as relaxed as possible. High muscle tone prevents limbs being straighter.

- It helps to be knowledgeable about trends in toys, books, music, television programmes and characters.
- It pays to watch children's television; use a child's own toys or take toys on visits with you.
- Positive reinforcement by praise, use of stickers, star charts, and certificates will further help with compliance and enjoyment.
- Descriptive commentary is an effective technique when working with children with underdeveloped language.
- The challenge with teenagers is maintaining their motivation.
- This can be achieved by incorporating sports or the Nintendo Wii into their routine to enable them to improve their skills and fitness.
- Encouraging exercise is important for their life after school and is a fun way to make friends.
- Paralympic competition in recent years has raised the profile of the variety of sports available, and access to special needs sport has improved (www.paralympics.org.uk).
- There may be support from a local disability sports officer in setting up local sports.

Equipment

- As an adjunct to the repertoire of techniques that the physiotherapist may use to achieve a child's goals, it is useful to consider the role of equipment.
- Equipment can assist the physiotherapist to position a child, for example, or to facilitate functional activity (Table 5.2).

Table 5.2 Equipment to assist in the treatment of children with neurological conditions

Equipment	Therapeutic use
Gaiters	To extend elbows or knees for a variety of reasons, including activation of more proximal joints
Gym ball or cushion	To provide an alternative base of support that in turn will induce different reactions within a body
Walking aids	Tripod or quadruped stakes, k-walkers with support from behind, to influence extension activity, with a rollator providing the support from in front
Stools	For working between sitting and standing
Ladders	A remnant from Conductive Education but providing functional support as a child attains standing (Peto Institute 2010)
Tricycles	Offers an alternative form of independent mobility
Wedges	Influence tone, alignment and ability level in prone
Kinesio taping	Aligning tissues, offering sensory, positional or mechanoreceptor stimulation

Orthotics

Background knowledge

- Physiotherapists working with children will encounter orthotics on a regular basis and therefore it is necessary to develop a basic knowledge of the types of orthoses and their application as they can be used as an adjunct to physiotherapy treatment and management.
- It is important to develop the knowledge and ability to identify why an orthosis may be of benefit to a child and then to refer the child to the nearest paediatric orthotist.

Function of orthotics

- Orthoses are externally applied medical devices used to modify the structural and functional characteristics of the neuromuscular and skeletal systems (International Organization for Standardization 2007).
- Orthotics are used to:
- Provide stability
- Correct alignment using force systems
- Minimise, correct or prevent further deformity
- Provide protection, e.g. protective helmets
- Improve function
- Facilitate and/or improve quality of movement/gait
- Reduce pain.

- There is a wide range of pre-formed orthoses available to use in the management of children.
- The following list includes a few examples of the most common orthoses that will be encountered during a period of working in community paediatrics (Figures 5.5–5.12).

Supportive orthopaedic footwear (Figure 5.5)

Trend for supply has reduced. Particularly useful for ankle instability which is delaying the child's development and/or affecting balance; however the weight of this footwear can make walking more difficult.

Insoles, functional foot orthoses (FFOs) (Figure 5.6)

Can be made from variety of materials depending on support required. Are used to improve foot position on weight bearing. These can be used to correct a variety of deformities, e.g. forefoot or hindfoot planus or cavus. Judicious use is required in relation to the bone growth potential of the child.

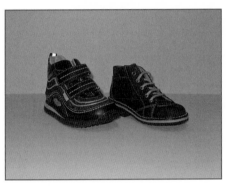

Figure 5.5 Supportive orthopaedic footwear.

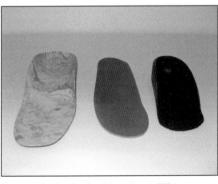

Figure 5.6 Insoles, functional foot orthoses (FFOs).

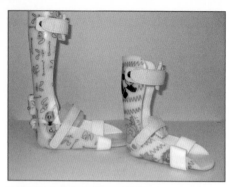

Figure 5.7 Ankle foot orthoses (AFOs).

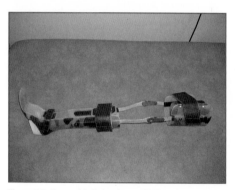

Figure 5.8 Knee ankle foot orthoses (KAFOs).

Ankle foot orthoses (AFOs) (Figure 5.7)

A plastic shell encompassing the posterior calf, ankle and foot. Applies three points of pressure to limit ankle dorsiflexion or plantarflexion. The splint may also be hinged if there is a need to limit only one of these movements. AFOs are commonly used in the management of the child with a neuromuscular condition. The same principle is used for night splinting to prevent the loss of extensibility in the calf muscles, e.g. in children with Duchenne muscular dystrophy.

Knee ankle foot orthoses (KAFOs) (Figure 5.8)

Most often used to compensate for week knee extensors. Are commonly used in the management of muscular dystrophy to prolong the ability of the child to achieve an independent gait.

Sitting Walking And Standing Hip orthosis (SWASH) brace (Figure 5.9)

This brace facilitates hip abduction when the hip is flexed. It was originally designed for a walking child, but has been adapted for use with children when they are sitting in order to improve their base of support and stability.

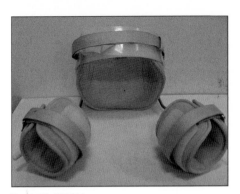

Figure 5.9 SWASH brace.

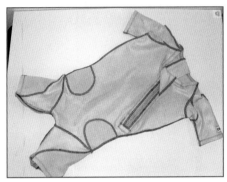

Figure 5.10 Dynamic elastomeric fabric orthoses (DEFOs).

Dynamic Elastomeric Fabric Orthoses (DEFOs) (Figure 5.10)

These are also known as Dynamic Movement Orthoses (DMOs) or Sensory Dynamic Orthoses (SDOs). They are made of a Lycra based fabric. Additional layers of reinforcing material add a biomechanical influence and encourage improved movement control and proximal stability.

The increased pressure on certain muscle groups is reported to improve proprioception.

Most common DEFOs are the suit, glove and sock.

Spinal jackets (Figure 5.11)

Provided to offer correction and/or support to the spine. They are used to minimise the development of a scoliosis where the child has inadequate trunk control to prevent a scoliosis.

Head protection (Figure 5.12a, b)

Provided for children who have a tendency to experience falls or who are likely to self-inflict injuries as a result of uncontrolled movements.

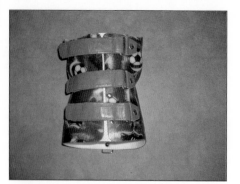

Figure 5.11 Spinal jacket.

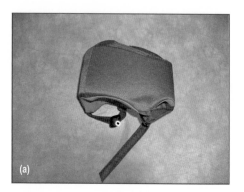

(a)

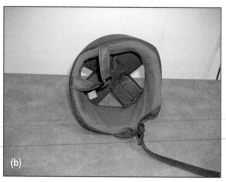

(b)

Figure 5.12 (a and b) Head protection.

Co-ordination difficulties

- Children may present with a wide range of difficulties with co-ordination.
- There are many reasons for poor or below expected age motor learning patterns including ligamentous laxity, learning difficulties, low muscle tone or prematurity and dyspraxia.
- The pattern of intervention may be very different depending on the child's diagnosis.

Ligamentous laxity

- The list of clinical findings seen in ligamentous laxity may include:
- Hypermobility
- Low muscle tone
- Slumped posture or poor ability to maintain a good posture for any length of time
- More physical effort to do things
- Poor stability around the pelvic or shoulder girdle affecting both balance, quality of running and gross motor tasks, and difficulties handwriting
- Poor anti-gravity abilities which can be assessed both in supine flexion, prone extension and during functional activity
- Difficulties with stability and compensatory fixation may lead to imbalance
- Postural background may be rigid to compensate
- May have flat feet and be 'heavy' when stepping, or may find it hard to jump or hop
- Unless the child has symptoms of pain or limited function they may not require intervention other than advice on supportive footwear, and on suitable sporting and play activities to maximise their potential. A more affected child will need therapy aimed at improving joint stability, core strength and possibly co-ordination and fitness. They may benefit from orthotics if foot pain is present.

Low muscle tone

- Children may show some of the following signs and symptoms:
- May have been slow in feeding
- Later than average standing and walking age
- Unsteady on feet longer than average
- Slumped posture
- Poor gait
- Tired after a short walk
- Poor concentration and easily distracted
- Tire over the week and over a school term
- May show difficulty in tasks involving (finger) strength.
- Children who need support from therapy should be worked in such a way that they increase their muscle tone, and then work different muscle groups for

short periods, changing positions and muscle groups before they tire too much.

Developmental co-ordination disorder (DCD)

- The existence of DCD and the impact it can have on the general well-being of the affected children has been widely recognised, although the underlying causes of the condition are unclear.
- DCD can be defined according to the following criteria:
- There may be marked delay in achieving motor milestones, e.g. sitting, crawling or walking, dropping things, 'clumsiness', poor performance in sports, or poor handwriting.
- The disturbances above interfere with academic achievement or activities in daily living.
- The disturbance is not due to a general medical condition, e.g. cerebral palsy, hemiplegia, or muscular dystrophy and does not meet the criteria for a pervasive developmental disorder.
- If learning difficulties are present the motor difficulties are in excess of those usually associated with it.
- The prevalence of DCD, estimated on the basis of the above-cited criteria, is as high as 6 % of all 5- to 11-year-old children (APA 1994).
- Many children may know by the age of 5 that they are unable to compete with their peer group, and may seek out ways to avoid physical activities they find difficult.
- This can include ignoring instruction, behavioural difficulties, joking and playing around or tears.
- Treatment should concentrate on functional behaviour.
- The therapist should aim to provide a motivational climate in which the CNS is forced to consider a proactive monitoring of movement execution in different tasks and environmental circumstances.
- Postural control deficits can hamper the efficient acquisition of motor skills, therefore the use of whole-body tasks is preferential to isolated motor exercises.
- Treatment should be directed towards 'functionality' but also teach the child to cope with 'dysfunctionality'.
- By offering children experiences of success and teaching them to deal with unsuccessful performance therapists can fulfil an important psychological role in the prevention of emotional problems (Deconinck 2005).

Management of children with respiratory disorders

- The management of children with respiratory disorders in the community can be considered to include management in the child's home and also during the time spent in the school setting.
- Children with long-term conditions may get respiratory infections or complications that require treatment.
- Central to maintaining the child at home are the parents or carers who will be able to monitor the child and seek help when they develop a respiratory problem.

- Parents will learn to identify problems and will either contact their GP for medication such as antibiotics or contact the paediatric service where the child is under consultant management for an urgent appointment.
- The role of the physiotherapist in the home setting in most cases is to assess, to provide education or to refer the child to other services.

Management of lower respiratory tract infection

- Physiotherapy intervention should be provided for the same reasons as those considered for the treatment of adults, i.e.
- The removal of secretions
- Management of conditions with chronic sputum production, e.g. cystic fibrosis
- To assist those with an ineffective cough, e.g. in neurological and neuromuscular conditions
- To assist those with a depressed cough, e.g. due to presence of pain
- Where the effort of breathing is very demanding
- Where a ventilation-perfusion mismatch occurs (Hardy 2007).
- Parents or carers should be taught assistive coughing, especially for children with reducing peak flow readings.
- The child may be taught glossopharyngeal breathing to assist air entry and enhance the effectiveness of coughing (Eagle 2007).
- As medical management has improved so too has the lifespan of children that would previously not have lived to the point where they develop respiratory complications.
- Increasingly, home ventilation is being required for children with Duchenne muscular dystrophy.
- Evidence now shows those being ventilated and having corrective spinal surgery living until 30 years and those being ventilated surviving until their early twenties (Eagle et al 2007).
- The community physiotherapist is now likely to encounter the interventions that were once the preserve of the intensive care environment in the acute hospital setting and the development of these skills is something that should be considered by a physiotherapist planning to work with children in the community.
- In the UK non-invasive ventilation is the preferred choice with nocturnal ventilation being used in the initial stages as the child begins to demonstrate signs of respiratory failure.
- Daytime ventilation is used as the individual gets older and respiratory function deteriorates.
- The maintenance of the power supply and a possible emergency power supply should be considered and put in place to provide adequate power supply to the ventilator in the event of a power cut.

The references for this chapter can be found on www.expertconsult.com.

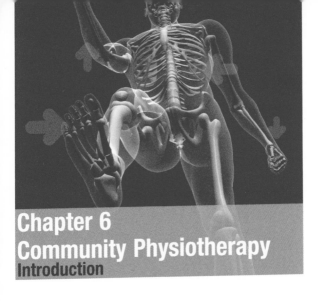

Chapter 6
Community Physiotherapy
Introduction

Treatment techniques/management approach

- For any treatment, as for assessment, there is the additional focus on improving function related to the patient's needs and their environment.
- The intervention can take place in a variety of settings, from privately owned or rented property, Council or Housing Association accommodation, supported housing (sheltered or special sheltered), a caravan, hostel, Residential/Nursing Home or Day Centre.

Patient choice and rights

- Careful consideration must be given to:
- the patient's choice DH (2001a)
- culture CRE (2002)
- privacy, dignity, confidentiality DH (2003) (including never leaving messages on answer-phones without the patient's permission).

Risk assessments

- Risk assessments should be carried out at the start of each treatment session as the environment may have changed since the previous visit. Risk assessment CSP (2002). Personal safety CSP (2009) (for the physiotherapist and the patient), Lone working CSP (2009).
- There will quite possibly not be any height-adjustable furniture or space for large pieces of equipment in the home environment. There could be environmental constraints when treatments take place in confined and cluttered areas, some of which may be unkempt or unclean.

- It may be difficult or impossible for a patient to manoeuvre, if they are becoming more dependent on a walking aid.
- Therefore, the environment may directly affect the choice of treatment. Moving and handling CSP (2009).

Consent

- Where consent is required for involvement with carers, either formal (through an agency) or informal (family and friends) this must be clarified in the treatment process (CSP, 2004; DH, 2001a,b,c; DH 2009).
- The involvement can be supporting the treatment regime through assistance with moving and handling, reinforcing exercise programmes, assisting with communication or helping to understand any cultural issues.
- Patients with a high level of anxiety can often be reassured by people who are familiar to them, especially when a physiotherapist is introducing alternative approaches to treatment or new activities.

Holistic assessment and treatment

- All patients should be assessed and treated holistically with functional treatments aimed at improving their independence, safety and quality of life.
- Assessment may have identified a need to involve other professionals in the treatment process and joint visits may be of benefit to the patients and physiotherapist.
- Treatment programmes or activities should always involve a good understanding of the rehabilitation ethos of enabling and handing over responsibility to the patient, wherever possible.
- If an assessment has highlighted a particular functional activity that the patient is unable to carry out independently or safely, the choice of treatment should be focussed on addressing this.
- As an example, toileting in the acute setting may require a patient to walk 10 or more metres on an uncarpeted floor to reach a toilet with adequate lighting and assistance if required.
- When this activity is attempted at home, a similar distance is likely to involve walking on different floor coverings, through doorways and in potentially poor lighting, so provision of a commode by the bed at night would improve patient safety.
- Practise getting out of bed, arranging their clothes, cleaning themselves and getting back into bed.
- To be able to go to the toilet safely and independently at night contributes greatly to an individual's quality of life and dignity and involves the coordinated action of different muscle groups, strength, balance, adequate range of movement and confidence to perform the task.
- There may also need to be provision of equipment for bed mobility to facilitate these activities.
- Another example of a functional activity would involve accessing a drink. In the acute setting, this is usually provided by staff. In the home setting a patient will need to plan how this is going to take place.
- The task will involve mobility, balance whilst multi-tasking, manual dexterity and transportation of the drink.

- This would apply to people of all ages and advice and exercises to address these activities should be incorporated into treatment programmes.
- Problem solving of the transportation for someone using a walking aid may include provision of a kitchen trolley or advising the use of a pocketed apron or shoulder bag in which to hold a bottle of liquid.

Pain management

- Treatments may involve the need for pain control, increasing range of movement, muscle strength, training on safe positioning, provision of appropriate equipment, improving balance and safety instructions.
- Repetition of activities may address some of these issues and can be carried out under the supervision of a delegated rehabilitation assistant or alternative carer.
- Treatments involving electrical and other equipment may be limited by the mode of transport used to travel to a patient and the environment of the patient.
- However, treatments can be carried out where appropriate using any of the following in the community: transcutaneous electrical nerve stimulator (TENS), portable ultrasound machine, pulse oximeter, interferential therapy, acupuncture, gym balls, Thera-Band and cuff weights for ankles and wrists.

Documentation

- All treatment interventions, conversations (with patients, formal and informal carers, family, friends and other colleagues and health professionals), giving advice and information must be carefully and accurately documented.
- If a patient chooses not to take your advice for whatever reason, this must also be documented (CSP, 2000).

Treatments specific to the speciality area

- The community is a speciality area using core skills that are enhanced by other specialities and skills specific to the environment.
- It should be recognised that it is not always possible to carry out a 'traditional' style of physiotherapy treatment and this may depend on the needs of a particular patient at a particular time in their unique setting.
- Invariably the treatment will involve problem-solving skills, using initiative, common sense and flexibility in approach.
- The physiotherapist may find that they are using a whole set of skills, apart from physiotherapy, as the treatment will be holistic and not just medical.
- The physiotherapist may need to draw on knowledge relating to other issues affecting the patient, for example, difficulty in accessing housing or other benefits, the involvement of young carers, may be of great concern to someone and until resolved, they may not be able to engage fully with their treatment plans.
- Following an assessment, the treatment will always take into consideration the specific abilities and needs of the patient.
- SMART goals will be agreed jointly between the physiotherapist and the patient (DH, 2001a).

Activities of daily living (ADL)

- The necessity or desire to perform functional activities of daily living will need to be addressed in the treatment plans.
- It is important to understand the daily routine of the patient and discover what it is reasonable to achieve.
- This may include:
- getting in and out of bed
- using the toilet
- getting washed and dressed
- managing to self-medicate
- getting on and off a chair
- preparing a meal/hot drink
- indoor and outdoor stair ascending/descending
- outdoor mobility over rough terrain and slopes
- tending the garden and other hobbies
- going to work
- going to the shops and/or post office
- using an ATM at a bank
- using public transport
- getting in and out of a car
- attending social activities
- visiting friends and family.

Patient confidentiality

- There are confidentiality issues if relatives, friends or neighbours are present.
- Just because a person is receiving their physiotherapy treatment within their own home does not alter the fact that they may not want anybody else present.
- Even if the neighbour is also their main carer, this does not automatically mean they are entitled to be present or contribute to the treatment session in any way, nor are they entitled to any information about the patient or their progress after a treatment session, unless the express permission to allow this has been given by the patient.
- Partners are also not automatically entitled to any information just because of their marital status (DH, 2003).

Cultural considerations

- Respect has to be given to cultural and religious beliefs in someone's own home, but expectations of the patient should not compromise the physiotherapist's rights, for example, taking off your shoes in someone's house.
- Is there a way to reach a compromise, maybe by covering your shoes with an acceptable material?

Treatments related to specific areas of the home

- It is important to look at the home as the treatment/rehabilitation base.
- Treatment should always be functional and when related to daily living and activities it will encourage more compliance and ongoing adherence to the treatment plan.
- The advantage of treating someone in their home environment is that it gives the patient an opportunity to talk about their condition/s and about any concerns that they may have and how to manage them, or any other related questions.
- It may be that the physiotherapist will not be able to 'cure' the problem, but will be able to talk through or demonstrate effective ways to manage it.
- Advice based on this information will provide lifelong benefits to the patient.
- The physiotherapist is a great source of information and knowledge to the patient and should ensure that relevant written resources are provided (these are often available from self-help groups and charities or from the internet).
- In each area of the home, it is necessary to consider:
- The environment
- Functional treatments in each area, incorporating safe use of fixtures and fittings and problem solving
- Adaptive equipment/exercises, to enable the patient to use everyday objects within the home
- Involvement of other agencies, professionals, informal and formal carers.
- There are some issues that need to considered during treatments in all areas, such as appropriate footwear, the potential use of assistive technology (including the use of a pendant alarm) and personal safety issues (for the physiotherapist, rehabilitation assistant or support worker, the patient and the carers).
- Patients should be encouraged to utilise as much of their environment as is possible to do safely and should resist the temptation to remain static, with the expectation that everything will be done for them (DH, 2001a).
- The community physiotherapist's work is fundamentally functional, therefore it is important to incorporate the patient's daily routine into the treatment plan. Therefore, a good place to start would be.

The Bedroom (upstairs or downstairs) (Figure 6.1)

Environmental considerations

- How much furniture or clutter is in the room? Are these forming obstacles? Can they be moved and re-positioned to improve the ability of the patient to mobilise and therefore reduce risk, if the patient agrees?
- Are there rugs or cables across the floor? Is it possible to tape down loose wiring and carpet edges and remove rugs, if the patient agrees? Can this be carried out by family members or the voluntary sector? Advise on risks, if the patient is unwilling or unable to adopt safer options.
- Is there adequate lighting/heating/ventilation (LHV)? Advise the patient to use a light if they need to get in and out of bed at night. When advising about the use of heating in the bedroom, it is an Act of Law that there should not be a working gas fire in a room where someone is sleeping unless it is a room-sealed appliance or it incorporates a safety control that will shut down the appliance to prevent a build up of combustible gas in the room concerned (GSR 1998 and HSE 1998).

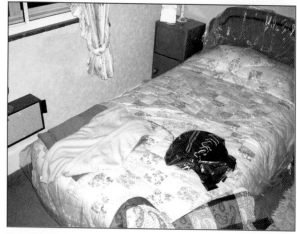

Figure 6.1 The bed area.

- Bed is not always height adjustable or as firm as the conventional physiotherapy plinth. The bed that is in situ may be the only option available to you that can be used as the place to do exercises for limbs, trunk, balance, posture and to practice sitting to standing and standing to sitting.

- Consider joint visits with or referral to an occupational therapist (OT). However, this may involve different time scales depending on whether there is an occupational therapist in your team or access to a 'Trusted Assessor' (a physiotherapist, nurse or support worker who, when trained, will be able to assess for and prescribe a simple solution or a basic piece of equipment to meet the needs of an individual) available. It may be necessary to make a referral to an OT in Social Services.

- A patient may have started to use a commode or walking aid that prevents safe access to the side of the bed on which they usually sleep. In this case if the patient has accessed the bed in a specific way that is no longer possible, then an alternative method has to be developed and practiced to ensure the patient is able to get onto and off the bed safely.

- Advise on appropriate footwear and where it is safely accessible.

- Remind the patient to put on their pendant alarm, if they use one, before getting out of bed.

Functional treatments

- Bed mobility:

- Patients with decreased mobility often find it difficult to move into a safe position in bed, especially if the mattress is soft or upper limb and trunk strength is reduced

- If there are no contraindications for a patient to be to turning onto their side or into prone lying in bed but ability to get into these positions has been reduced, treatment would involve showing them how to roll over or move to the edge or centre of the bed by bridging

- Techniques can be shown to carry out these activities and reminders given that first thing in the morning their joints/muscles may feel less flexible until their analgesia is effective
- Sitting up over the side of the bed using the correct technique may be facilitated by the use of equipment if they have sufficient upper limb strength.
- Transitional activities:
- It is important to teach or reinforce the correct techniques for lying to sitting and sitting to standing and these should be used as life-long methods
- They should be demonstrated and practised with informal carers to avoid carer strain as patients often have unreasonable expectations of how their informal carers should assist them
- It may be necessary to consider a mattress variator or profiling bed if therapy has not enabled the patient to manage by any other means
- It is important to measure the compressed bed height (that is, when the patient is sitting on the side of the bed) before recommendation and provision of equipment.
- Transfers:
- If a commode is being used, it will be necessary to practise the technique for getting out of bed and onto the commode and also getting off the commode and back into bed safely
- A commode always needs to be positioned appropriately against a solid, static object.
- Exercise:
- Patients can use the bed for exercise at any time during the day
- After lunch, rather than falling asleep in the chair, it is worth encouraging patients to have 'siesta time' lying on the bed
- This positioning can maintain joint range and prevent potential postural deformities that may lead to contractures
- It also has the added benefit of reducing damage to pressure areas from constantly sitting and assists venous return and the reduction of dependent oedema
- Patients should be made aware that this is not an indulgence, but a way of maintaining energy levels during the day.

Adaptive equipment/exercises

- To assist the physiotherapist to adapt to this different working environment, the following will provide suggestions of alternatives to the equipment more commonly encountered in a hospital/clinic setting.
- Physiotherapists will find that they have to be creative and adaptable within a community environment, often using available resources such as:
- Sliding board – using an upturned tea tray, plastic bags or black bin liners
- Wall bars – utilising a headboard to attach the Thera-Band to
- Treatment roll – use towel rolled up in an old stocking or tied with string
- Walking stick – for double arm stretches in lying or sitting.

Involvement of other agencies and informal carers

- An equipment assessment with an occupational therapist could facilitate the treatments and personal activities of daily living with provision of bed equipment, bed raises or a commode.

- A community nurse can order a specialist bed, if required for nursing management, such as a height-adjustable/profiling bed with a pressure relieving mattress.
- The informal carers should be involved in the treatment process (with the patient's consent) and shown specific techniques to avoid carer strain, such as using sliding sheets.
- Suppliers of assistive technology such as a pressure pad on the floor that switches the light on when the patient stands on it.

The bathroom and toilet (Figure 6.2)

- If it is a goal, the patient will expect to access the bathroom; however, not all patients need to access the bathroom to wash as they may just use a bowl in another room.

Environmental considerations

- What type of floor covering and what state of repair is it in?
- Ensure floor coverings are safe, i.e. not loose or slippery.
- Are there any obstacles?
- Can they be moved and re-positioned to reduce risk, if the patient agrees?
- Is there adequate LHV?
- Ensure lighting is accessible and sufficient, especially if the patient needs to move around the home at night.
- Is there already equipment in situ and is it appropriate and safe for purpose.
- Advise on use or misuse of fittings already in situ, e.g. it may be possible to pull up from the toilet using a secure towel rail, but not using the toilet roll holder.
- Always advise against using a radiator to pull up on as this could lead to burns. Consider a joint visit with an OT or referral to an OT in a community or Social Services team.
- Is there sufficient access through the doorway for a walking aid?

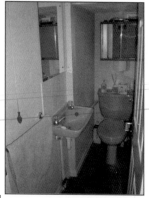

Figure 6.2 Access to the bathroom.

- Is there room for a walking aid inside the bathroom/toilet?
- Is there floor space for equipment if needed, e.g. a perching stool?
- Is there space for a carer to be present?
- Does the patient become short of breath performing certain personal care activities? If appropriate, a perching stool or another suitable item of equipment can be supplied.
- If a pendant alarm is used, remind patient to always replace it around their neck after washing.

Functional treatments

- Transfers:
- A treatment goal may include getting on or off the toilet
- The patient should practise sitting to standing and standing to sitting using the correct technique
- Appropriateness of equipment needs to be considered
- A toilet seat raise may not be acceptable if it is impractical to remove and replace if other family members need to access the toilet Alternatives are available. (Figure 6.3).
- Personal care activities:
- Functional activities can be used to increase range of movement and muscle strength, to enable the patient to wash and dry themselves, dress and undress themselves, turn taps on and off and use the toilet
- Personal care activities may also be carried out in the bedroom or kitchen if this is more appropriate.
- Balance exercises:
- To ensure the patient is safe to perform activities in sitting and standing
- It may be necessary to alter their sitting postures to wipe after using the toilet and/or to maintain an unsupported stand whilst washing and dressing and cleaning after using the toilet.

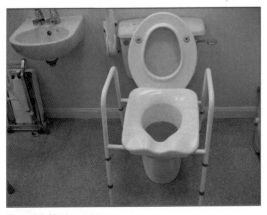

Figure 6.3 Mowbray toilet.

- Bath mobility:
  - This could be either stepping into the bath to shower or sitting on the bottom of the bath or getting on and off a bath board
  - The assessment will have identified areas of weakness, safety and what equipment may be required
  - Exercises can be carried out to improve range of movement and muscle strength of the relevant joints and muscle groups
  - Appropriate equipment can be recommended or supplied, e.g. bath board, non-slip mat, grab rails, bath seat, tap turners
  - Patients need to be as independent as possible, as formal carers will not assist patients to get out of a bath and it is not advisable for family members to assist either.

Adaptive equipment/exercises

- Functional exercises/activities may involve:
- Forearm pronation/supination and strengthening of grip by wringing out a flannel
- Shoulder medial/lateral rotation and flexion/extension can be increased by drying the back with a towel
- Trunk flexion/extension will occur when the patient dries their feet with a towel.

Involvement of other agencies and informal carers

- An equipment assessment with an occupational therapist could facilitate the treatment and personal activities of daily living through the provision of equipment, such as a toilet surround or bath board and grab rails (Figure 6.4).
- The informal carers should be involved in the treatment process (with the patient's consent) and shown specific techniques to avoid injuring themselves, with an emphasis on safety.

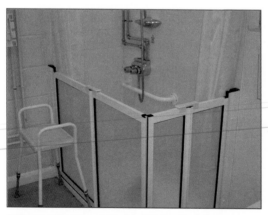

Figure 6.4 Equipment and potential adaptations to a bathroom.

- Suppliers of assistive technology for example can be involved, to provide monitoring equipment to prevent the bath from overflowing, if the taps are left running.

The stairs and hallway (Figure 6.5)

- This is a high risk area where additional handrails may need to be considered.
- The physiotherapist needs to be aware that a patient may be particularly anxious about using the stairs if they have fallen on them previously.

Environmental considerations

- How much furniture or clutter is in the hallway?
- Are there any obstacles? Can they be moved and re-positioned to reduce risk, if the patient agrees?
- Are there rugs or cables across the floor or stairs?
- Is the floor covering loose, worn or slippery? Is it possible to tape down loose wiring and carpet edges and remove rugs, if the patient agrees? Can this be carried out by family members or the voluntary sector?
- Advise on risks if unable to adopt safer options.
- Is there adequate LHV? Ensure lighting is accessible and sufficient.
- Are there already handrails in situ? Are they in the right positions and safe to use? If not and it is appropriate, measure for handrails or refer to an occupational therapist.
- Consideration must be given to:
- The ownership of the property (Is it privately owned or housing association or private landlord?). The owners or landlords may not wish to have handrails attached to the walls.
- Are the walls sufficiently strong to support the attachment and use of handrails?
- Is the flight of stairs straight or does it go round a corner?
- If a patient suffers from shortness of breath or reduced muscle strength, it may be beneficial to locate a chair at the top or bottom of the stairs as a resting place.
- If a patient is using walking aids to mobilise, it is worth considering if they would benefit from having identical aids at the top and bottom of the stairs to avoid them needing to carry them on the stairs.
- Advise the informal carer on the safest way to assist the patient whilst negotiating the stairs. They should not push or pull the patient. Suggest where they can stand so both are safe.
- The patient may need advice on appropriate types of footwear to use on the stairs.
- If patient is unable to access the front door, consider referral for the fitting of a door entry system, if appropriate.
- Can the front door be accessed easily?
- Does it have a door chain or peephole fitted for personal safety? If not, these can be fitted privately or by the voluntary sector.
- Can the patient pick up the post? If not, it may be possible for someone to fit a collection box on the back of the front door or provide a Helping Hand with which to pick up letters.

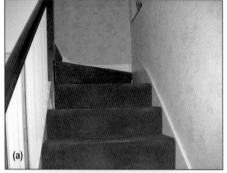

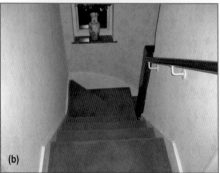

Figure 6.5 (a and b) stairs.

- Is there a smoke alarm fitted and working? If not, this could be organised privately or arranged through the local Fire Service.

Functional treatments

- Ascending/descending stairs:
- Advise on single step or reciprocal method
- Demonstrate the correct techniques appropriate to the individual patient, using equipment and walking aids as appropriate.
- Walking practice:
- The hallway is often the longest and least cluttered floor space in which to progress mobility.
- Exercise tolerance:
- Patients who suffer with limited exercise tolerance can count the number of stairs they will need to climb for the whole flight and start with step ups on the bottom step to gauge their exercise tolerance
- This avoids getting half way up the stairs before realising that the patient does not have the exercise tolerance to complete the flight

- Gradually increase the number of step ups on the bottom step until the required number is achieved.

Adaptive equipment

- Wall bars:
- Use stair spindles to increase shoulder elevation/flexion by reaching up the spindle and sliding the hand down the spindle
- Also for hand grip/release exercises
- Use stair spindles for the attachment of Thera-Band or for the use of pulleys.
- Steps:
- Use the bottom step for foot placement, with foot positioned properly on the step
- Use the bottom step for step-ups and dips for quads strength, with the newel post for support
- Standing on the bottom step, the patient can lower their heels down to perform calf/heel stretches
- Bottom stair can be used for step ups to ascertain the exercise tolerance needed to complete a flight of stairs.
- Walking practice:
- The hallway (with a chair in it) can be used for a measured walk, or Timed Up And Go (TUAG), if appropriate, as part of an outcome measure, possibly adapted (Mathias et al, 1986)
- Raised strips at each doorway to practise stepping over and lifting the feet properly to avoid trips (Figure 6.6).
- General mobility and dexterity:
- Use front door locks and the placing of a key in the lock along with the locking and releasing of high and low bolts for practising hand dexterity and strength, reaching ability and trunk flexion and extension

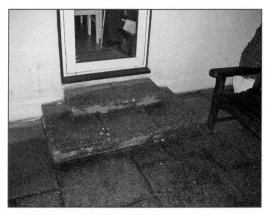

Figure 6.6 Steps, potential hazards for trips.

- Practise front door opening and closing, to improve balance, muscle strength and co-ordination
- Coat hooks can be used for hanging coats on to achieve trunk extension, shoulder elevation and flexion.

Involvement of other agencies and informal carers

- An equipment assessment with an occupational therapist could facilitate the treatments and personal activities of daily living by the provision of equipment such as hand rails and grab rails.
- The informal carers should be involved in the treatment process (with the patient's consent) and shown specific techniques to avoid carer strain, with an emphasis on safety.
- Voluntary organisations can be involved with fitting a mail collection box or a door chain and peephole to the front door.
- Fire service for installation of a smoke alarm.
- Local crime prevention officer for advice on personal safety.

The lounge and dining rooms

- This may be where the patient is living day and night, with the bed, chair, commode/urine bottle and other essential items all in one place (a microenvironment).
- This may be an optimum solution for independent living from the physiotherapist's point of view; it may not be what the patient wants.
- This is not a suitable arrangement for everyone as people can be self-conscious about maintaining their dignity with the presence of equipment related to personal use, especially if they have visitors.
- Also, shared living space with several generations may prove a hindrance to adapting the environment appropriately.

Environmental considerations

- How much furniture or clutter is there? Are there any obstacles? Can they be moved and repositioned to reduce risk, if the patient agrees?
- Are there rugs or cables across the floor? Is the floor covering loose, worn or slippery? Is it possible to tape down loose wiring and carpet edges and remove rugs, if the patient agrees?
- Can this be carried out by family members or the voluntary sector? Advise on risks if unable to adopt safer options.
- Is there adequate LHV? This is especially important as patients often spend the majority of their day (and possibly night) in this area.
- Does the gas fire need to be capped off? Remember there should not be a working gas fire in a room where someone is sleeping unless it is a room-sealed appliance or it incorporates a safety control that will shut down the appliance to prevent a build up of combustible gas in the room concerned (GSR, HSE, 1998).
- Is the patient sleeping in an armchair at night instead of going to bed?
- Discuss the option of a riser/recliner chair for patients who sleep in the armchair so that their legs can be elevated.

- Is there sufficient room to use walking aids? Supply appropriate walking aids that can be used safely.
- Many patients use the furniture in the lounge and dining room areas as a support ('furniture walking'). If this has been assessed as a safe method of mobility, there is no reason why it should not continue.
- Can the patient carry items from room to room? Discuss the option of safe transportation of items to and from the kitchen and other areas of the accommodation on the same floor level, providing the door thresholds are not raised, e.g. using a trolley or caddy.
- Is the height of the furniture (sofas/chairs) correct for safe use? Raise it if appropriate and possible. If not, discuss an acceptable alternative.
- Can the patient open and close the curtains safely? This could be assisted by the provision of a simple piece of equipment such as a Helping Hand.
- Is it possible for the patient to independently operate the telephone, television and door entry?
- Always make sure the controls for these are within easy reach.

Functional treatments

- Sit to stand and stand to sit:
- Reinforce correct techniques and use these as activities to increase muscle strength
- Always check the compressed chair height (that is, when the patient is sitting on it) to ascertain the need for chair raises. If chair raises are not acceptable, the physiotherapist would have to work on techniques and strengthening exercises to improve the patient's ability to stand up from a lower height, e.g. upper and lower limb exercises in sitting and standing and weight transference and balance in sitting and standing
- If the patient is unsafe in an unsupported stand position, a solid chair back, sideboard or dining table can be used as support, if it is safe to do so.

Adaptive equipment and exercises

- A chair is not just for sitting on!
- It can be used as a tool for exercising for the trunk, neck, upper and lower limbs.
- Leaning over the side of the chair on one side and then the other side, for trunk side flexion.
- Weights:
- The upper limbs can be exercised by using plastic bottles filled with liquid/sand/lentils as weights or by using a walking stick held in both hands for bilateral stretches
- The lower limbs can be exercised by using oven gloves with baked bean tins in or a bag of potatoes as weights
- It is also possible to purchase weighted bracelets and anklets in sports shops.
- Towels:
- An old scarf can be used to improve medial and lateral shoulder rotation by holding it behind the back and using a 'drying the back' action.

- Table:
  - At the dining table, polishing with a duster can improve shoulder range and mobility
  - Also use as a surface to carry out hand activities, such as using playing cards, to increase manual dexterity.
- Radio and television:
  - Rhythmical exercises can be performed to music on the radio or television
  - Advert breaks or programme changes on the radio or television can be used as a prompt to get up and walk or exercise.
- Patients should be encouraged to get out of their chairs and walk to the dining table for meals, if this was part of their previous routine.

Involvement of other agencies and informal carers

- An equipment assessment with an occupational therapist could facilitate the treatments and personal activities of daily living by the provision of equipment such as chair raises or a trolley.
- The informal carers should be involved in the treatment process (with the patient's consent) and shown specific techniques to avoid carer strain, with an emphasis on safety.

The kitchen

- Not all patients want or need to access the kitchen, as meals may be supplied for them by 'meals on wheels' or formal/informal carers.
- It may be appropriate to discuss the patient's appetite and nutritional needs.
- Some patients will have a treatment goal to prepare a hot drink and others to prepare a snack or meal (Figure 6.7).

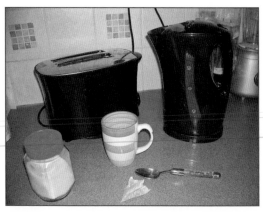

Figure 6.7 Hot drink practice, preparation of equipment required.

Environmental considerations

- How much furniture or clutter is there? Are there any obstacles? Can they be moved and re-positioned to reduce risk, if the patient agrees?
- Are there rugs or cables across the floor? Is the floor covering loose, sticky, greasy or slippery?
- Is it possible to tape down loose wiring and carpet edges and remove rugs, if the patient agrees?
- Can this be carried out by family members or the voluntary sector?
- Advise on cleaning and risks if unable to adopt safer options.
- Is there adequate LHV? Lighting and ventilation are of particular importance in the kitchen.
- Is it safe and appropriate to use walking aids in the kitchen?
- Work tops in galley type kitchens often provide adequate support.
- Is there room for equipment such as a trolley or perching stool?
- Discuss option of equipment for safe transportation of items to and from the kitchen to other areas of the accommodation on the same floor level.
- Are the work surfaces the right height?
- Is there a step up or down into the kitchen area? Discuss grab rails.
- Does the cooker need to be capped off? This may be applicable for patients who have been assessed under the Mental Capacity Act 2005 as not having the mental capacity to manage the hazards associated with having to use a gas appliance.

Functional treatments

- Sit to stand and stand to sit:
- Reinforce correct techniques and use these activities to increase muscle strength using a kitchen chair or perching stool.
- Practise upper and lower limb exercises in sitting or standing and weight transference and balance practice in standing.
- If the patient is unsafe in an unsupported stand position, the kitchen table and sink unit can be used as support, if it is safe to do so.

Adaptive equipment/exercises

- Exercises can be carried out in sitting at a table or perching at a work top.
- A perching stool can be a useful piece of equipment to help when undertaking domestic activities of daily living (DADLs).
- As the patient improves, the exercises can be progressed and carried out with them in standing.
- Sitting: assisted exercises:
- Preparing vegetables can improve manual dexterity
- A rolling pin can be held in both hands and used to assist bilateral shoulder exercises into elevation and flexion
- Opening cans, using the tin opener and unscrewing bottle tops to improve hand strength and dexterity
- Washing up (including turning taps on and off and wringing out dishcloths) to improve manual dexterity

- Weight transference/balance
- Wiping or polishing work surfaces improves balance, and upper limb range of movement.
- Standing:
- It is acceptable to use fixed worktops and the edge of the sink as support when mobilising, especially if a walking aid is more of an obstacle than a support in a confined area.
- Balance:
- Weight transference using the sink or kitchen table for support. The patient can practise open and closed chain exercises
- Reaching towards wall and base units to improve balance and shoulder range of movement, progressing to functional activity when safe
- Strengthening:
- Moving items, tins, equipment or bags from one place to another safely to improve muscle strength
- Complex coordinated movements
- Using kitchen equipment such as pressing the cooker/oven ignition and stooping to check the gas has lit, if appropriate and safe to do so.

Involvement of other agencies and informal carers

- An equipment assessment with an occupational therapist could facilitate the treatments and domestic activities of daily living by the provision of equipment such as a trolley, tap turners, kettle tipper and adapted cutlery.
- Assistive technology to prevent misuse of the gas cooker and monitor frequency the fridge is accessed, where there are concerns about a patient's nutritional status.

The floor

- To reduce the fear of falling, patients should be given advice on causes and prevention of falls and contingency plans if it should happen, as part of a treatment plan (DH, 2001a).

Environmental considerations

- How much furniture or clutter is in the room? Are there any obstacles? Can they be moved and re-positioned to reduce risk, if the patient agrees?
- Are there rugs or cables across the floor? Is it possible to tape down loose wiring and carpet edges and remove rugs, if the patient agrees? Can this be carried out by family members or the voluntary sector? Advise on risks if unable to adopt safer options.
- Is there adequate LHV? Heating is important if a patient has fallen and is unable to summon assistance as hypothermia is one of the complications of a long-lie.

Additional considerations

- Has the patient been feeling unwell or had an infection?
- Make the patient aware that they may lose their balance more easily if they are feeling unwell or have had a recent infection or if they are very tired.

- Has there been a change of medication?
- Advise the patient that a change in some types of medication could affect their balance.
- Some medications can affect blood pressure leading to postural hypotension, so patients may feel 'dizzy'.on sitting up or standing up.
- Remind them that they will need to let this feeling pass and support themselves in standing before mobilising.
- This is particularly important if they have a tendency to get up quickly to answer the door fearing that the visitor will leave.
- Foot health needs to be considered, as many patients are unable to reach their feet, which then become neglected. Corns, ingrowing or very long toenails, calluses and ulcers can all cause pain and difficulty in mobilising. Referrals can be made to the podiatrist with the patient's consent.
- Are they wearing inappropriate footwear? Advice on footwear is important as ill-fitting (too loose or too tight) shoes and slippers can contribute to a fall.
- Have they had their eyes tested in the last year? Poor vision can contribute to a fall and many patients are unable to visit the opticians.
- If this is the case, some opticians can be contacted to visit at home or transport may be arranged to take a patient to the opticians.

Functional treatments

- The floor as a treatment area:
- Use the floor as a treatment area although this will vary greatly in size or suitability, depending on location
- Patients may have their own exercise mat, but a duvet/blanket can be used for exercise on the floor.
- They need to be taught the safest and easiest way to get down onto the floor using an appropriate technique.
- Some patients fall often with no diagnosed cause.
- These patients could benefit from:
- Being taught how to 'backward chain' (i.e. Get up from the floor using a specific technique, providing they are unhurt)
- Discussing the benefits of using a pendant alarm.
- Devise contingency plans, if they fall and are unable to get up from the floor, which could include:
- Keeping a blanket, cushion and towel at a low level in different rooms that would be accessible from the floor and could be used respectively to either cover the patient (to avoid hypothermia) or to lie on top of (to prevent pressure sores developing) or to use as a pad (if the patient needs to pass urine whilst still on the floor) to increase comfort in the event of a long lie.
- Informal carers should be shown how to assist a patient with 'backward chaining' but advised not to try and lift a patient from the floor unaided.

Adaptive equipment/exercises

- The floor is the equipment and the treatment area. It can be used for:
- Balance work
- throwing and catching exercises
- Practising foot placement using the patterns on the floor coverings or laying ribbons, tape or sticks on the floor to step over
- Multi directional stepping and other supervised, dynamic balance work
- Improving confidence
- Progression in the use of walking aids to walking independently across the floor, if appropriate.

Involvement of other agencies and informal carers

- Liaise with GP or community nurses if there are problems with medication or you suspect the patient may have an infection.
- Refer to the podiatrist, if appropriate and with the patient's knowledge and consent.
- Refer to an optician, if appropriate and with the patient's knowledge and consent.
- The informal carers should be involved in the treatment process (with the patient's consent) and shown specific techniques to avoid carer strain, with an emphasis on safety.
- Refer for supply of a pendant alarm, if the patient agrees.

The garden (front and back)

- Not all people live in accommodation that has a garden, but most will need to access their properties by the front path and front door.
- Some people have a garden that they do not need or want to access and others like to walk or sit in their gardens or even perform gardening activities, if they are safe and able to do so.
- Accessing the outside can often have a positive effect upon a patient's mood, morale and progression of activities.
- Treatment goals can be set to achieve any of the above, if they are realistic.

Environmental considerations

- Is the access to the front/back door by one step, a flight of steps, or a slope?
- Are there rails/ grab rails already in situ? Are they appropriately positioned and safe to use?
- Recommend and refer for supply of safe and well-positioned rails and grab rails, if appropriate and if the patient/landlord consent.
- How rough is the terrain? Is the ground very uneven to walk on? Is there broken paving or are there mossy paths? (Figure 6.8)
- Is there somewhere to sit and rest in the garden?

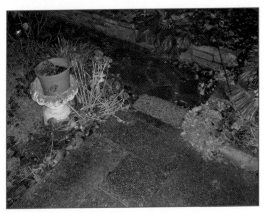

Figure 6.8 Steps and pathway in a garden at night in the rain.

- Are they alone when accessing the garden or will they have someone with them?
- Demonstrate and advise on how to access the garden. This may involve informal carers.

Functional treatments

- Teach an exercise programme to increase joint range and muscle strength to enable the patient to access the garden.
- Practice with informal carers or rehabilitation assistants.
- Mobilise around the garden, recommending the safest and most practical walking aid, as appropriate.
- This may be different from the walking aid used indoors as the terrain may be uneven and rough.
- Advise the patient that different walking aids may have to be privately purchased for outdoor use.
- Facilitate gardening activities by referring to voluntary groups.

Adaptive equipment/exercises

- Putting rubbish in the bin is a functional activity to improve balance, co-ordination and strength.

Involvement of other agencies and informal carers

- Refer to the occupational therapist for the provision of outdoor rails.
- Refer to a voluntary organisation that assists patients to carry out gardening activities within their abilities.
- The informal carers should be involved in the treatment process (with the patient's consent) and shown specific techniques to avoid carer strain, with an emphasis on safety.

The big outdoors

- Not all patients will want to or need to go outside their property.
- However, this may be a very realistic treatment goal for patients who would like to and are able to resume a more active lifestyle.
- Some patients may be able to achieve a level of independence to allow them to manage their domestic, travel and financial arrangements themselves
- However, safety must be the over-riding consideration.

Environmental considerations

- Has an event occurred to cause the patient to lose confidence?
- The patient needs insight into the risks of being outdoors.
- Point out hazards that the patient may encounter, such as uneven ground, people bumping into them; the speed with which they need to cross a road, ability to assess the speed of traffic, erratic bus movements that could cause a loss of balance.
- Very light or very dark conditions or sudden changes in light (especially for patients with visual impairments).
- Weather conditions especially extreme heat or cold, snow, ice, strong winds.
- Uneven terrain (on the patient's property and in the street).
- Need to negotiate steps, stairs, kerbs, slopes, etc.
- Can the patient communicate effectively to seek help?
- Will a different walking aid be required?
- Does the patient need to get in and out of a car?
- Does the patient want to use public transport (train, bus, etc.)
- Negotiating sensory surfaces at the edge of the kerb.
- Do they want to walk/travel a long distance?
- Will they be shopping, using an ATM, going to a friend's house, going to the pub?
- Will they return to work?

Functional treatments

- Patients may need an appropriate walking aid for outdoor use and advice on how to purchase one privately.
- Demonstrate and practise how to negotiate stairs, steps and slopes.
- If the physiotherapist is going to take a patient outside, the patient may need to have a contingency plan for communication, if they have lost confidence or have a communication problem.
- It may be necessary to practise a simulated conversation with a shopkeeper for example.
- If the patient will be using money, practise hand dexterity exercises
- Give a regime of exercises to help increase exercise tolerance.
- Give advice on fatigue management.
- Remind patients that whatever distance they travel, they will need to return.

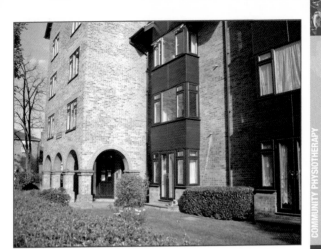

Figure 6.9 Sheltered accommodation.

- Encourage them to plan a route where they may be able to rest (on a bench or at a friend's house).
- Consider the size of a supermarket and how much walking that would involve.
- Arrange for family, carers or rehabilitation assistants to accompany the patient, either to give physical or moral support and encouragement.
- Practise getting in and out of a car, using the correct techniques for safety and to minimise risk.

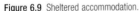

Adaptive equipment/exercises

- Locate different height steps to practise stepping up and down.
- Slopes can be used to improve balance and muscle strength, both when ascending and descending.
- Use trees, lamp posts, etc. as markers to set goals and identify distances covered.
- Practise advanced balance exercises to prepare for a bus journey.
- Use a trolley as a support/walking aid in the supermarket.

Involvement of other agencies and informal carers

- Refer to the occupational therapist for potential aids and adaptations for use in the car.
- The informal carers should be involved in the treatment process (with the patient's consent) and shown specific techniques to avoid carer strain, with an emphasis on safety.
- Refer to 'Dial A Ride' to facilitate transport.

- Refer to voluntary organisations to accompany patient when they are mobilising outdoors.
- Access to a wheelchair for outdoor use over long distances will be dependent on local provision/services.
- Refer for the Blue Badge scheme, if appropriate (DOT, 2010).
- Physiotherapists may be consulted regarding the appropriateness of accommodation or the level of input needed to remain safe and supported (Figure 6.9).

The references for this chapter can be found on www.expertconsult.com.

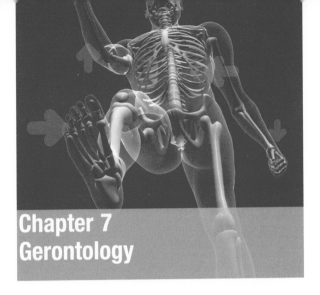

Chapter 7
Gerontology

Clinical reasoning and treatment choice based on assessment findings

- In principle, the same treatment techniques are used within older peoples' rehabilitation as are used with younger people.
- The physiotherapist may need to adapt the treatment techniques taking into account the older person's past medical history.
- More time should be given for learning exercises and practising skills.
- Assessment may identify multiple impairments that contribute to an older person's functional problem. For example: difficulty in standing up from a chair may be due to reduced muscle power, poor balance and painful joints. The physiotherapist can apply a range of interventions as part of the treatment plan to address each of these impairments, e.g. Exercise therapy, practice of the task and MSK treatment techniques to reduce pain.
- If the treatment plan proves only partially successful, then compensatory strategies may enhance the outcome of treatment. eg: raising the height of the chair to compensate for reduced muscle power.

General principles of exercise prescription

- Exercise prescription should include the frequency, duration, intensity and type of activity dependent upon the ability of the person.
- For all older people, exercise sessions should start with a gradual warm up and cool down.
- Pre-exercise assessment should include the older person's:
- Health history
- Functional abilities

- Activity history
- Current interests
- Preferences
- Social and economic needs
- Motivation and readiness to exercise.

- Older people with existing medical conditions or those with a recent injurious fall, without a medical assessment and those who are unsure about their safety during physical activity, should first consult an appropriately qualified health care professional, before embarking on a physical activity programme (DOH 2001a).

Physical activity guidelines

- The CMO (2011) guidance for physical activity in older adults recommends that:
- Older adults should engage in 150 minutes of moderate intensity activity in bouts of 10 minutes or more over a week.
- For those who are already regularly active at moderate intensity, 75 minutes of vigorous activity spread through the week is comparable.
- Older adults should engage in physical activity that improves muscle strength on at least 2 days per week
- Older adults at risk of falls should incorporate physical activity to improve balance and co-ordination at least 2 days per week.
- Older adults should minimise the time they spend sitting for prolonged periods.

- The British Heart Foundation acknowledges that any activity is better than none at all, and (especially older) sedentary people should be encouraged to start at a level of activity with which they are comfortable.

- This may be as little as 5 minutes of activity to begin with, with the aim of gradually increasing in duration and intensity (British Heart Foundation 2008). Older people require clear messages about how much physical activity is beneficial for their health, but they also need reassurance that they are unlikely to over-exert themselves.

- The physiotherapist should educate the older person in the early recognition of symptoms that might indicate an exacerbation of a chronic problem, e.g. an increase in pain, swelling or stiffness of an osteoarthritic knee.

General treatment considerations

- Footwear:
- Appropriate footwear is a key part of older peoples' rehabilitation.
- Every effort must be made to bring the person's footwear into hospital.
- Footwear may compensate for impairments, e.g. heel raise for leg length discrepancy.
- An individual may be immobile until their footwear is available.
- Foam disposable slippers are not suitable for older people who have balance/gait impairment as the soles tend to stick to the floor.

- If the older person has significant swelling of the lower limbs ± bandages, a referral to surgical appliances may be required to assess for suitable long-term footwear.
- Continence:
- The older person may wish to use the toilet prior to a therapy session especially if they have urinary frequency.
- If the person has a catheter, remember to check that it is not too full and that it is secured to their leg.
- Do not let the older person carry the catheter bag at the hand grip of a walking aid (risk of back flow) and always think about the older person's dignity.
- Check that incontinence pads are securely in place prior to treatment.
- Try to keep a spare pair of gloves in your uniform pocket (infection control).
- Level of effort:
- An older person's exercise tolerance is likely to be lower than a younger person.
- However, it is essential that the patient works sufficiently hard during a physiotherapy session otherwise the treatment will be ineffective.
- The person may need lots of rests while working towards their goals, but they also need lots of practice in order to achieve them.
- Watch their work of breathing, as an indicator of exertion and ensure adequate rest/recovery periods with treatment.
- Encourage the person to monitor their own level of effort by using a scale of 0–10 where sitting is 0 and 10 is all-out effort.
- Aim for a level of 5 (moderate intensity) where the older person is still able to have a conversation but is breathing slightly harder.
- Ensure that inhalers, GTN spray or other medication is readily at hand.
- Effects of bed rest:
- Prior to moving from lying to sitting, ask the person to perform leg exercises to increase their circulatory flow.
- Break down the bed transfer into stages.
- Encourage the person to move slowly from lying to sitting over the edge of the bed.
- Observe for signs of postural hypotension. Symptoms may include dizziness, light headedness, weakness and/or pain across the shoulders and neck.
- Carers:
- Encourage relatives/carers to be involved in the rehabilitation programme and update them of progress made if the older person wishes.
- Involving the carer early in rehabilitation ensures that there is ample opportunity to discuss concerns and plans for discharge.
- Personal autonomy:
- There are few opportunities for choice when in hospital.
- The physiotherapist should offer, where possible, choice, e.g. time of the treatment session or choice of at least two different activities during the treatment session that the older person wishes to work on.

- Declining treatment:
  - Listen to the person and spend time exploring the reasons behind the refusal.
  - There are many reasons that contribute to loss of confidence and reluctance to participate in rehabilitation.
- Reasons for reluctance to participate in treatment
  - Lack of practice and/or familiarity
  - Impairment, e.g. weakness, loss of sensation, pain, unsteadiness, tightness, stiffness, breathlessness
  - Beliefs about illness and/or condition
  - Anxiety, e.g. sense of loss of control over the body, sense of imminent disaster in specific circumstances such as a sense of knee giving way, loss of balance when not using a walking aid
  - Low perception of control
  - Low self-efficacy.
- Outcome measures
  - Choose the outcome measure that is valid, sensitive and specific to the person's needs.
  - Avoid using an outcome measure as an assessment tool; this can detract from assessing the specific impairments underlying the patient's functional problems.
  - Tables 7.1–7.6 provide examples of outcome measures that can be used for specific impairments.
- Treatment environments
  - Acute care rehabilitation is the start of the rehabilitation pathway for hospitalised patients with an acute illness or injury.
  - Patients may have less time to reach their rehabilitation goals while in acute care and risk being discharged as soon as they are able to cope at home rather than having the opportunity to achieve wider safety margins or developing reserves of coping ability.
  - A US study by Sager et al (1996) found that a third of elderly medical inpatients experienced a decline in function whilst in hospital, therefore efficient use must be made of the limited time in the acute care setting.
  - Brief but intensive rehabilitation programmes should be targeted at improving muscle strength, functional mobility and endurance in order to widen the patient's safe functional abilities.
  - Adequate practice opportunities throughout the day are crucial to achieving effective acute rehabilitation, e.g. delegating to physiotherapy assistants, working with nursing staff and health care assistants.
  - The importance of exercise provision is highlighted by a systematic review completed by de Morton et al (2007) that found multidisciplinary intervention including exercise improved patient and hospital outcomes for hospitalised older medical patients.
  - Regular liaison with the multidisciplinary team (MDT) regarding the estimated date of discharge (EDD) is essential so that the necessary assessments are carried out in a timely manner.
  - A useful question to consider is: 'Are the person's goals likely to be met before the EDD?'
  - If the individual is making progress on a daily basis and is likely to reach their pre-morbid function at the same time as the EDD, consider referral to

Table 7.1 Evaluating therapy interventions – balance

Outcome measure	Reasoning	Testing tips
Timed Unsupported Steady Standing (TUSS)	This is a simple test of static steady balance for frail older people (Simpson et al 1996).	The end point is 60 seconds. It can be made more challenging by assessing with feet together (TUSSTOG) and feet in tandem (TUSSTAN).
TURN 180	This is a staff-rated performance based test of dynamic postural stability when turning 180° (Simpson et al 2002, Fitzpatrick et al 2005).	It can also be used as a screening test for risk of falling. Taking 5 steps or more to TURN 180 increases the relative risk of falling in the following year by 1.9 in community dwelling older people (Nevitt et al 1989). The older person needs to be able to stand unsupported for one minute in order to perform the test. It is not appropriate for older people with weight bearing restrictions, pain, anxiety or severe confusion.
Berg Balance Scale	This is a scale designed to measure balance by assessing the performance of 14 functional tasks in older people with balance impairment (Berg et al 1989).	It can be used in a variety of settings. It can be used as a screening test for risk of falling. A score of less than 45/56 has been shown to be predictive of falls (Berg et al 1992, Gillespie et al 2000). It can be quite tiring for frail older people or those recovering from an acute illness.
Functional reach	This test measures the maximum distance a person can reach forward beyond arms length with a fixed base of support in standing (Duncan et al 1990).	It can be used in many clinical settings; however the older person must be able to stand unaided and the test performance may be affected by fear of falling. It is not appropriate in patients with significant spinal deformities and may be difficult in those with marked dementia. It can also be used as a screening test for risk of falling (Duncan et al 1992).

Continued

Table 7.1 Continued

Outcome measure	Reasoning	Testing tips
Lateral reach test	This is a test of ability to reach directly left and right as far as possible from a fixed base of support in standing (Brauer et al 1999).	Lateral reach assesses a distinct component of postural stability. The older person must be able to stand unaided and the test performance may be affected by fear of falling.
One leg stance	This test measures the time in seconds of ability to balance while standing on one leg (Bohannon 2006a).	The test can also be used as a predictor of injurious falls in older people (Vellas et al 1997a). Inability to stand for 5 seconds on one leg is suggested as a marker of risk (Jonsson et al 2004). Impaired one leg stance is also a marker of frailty (Vellas et al 1997b).
Four step square test	This test is a timed performance based test that assesses dynamic standing balance (rapid stepping and obstacle avoidance) in active older community dwelling older people (Dite & Temple 2002)	The physiotherapist should have a clear view of the patient as they step. Have a second person to closely supervise the patient as they perform the test. This test is cognitively challenging as the older person has to understand and incorporate the stepping sequence. A cut-off time of greater than 15 seconds is associated with increased risk of recurrent falls.

Table 7.2 Evaluating therapy interventions – gait

Outcome measure	Reasoning	Testing tips
Get up and go test	This is a test of sit to stand, walking and turning ability for frail older people (Mathias et al 1986).	This is a staff-rated performance based test rated on a five point scale where 1 = normal and 5 = severely abnormal. A score of 3 or more is at risk of falling.
Timed Up and Go (TUAG)	This is a test of timed sit to stand, walking and turning ability for frail older people (Podsiadlo and Richardson 1991)	The test correlates well with every day function. The chair used should have a seat height of 44-47cms and arm rests as a lower chair may affect the validity of the test (Siggeirsdóttir et al 2002). Try to avoid talking to the person during the test as this may distract them from the task. The test can be used as a screening tool to see if further in-depth assessment of mobility is required. For community dwelling older people a TUAG of 12 seconds is regarded as normal. There is some variation according to age (Bohannon 2006b). TUAG can be used as a falls screening tool but its predictive validity and sensitivity has been variable upon the populations studied, setting and the research methodology (Shumway-Cook et al 2000, Chui et al 2003, Thrane et al 2007, Lindsay et al 2004, Large et al 2006, Kristensen et al, 2007).
6 metre timed walk	Distances limited timed walking tests are useful indicators of functional mobility of older people. Gait speed is important for safe community mobility, e.g.: crossing a road.	A 2 metre distance before and after the course minimises the affects of acceleration and deceleration. Normative data are available (Butler et al 2009)

Table 7.3 Evaluating therapy interventions – combined functional performance

Outcome measure	Reasoning	Testing tips
Elderly Mobility Scale	This is a standardised scale for assessment of mobility, gait, balance and key position changes in frail older people in an acute hospital or day hospital environment (Smith 1994, Prosser et al 1997).	The test correlates well with function. The test has a ceiling effect for older people who are more able. The functional reach scale differs from the original research paper.
Lindop Parkinson's Assessment Scale	This is a functional assessment scale designed to measure bed and gait mobility in patients with Parkinson's disease (Pearson et al 2009).	The bed mobility section should be performed without shoes on.

Table 7.4 Evaluating therapy interventions – endurance

Outcome measure	Reasoning	Testing tips
6 minute walk test	This is a useful measure of exercise capacity in older people (Mangan & Judge 1994).	Ideally the test should be conducted in a quiet hallway with cones placed at the beginning and end of 30 metres. The goal is for the individual to walk as far as possible in 6 minutes. The individual is allowed to self-pace and rest as needed as they traverse back and forth along a marked walkway. Encouragement increases the distance walked (Harada et al 1999).

Table 7.5 Evaluating therapy interventions – quality of life

Outcome measure	Reasoning	Testing tips
SF12/36	These generic scales measure functional health and well-being from the patient's point of view (http://www.sf-36.org/tools/SF36.shtml).	They can be self-administered or completed by interview
EQ-D5	This generic scale measures health related quality of life consisting of five dimensions (mobility, self-care, usual activities, pain and anxiety) plus the individual's rating on a Visual analogue scale of their current health status (Szende A et al 2007)	Self-administered or completed by interview.
PDQ-39	The Parkinson's Disease Questionnaire is designed to address aspects of functioning and well-being for those affected by Parkinson's disease (PDQ-39 – Isis Innovation Ltd, Ewert House, Ewert Place, Summertown, Oxford OX2 7SG UK **T** +44 (0)1865 280830 **F** +44 (0)1865 280831 **E** innovation@isis.ox.ac.uk)	Self-administered.

Table 7.6 Evaluating therapy interventions – fear of falling

Outcome measure	Reasoning	Testing tips
Falls Efficacy Scale-International (FES-I).	This is a test to measure level of concern of falling during a range of physical and social activities that is suitable for use across a range of cultures and languages (Yardley et al 2005, Kempen et al 2008).	To obtain a total score for the FES -I add the scores on all the items together, to give a total that will range from 16 (no concern about falling) to 64 (severe concern about falling).
Activities Balance Confidence Scale (ABC)	This is a test to measure confidence in doing a range of activities on a scale from 0-100% (Powell et al 1995).	If the older person normally uses a walking aid, ask them to rate themselves as if they were using the aid.

community services for further rehabilitation if indicated, e.g. day hospital or community physiotherapy.

– If the individual has experienced a significant change in their function, discuss the options for further rehabilitation in the community, e.g. bed-based community hospital or intermediate care with the patient and in collaboration with the MDT.

Exercise interventions to prevent falls in older people at high risk or who have fallen

- The following risk factors for falls can be improved by physiotherapy intervention:
- Muscle weakness
- Impaired balance
- Impaired gait
- Reduced reaction times.
- Exercise prescription will differ depending upon the individual's history of falls, medical conditions and functional capacity.
- In older people with poor balance, some preparatory strength, co-ordination and flexibility training may be required before unsupported dynamic balance exercise starts.
- Safety is paramount, less challenging balance exercises may need to be prescribed initially, particularly if the older person is exercising at home unsupervised.
- Exercise programmes to prevent falls should include dynamic balance, strength and functional floor activities. They should also aim to include bone loading, power, flexibility, posture, gait training, supported endurance work and tasks to improve visual, vestibular and sensory input (DOH 2009).
- Evidence:
- Recent reviews and guidance recommend that falls intervention, including exercise, should be considered alongside osteoporosis management to reduce both the number of falls and falls-related injuries (NICE 2004, DOH 2001b, DOH 2007, Skelton and Todd 2004, Sherrington et al 2008).
- Studies of strength and specific balance training have shown falls reduction in intervention groups when evaluated at the end of one year (Tinetti et al 1994, Campbell et al 1999, Province et al 1995).
- A randomised controlled trial (RCT) of group based exercise over one year found that the intervention group (community dwelling older people $n = 551$) had a 22% lower rate of falls than the control group and 31% fewer falls in those who had fallen in the past year (Lord et al 2003).
- A UK study of community dwelling older people with a history of falls, halved their risk of falls with 9 months of weekly group balance and strength exercise combined with twice weekly home exercises (Skelton et al 1995). In this study the exercise intervention consisted of progressive resistance, gait, balance, functional activity, floor work, endurance and flexibility training. The exercise was individually tailored in type and intensity with most exercise in weight bearing positions, reducing upper limb support.
- In New Zealand, an RCT of home-based individually tailored exercise (OTAGO) including a warm up, muscle strength and balance exercises plus a walking programme three times per week for one year was found to be effective in

reducing falls and injuries in community dwelling older women over 80 years old (Campbell et al 1999). During the study the physiotherapist visited each individual in the intervention group 4 times in the first 2 months followed by regular telephone contact.

- There have been several studies investigating the effects of Tai Chi on falls. There is some evidence that Tai Chi is effective as a preventative group exercise for older people with impaired balance and strength who have not fallen (Wolf et al 1996). However modified Tai Chi has not been found effective in frail older people (Wolf et al 2003). A review paper by Harmer et al (2008) recommended that longitudinal studies with consistent intervention parameters and clinically meaningful outcomes were required in order to establish the role of Tai Chi in falls prevention.

Long-term physical activity and exercise opportunities

- A major challenge is to ensure a continuum of exercise provision and to make a successful transition from a health care setting (one to one or small group basis) to a community based setting.
- Sherrington et al (2008) showed that the greatest relative effects of exercise on falls rates is seen in programmes that include a combination of a higher total dose of exercise (>50 hours over the trial period) and challenging balance exercises.
- It is important to provide a choice of exercise opportunities to ensure individual need and preference are met, as this is more likely to improve participation and uptake.
- Effectiveness will be determined by how receptive the individual is to the recommendations and by how capable they are when carrying out the exercises independently, safely and effectively (Dinan 2001).
- Evidence suggests that older people will be more receptive and more likely to undertake an exercise programme if the information provided discusses the wider benefits of exercise to well-being and maintenance of independence, rather than just to prevent falls (Skelton & Todd 2004, Yardley et al 2007a, Yardley et al 2007b).

Progressive Resistance training

- Resistance training aims to increase the ability of a muscle or group of muscles to generate force.
- To increase strength, a resistance should be used that allows 6–8 repetitions for each exercise. Aim for a resistance of 65–75% of 1RM. Make sure that the older person has a 1–3 second rest between repetitions and a 90–120 second rest between sets. Aim for 1–3 sets of each exercise using the major muscle groups 2–3 days per week with 48 hours between sessions. The level of effort should be moderate to high.
- On a 10 point scale, where no effort is 0 and maximal effort of a muscle group is 10, moderate intensity is 5–6.
- With frail older people, using body weight is often a sufficient training stimulus initially. Exercise intensity can be altered by adjusting the performance of the exercise, e.g. reducing the use of the upper limbs when practicing sit to stand or increasing the repetitions.
- Using lighter weights and a higher number of repetitions, particularly if the patient has musculoskeletal disease, will assist the development of endurance and power required for functional activity.

- Gradual progression in weight and repetitions should be made on a regular basis to maintain overload.
- Overuse injuries can occur during resistance training. To reduce the risk, precise teaching instructions and skilled demonstration together with observation of the person and feedback are required.
- Evidence:
- The greatest strength gains occur in programmes of moderate to high intensity where exercises are performed at 50% or more of the patient's one repetition maximum.
- Some studies have shown that progressive resistance training programmes improve performance in functional tasks (Jette et al 1999, Fiatarone et al 1990, Vincent K 2002).
- Other studies have found large strength gains, but no or small improvements in physical performance or function (Jette et al 1996, Judge et al 1994, Skelton et al 1995).
- A Cochrane review by Liu and Latham (2009) found that resistance training conducted two to three times a week, at moderate to high intensity, with free weights, exercise machines or elastic bands increased strength in older people and had a positive effect on performance of activities such as standing up from a chair more quickly, walking and stair climbing. In addition progressive resistance training improved older peoples' ability to perform more complex functional tasks such as preparing a meal. However the reviewers advised caution when transferring the research into practice as adverse events were not adequately reported in the studies.
- An RCT of home-based exercise ($n = 29$) that included progressive resistance training, balance and general physical activity over a 6 month period found that functional performance, dynamic balance, muscle strength and aerobic fitness improved significantly in the intervention group (Nelson et al 2004).
- An RCT of 3 months low intensity exercise programme versus unsupervised home based flexibility activities in frail older people ($n = 84$) found significant improvement in the exercise group on frailty markers such as strength, gait speed and balance (Brown et al 2000).
- Weighted vest exercise has been used safely in older people and has been found to be effective in improving balance, strength and bone mass (Shaw & Snow 1998, Bean et al 2004, Snow et al 2000).
- Research has also studied frail older people living in care homes although the sample numbers have been small. Fiatarone et al (1990) found that an 8 week high intensity strength training ($n = 10$) improved muscle strength and tandem gait speed in nonagenarians in care homes. Ikezoe et al (2005) found that a 12-month low-intensity exercise programme was effective in increasing strength and maintaining balance and mobility in frail older people residing in care homes ($n = 28$). Sauvage et al (1992) conducted an RCT of a 12 week (3 times per week) programme of PRT and stationary cycling ($n = 14$) on older men living in a care home. This resulted in significant although limited improvements for clinical mobility scores, strength, muscular endurance and gait velocity.

Endurance training

- Every functional activity has a certain level of cardiovascular fitness required in order to achieve it successfully.

- Older people may be able to carry out activities of daily living (ADL) yet they may have reduced physiological reserve and be close to their maximum aerobic capacity.

- When faced with a more challenging task, they may be unable to meet these extra energy needs and their level of fitness then becomes apparent.

- The relative intensity of moderate physical activity (still able to maintain a conversation, but breathing slightly harder than normal) will depend on the age and fitness of the older person. It is helpful to educate the older person to listen to their body using the Borg scale of perceived exertion (Borg 1998).

- For some people this may require sustained activity, e.g. cycling on a stationary bike; for others with lower levels of fitness, it may mean walking at quite a slow pace.

- For frail older people a 10 minute walk may be beyond their functional capacity and they will have to begin with shorter bursts of activity.

- Evidence:

- Research has shown that older people can benefit from endurance training. Buchner et al (1992) in a review of 22 studies found that 3–12 months of aerobic exercise improved aerobic capacity by between 5 and 20%.

- An RCT of a 4 month programme of aerobic training, yoga and flexibility and a waiting list group ($n = 101$ older men and women (mean age 67)) found that aerobic training produced an overall 11.6% improvement in peak VO_2 and a 13% increase in anaerobic threshold (Blumenthal et al 1989).

Functional strength training

- Reduced muscle power is one of the underlying mechanisms of reduced functional ability.

- Studies focusing on increasing muscle power have not always translated into improvements in functional tasks in older people.

- It has been suggested that this may be due to insufficient specificity between the mode of training and the desired mobility task.

- Evidence:

- Skelton et al (1996) carried out an RCT that involved patients in an 8 week moderate intensity exercise programme ($n = 19$) involving community dwelling older women. The study found that there was training associated improvements of 9–55% in quadriceps and handgrip strength, flexibility, balance and selected tests of functional ability. Exercise comprised one supervised session (progressive resistance training and functional strength training) and two unsupervised home sessions of resistance exercise per week.

- An RCT of a 12 week (3 times weekly) functional task exercise programme in community dwelling older women ($n = 98$) was more effective than resistance exercises at improving functional task performance at 3 and 6 months (de Vreede et al 2005).

- An RCT of 12 week task-specific resistance training in community dwelling older people ($n = 161$) showed a significant training effect for bed and chair rise tasks (Alexander et al 2001).

- McMurdo and Johnstone (1995) conducted a RCT of a daily 6 month home exercise programme (health education or mobility training or PRT) on community dwelling older people with limited mobility and dependence in at least one ADL. The results showed a trend towards improvement in both exercise groups in the sit to stand test and timed up and go tests.

- Gill et al (2002) conducted an RCT of a 6 month home based intervention programme that included daily balance, muscle strength, transfer training and gait re-education ($n = 188$) of frail community dwelling older people designed to prevent functional decline. Participants in the intervention group had less self-reported disability at 7 and 12 months and the most benefit was observed among those with moderate frailty. This was not the case with participants with severe frailty.

- A further trial by Gill et al (2004) considering a home-based programme, focused on improving underlying impairments in physical ability in frail community dwelling older people. Subjects in the intervention group had reductions in Instrumental ADL disability and gains in mobility and physical performance at 7 and 12 months.

- The research suggests that a combination of strength training and functional strength training results in functional gains in frail older people. The association between strength and function may be curvilinear: a critical amount of strength is required for 'normal' performance of specific activities. Above this threshold level of strength, further increase will not enhance the performance of the task. But below this threshold, there should be a stronger relation between strength and change in performance (Buchner et al 1996).

Balance re-education

- Balance exercises must be task and context specific.
- Actions may need to be modified initially so that the postural adjustments required are relatively small, e.g. sitting unsupported, reaching out with one hand at a time to touch the physiotherapist's hand.
- Actions can be made more demanding by:
- Changing the shape and base of support
- Increasing the movement amplitude by increasing the distance of the object to be reached
- Increasing speed
- Increasing weight of the object
- Using both hands
- Requiring a quick response, e.g. catching a ball
- Introducing simultaneous performance of two tasks.
- When a person is practicing a specific balance activity, feedback from the physiotherapist must be immediate and specific.
- The older person has to learn to assess and correct his own performance.
- The activity has to be challenging enough to test their balance and postural stability; however care must be taken to ensure the safety of the older person practicing the task.

- Evidence:
- A Cochrane review by Howe et al (2007) found that exercise has statistically significant positive effects on balance as opposed to usual activity for older people. Interventions that appeared to have the greatest impact were walking; balance; co-ordination and functional exercises; muscle strengthening; and multiple exercise types. Improvements were seen in the ability to stand on one leg, reach forward without overbalancing and walking. However the majority of the studies only had short follow up times.
- Wolf et al (2001) investigated the effect of a 12 sessions of individualised exercise programme on balance dysfunction in older people in a randomised multi-centre trial (*n* = 94). Subjects in the exercise group had significantly improved functional balance at the four week follow up but the effect had worn off by one year.
- An RCT of a 6 week balance training programme consisting of repetitive tasks of increasing difficulty specific to the functional problem in community dwelling older people with balance impairment (*n* = 199) was effective in improving balance and gait speed at 6, 12 and 24 weeks after intervention. The control group received physiotherapy for mobility problems and also improved.

Walking aid provision

- Walking aids are commonly prescribed to increase an older person's walking ability and decrease the risk of falls.
- The main indications for a walking aid are:
- Excessive pain on weight bearing (Deathe et al 1993)
- Decreased leg muscle strength and control (Tyson and Ashburn 1994)
- Instability (Deathe et al 1993)
- Shortness of breath
- People with chronic airflow limitation and other respiratory or cardiac conditions may find a wheeled walking aid helpful. Some studies have found that using a walking aid can increase walking distance (Chrisafulli et al 2007, Roomi et al 1998).
- Poor vision
- Poor distal lower limb proprioception (Deathe et al 1993)
- These impairments may be associated with acute events such as major illness or surgery, or with chronic conditions leading to a more gradual decline in physical ability.
- A walking aid should be prescribed only after thorough assessment of the person's physical problems and clinical reasoning about the causes. Provision of a walking aid should not be seen as the sole solution to the impairments identified during the assessment process. Strategies to address the specific impairments should be implemented as part of the treatment plan.
- When a walking aid is used, the individual is essentially using their upper limbs to support the lower limbs in the maintenance of an upright posture. If a patient becomes reliant on a walking aid, they may become more unsafe during sit to stand or when reaching out of their base of support during everyday tasks (Simpson et al 2002). Older people who use a walking frame should practise standing unsupported with a sturdy support in front of them, several times a day.

- The older person's abilities and skills to use the walking aid along with the environment including steps, position of furniture, and type of floor coverings must be taken into account when prescribing a walking aid. Early assessment of the environment and the suitability of a walking aid should be made by a physiotherapist and an occupational therapist if a new walking aid is being considered. Referral to community therapy services should be made if the physiotherapist feels that further review is necessary after discharge from acute care.
- Common scenarios and walking aids.
  - A inpatient who is anxious when mobilising across the bay in an acute hospital environment may request a wheeled Zimmer frame so that they can mobilise independently and confidently. On a home visit, they disregard the frame and walk safely around their property using the furniture.
  - A person with dementia may be able to use a walking aid appropriately when prompted or supervised. The nurses report that they have observed the person carrying the walking aid while walking. The physiotherapist needs to consider the potential for the long-term use of a walking aid.
- Ensure that the older person and/or carer are taught how to maintain the walking aid. It is not uncommon to see worn ferrules or loose fixings.
- Some older people may be reluctant to use a walking aid as the use of an aid may be perceived as a sign of frailty or aging. The physiotherapist needs to be mindful of these issues when suggesting a walking aid. Always discuss the reasons behind the recommendation of a walking aid to the person.

Gait re-education

- Parallel bars can be a useful piece of equipment to use to initiate walking, especially if the individual is fearful of falling or weak from an acute illness, prior to walking on the ward or an open area.
- Once standing, encourage the person to move the upper limbs in turn forwards and backwards on the bars.
- Weight transfer:
  - Practise weight transference from one leg and arm to the other.
  - Facilitation at the pelvis and use of a mirror can be helpful in encouraging adequate transference of weight prior to stepping practice.
- Stepping practice:
  - Standing: stepping over an external visual cue, e.g. lines on the floor, foot printed shaped mats.
  - Stride standing: the person transfers their body weight from the back leg to the leading leg, stepping through with the back leg.
  - A visual target on the floor can be used to encourage a normal step length.
- Gait re-education
  - Ask the person to walk inside the parallel bars, using the bars for support initially.
  - Again a mirror can be helpful in providing feedback.
  - Give immediate and specific feedback to the person.
  - The physiotherapist can increase the difficulty by asking the person to walk holding onto one bar.

- Gait re-education in a ward/rehabilitation area:
- Always set a target distance and place a seat clearly in view.
- Encourage the older person to set their own target distance.
- This target should be frequently revised.
- Allow frequent rests if the person is fearful or weak.
- As they improves, increase the distance and reduce the number and length of the rest periods.
- Place chairs at strategic places.
- Turning must be taught early.
- For an individual to be able to function in a complex environment, practice should include walking around obstacles, carrying an object and dual tasking.

Teaching a patient how to get off the floor and coping strategies

- If an older person has a history of falls, exercise should retrain or maintain the ability to get up from the floor to avoid a 'long lie'.
- A long lie (more than 1 hour on the floor) and the resultant complications can be more severe than the initial fall itself.
- Wild et al 1981 found that 50% of those who lie on the floor for an hour or longer die within 6 months, even if there is no direct injury from the fall.
- Vellas et al (1987) found that more than 20% of patients admitted to hospital because of a fall had been on the ground for an hour or more.
- Tinetti et al (1993) found that 148/313 (47%) of non-injured fallers were unable to get up following a fall.
- McCabe (1985) found that 75% of housebound older people were unable to get up from the floor.
- Some of the difficulty in getting up from the floor may be due to shock or injury, or anxiety of further injury to the body, but for many lack of physical fitness is an important cause (Skelton et al 1999).
- Therefore the physiotherapist must teach coping strategies that the older person can use if they do fall again and teach them an appropriate method to get off the floor if possible.
- There is minimal research in this area. A small randomised controlled trial ($n = 48$) suggested backward chaining was the most successful method for teaching patients to get on and off the floor (Reece and Simpson 1996).
- Backward chaining is a method for teaching a patient to perform a functional task by breaking the task down into smaller stages. The chain of subtasks is taught sequentially beginning with the last step in the sequence. As this step is mastered, the preceding step is taught and the step preceding that until the whole chain has been learnt. If the patient experiences difficulty in mastering a subtask, then it is broken down into even smaller steps.
- Reasons for teaching a person to get onto and off the floor may include:
- Patient may be at risk of falls
- Allowing a person to carry out floor work on mats by providing a safe and simple method of getting up and down
- Increasing confidence and functional independence
- Provide the person with coping strategies once on the floor.

- Hazards and risks
- Individuals with orthostatic hypotension
- Patient groups with reduced joint range in hips, knees and ankles and/or reduced upper limb/body strength e.g. hip replacement, osteoarthritis, rheumatoid arthritis, severe osteoporosis, moderate to severe stroke
- Cognitive/perceptual/behavioural/communication impairment
- Patients who are fearful of getting onto the floor
- Patients unable to lie supine; postural impairments, orthopnea, hiatus hernia and pain
- Moderate to severe tonal changes
- Unprotected hemiplegic shoulder with : marked reduction in muscle tone, glenohumeral/radiocarpal joint subluxation, poor voluntary control/functional movement in the upper limb, inattention or neglect
- Patients with painful soft tissue or joints
- General frailty
- Severe dyspnoea at rest or with minimal exertion
- Recent hip surgery within past 4 months.

- Preparing the environment
- Ensure sufficient space
- Mat on floor
- Ensure hoist and sling is available and functioning, e.g. battery is charged
- Patient to be wearing appropriate clothing
- Adjacent furniture is stable ie: plinth, chair, bed
- Have pillows, wedges, blocks, stools available that can be incorporated into the training.

- Methods and positions for patients to practise:
- Stride standing to half-kneeling

  Patient holds onto a chair or plinth (static furniture) with both hands and lowers back knee onto a mat or wedge cushion, then rises back to stride standing. This movement can be graded using varying heights of cushions and is complete when the patient is fully weight bearing. The physiotherapist supports the patient's pelvis from the side and slightly posterior and follows the movement of the patient.

- Standing to High-kneeling (Figure 7.1):

  Patient holds onto a chair or plinth (static furniture) with both hands and lowers back knee onto a mat or wedge cushion, then front knee onto the floor (high kneeling) then back to half kneeling and back to standing.

  The physiotherapist supports the pelvis from the side and slightly posterior and follows movement of the patient.

- 4 point kneeling (Figure 7.2):

  As for previous two methods, patient puts one hand down onto the floor followed by the other hand (4 point kneeling) then lifting one arm at a time rising up as per high kneeling.

  Physiotherapist supports from mid chest point whilst kneeling next to patient to help assist patient lowering and raising thorax to place and remove hands on the floor.

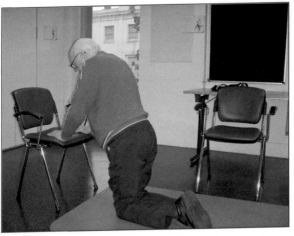

Figure 7.1 High kneeling.

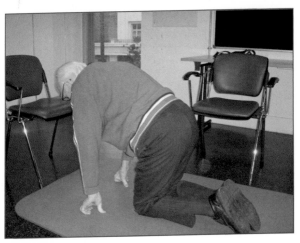

Figure 7.2 Four point kneeling.

– Side sitting (Figure 7.3):

Patient gets into position of 4-point kneeling, maintaining extended arms, the patient side flexes and lowers pelvis to rest greater trochanter on one side onto a mat or wedge/cushion. The return moves the patient into 4-point and then into standing via high kneeling.

The physiotherapist kneels by the side of the patient and guides the patient's pelvis towards them and onto the mat or wedge/cushion.

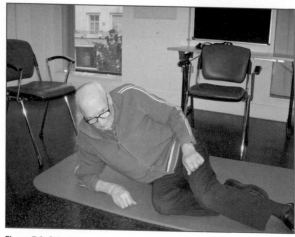

Figure 7.3 Side sitting.

– Side lying:

  As for side sitting the patient lowers themselves down onto weight bearing side onto a mat using one or two arms. The return raises them back into side sitting, then 4 point kneeling and high kneeling and back into standing.

  The physiotherapist moves in front of the patient (still kneeling), supporting with one hand on the pelvis, and the other hand under the rib cage. The physiotherapist assists with lowering the trunk onto the mat.

– Supine lying

  As for side lying then the patient rolls from side lying to supine, then back into side lying and follows the steps back through to standing.

  The physiotherapist (still kneeling) supports from the pelvis and shoulder girdle to assist with the movement

- Safety note: If the patient is unable to raise themselves from the floor a hoist will be required to achieve this.

- The physiotherapist must take care of their own joints when facilitating the movement of a patient onto and off the floor.

- The importance of back and general posture must be a priority.

- Modifications:

– Starting positions may include sitting on the edge of a chair, side sitting on a plinth or bed or using additional supporting surfaces in front.

– Older people who lack joint flexibility, have severe shortness of breath or are too frail to be taught, should discuss how they would summon help in the event of another fall and in case help is slow to come, how they would prevent the complications of a long lie.

- Patients should also be taught how to move about the floor, to reach for a telephone (placed at a low level) or alarm cord, to reach a blanket or something else to keep warm (kept in a bottom drawer or other place accessible near the floor).

- Simpson and Mandelstam (1995) found that some older people do not face up to the risks of falling, often having unrealistic expectations of their own abilities to get up or summon help. The physiotherapist should ask the patient to demonstrate their coping strategy.
- Don't assume that the patient who has an alarm system actually knows when and how to use it or when they should wear the alarm. When older people are in acute care, the physiotherapist should initiate these discussions in collaboration with the MDT and if necessary ensure that they are reinforced when they return to the community.

Functional transfer training

- Physiotherapy should provide opportunity to practise every day tasks such as techniques for efficient and safe transfers in and out of chairs, beds and cars.
- Standing up from a seated position is a critical preliminary to walking and therefore to independence.
- Once the person has moved forward to the front of the chair, ensure that they place the feet back, so that initial ankle dorsiflexion is approximately 75°. The hands should be placed on the chair arms. Discourage the person from pulling up on a walking aid. It may be helpful to place the walking aid a little further away. Encourage them to lean forwards 'nose over your knees' and 'push up to standing'. A rocking forward motion can give momentum to the movement.
- A common observation is the person's feet sliding forward. This can happen if the feet aren't back far enough, if they are not forward enough in the chair or they do not lean far enough forwards. Avoid blocking the person's feet with your own (risk of injury to feet).
- Encourage forward momentum before extension of the trunk (place a non-slip square of material under the feet, if the feet slip). Check the length of the soleus/gastrocnemius muscles, which can become shortened with disuse and physical inactivity. Strengthen the lower limb extensors and the anterior tibialis muscles.
- Clarify the specific heights and any equipment used in the home environment with occupational therapy colleagues and/or carer (task specificity).
- Don't forget to practise stand to sit. Some patients will start to turn around while some distance away from the chair resulting in an unsafe transfer, especially if they are tired after mobilising. The physiotherapist should teach them to walk up to the chair and only start turning when they are close enough.
- Some frail older people may have assistance to get into bed by carers/family members. However, bed transfers should still be taught especially if the person needs to go to the toilet during the night.

Techniques for promoting movement in older patients with cognitive impairment

- Consider the environment. Close curtains around the bed side to minimise distractions and to maintain the person's dignity.

- Is there an alternative environment if the person is distractible?
- Joint sessions with family/carers can be helpful to increase participation.
- General points to consider:
- Seating
- Footwear and clothes
- Hearing aids and dentures
- Spectacles.
- Suggested strategies: Moving from sitting to standing.
- Put a chair (or walking aid) in the space in front of the person
- Ask them to stand up either firmly and politely, or lightly and casually to suggest the ease of the task
- Use a gesture to indicate the need to stand up
- Use a stationary touch cue or sweep your hand up the person's back
- Place their hands on the chair arms as a cue to the movement
- Use a goal based cue: 'Get your nose over your toes'
- Sit beside the person and lean forwards in an exaggerated way to show them what they have to do
- Provide a firm pillar of support for the person to push against: for example, providing the individual with bed blocks as a substitute chair arm
- Use the palm to palm thumb hold (or a suitable alternative) to stop the person from gripping the arms if getting out of a chair
- Keep your hand soft and relaxed
- Remember that if two people go to assist, this may convey to the person that you expect the movement to be difficult- so start with just one assistant
- Throughout the process ensure there is adequate: time, repetition and reassurance
- Never pull a person out of their chair
- Approaching a chair: aim to reduce anxiety and anticipate and manage misjudgements.
- Suggested strategies:
- Assist at the person's side so that you are both facing and moving in the same direction. Encourage the person to approach the chair across its front using a curved pathway, especially if they use a walking aid
- Encourage the person to get their feet beyond the mid-line point on the ground, between the front legs of the chair, with the walking aid positioned even further ahead, before starting to sit down
- Make sure the person to keeps the chair in sight and sits down sideways on it
- Give little taps to the person's hips to turn them towards the chair (a directional cue)
- Use your own thigh or knee to guide the person's hips safely into the chair.
- Always avoid blocking the person's view of the chair.
- If someone is recovering from a recently repaired hip fracture, they must not sit down sideways-instead the chair needs to be directly behind them. Because this means that they cannot see the seat, they may need more reassurance than usual before they sit down.

Walking

- General points to consider:
- Footwear
- Clothes/incontinence pads
- Drainage bags, catheters.
- Suggested strategies:
- Assist at the person's side, so that you are both facing and moving in the same direction.
- Aim to cover a short distance to a seat that the person can see
- Give the walk a purpose for example to eat a (meal, watch TV, see a visitor, go to the toilet, or do some exercise)
- Give effective physical support or use a walking aid. Use the back of a row of chairs for support and practice
- Add to the sound of the person's footsteps with your own (providing a sound cue)
- If the person tends to grab the furniture, walls, you or other people, give them something to hold in their free hand
- Give them the opportunity to walk for longer distances so they have time to get into the rhythm of walking
- Reassure the person about the surroundings (hard to soft floor coverings, dark to light etc)
- Encourage longer strides by using a 'goose-step' (providing a visual cue)
- If the person's feet shuffle, encourage marching and/or sing a maching tune
- If the person's feet 'stutter', stop and restart by 'stepping'
- If the person threatens to sit down on an imaginary chair, tell them firmly 'Stay standing – stand up' rather than 'Don't sit down'
- When guiding a falling person on to the floor, follow the technique of sliding a falling person down your body
- Learn the technique of sliding a falling patient down your body onto the floor
- Make walking an enjoyable experience by conversing with them and paying them plenty of attention
- Be aware that the person's abilities may change from hour to hour or during the day.
- Never tow a person

Steps and stairs

- General points:
- Good lighting is needed
- Encourage the person to place their whole foot on each tread
- Make sure that an unsteady or breathless person places one foot onto the tread, then the other (two feet on the same tread) in order to slow the movement down and allow for better control.
- Suggested strategies:
- Step down the step just ahead of the person to show the change in level (visual cue)

- Step down the flight of steps or stairs slightly in front of the person, to partially block the space ahead (gap-filling)
- Or encourage the person to use both hands on one rail and come down sideways
- Paint the edge of concrete steps with a wide stripe in a contrasting colour.
- Even if a person does not need to be able to go up and down stairs, they often need to be able to manage steps.

Transfers

Chair

- The 'receiving' chair should be positioned close to and at about 90° to the chair that the person is sitting on.
- Suggested strategies
- Place an extra (third) chair in the space in front of the person (as a gap-filling strategy)
- Demonstrate the side to side rocking motion if the person needs to move to the front of the chair (providing a visual cue)
- Tell the person to 'Sit here please' and slap the seat of the chair (providing a sound cue)
- During the transfer, lightly tap the person's hips in the direction of the receiving chair (providing a touch cue)
- If you are assisting the person on your own, stand in the space between the backs of the two chairs to help the person's hips across more easily
- If there are two of you assisting, one of you can help at the person's side while the other stands in the space between the backs of the chairs.
- The most common patterns for transferring are to reach across and transfer, or to stand up and then transfer. Alternative methods of transferring include using a slide board, and then sliding the person across it, or using a weight-bearing hoist if necessary

Bed

Moving from lying to sitting on the edge

- This involves major changes of position, so that the person needs reassurance and time to adjust to each change.
- Suggested strategies:
- 'Get up please' with a rising gesture (providing a visual cue)
- 'Sit on the edge please' (providing a goal based request)
- Make sure the person is lying with their knees bent up, Then encourage them to roll onto their side by asking them to look at you, and to reach for the edge of the bed or your hand
- Prevent the person from seeing the drop to the floor by using a gap filling strategy. At the level of their head, you can either use your own body to block the view or place a; pillow lengthways along the edge of the bed or position a chair with its back against the side of the bed.

Sitting on the edge of the bed to lying down

- This is a major change in position.
- Suggested strategies:
- Use the command 'Lie down please' and slap the pillows (providing sound cues)
- To encourage the person to lie down along the length of the bed say 'Here's the pillow' and help the person to feel it, (providing a touch cue)
- Ask the person first to lift their legs onto the bed and then to lie down.

Moving across the bed

- Suggested strategies:
- 'Move across here, please' with a sliding gesture (providing a directional cue)
- Offer guidance with touch cues
- Use a slide-sheet to help the person move their hips across.

Moving along the edge of the bed

- Suggested strategies
- 'Move along please' accompanied with a gesture (providing a directional cue)
- Sit beside the person and encourage them to use a bed block as a substitute chair arm: this enables them to raise their hips higher and move sideways more easily
- Sit beside the person and move up very close against them. Move even closer moving into their personal space, and ask them to 'Move up/along/across please'
- Alternatively sit away from the person and pat the bed to encourage them to move towards you, saying 'Come and sit beside me'.
- Note: If the person seems to be afraid or unwilling to move, place a chair in the space in front of them, with its back towards them (as used during standing or transferring).
- Older people with both a mobility problem and dementia can be perceived as a poor rehabilitation prospect. However clinical reports suggest that functional improvements can be made, despite cognitive impairment, if the practice of independence skills is encouraged and specific stimulation is directed at improving mobility skills (Oddy 1987).
- Although the evidence is limited, the research that does exist suggests that older people with dementia can respond to rehabilitation. Pomeroy (1993) conducted an RCT of 24 subjects resident in a long-term care facility, who had severe dementia (age 65–91). It was found that there was a significant improvement in mobility skills following a period of physiotherapy input (90 minutes per week for 6 weeks).
- Huusko et al (2000) performed a subanalysis of an RCT to evaluate the effect of intensive geriatric rehabilitation on patients with dementia following hip fracture. Three months after surgery, in the intervention group 91% of the patients with mild dementia and 63% of those with moderate dementia were living independently. In the control group, the corresponding figures were 67% and 17%. There were no significant differences in patients with normal mini-mental state or severely demented patients. They concluded that hip fracture patients with mild to moderate dementia can often return to the community if they are provided with active rehabilitation programme to facilitate this.

Falls interventions for older people with dementia

- An RCT by Shaw et al (2003) investigated the effectiveness of multifactorial intervention after a fall in 274 older people with cognitive impairment and dementia attending the A&E department. There were no significant differences between the intervention and control groups in the proportion of people who fell during 1 year follow up. The authors concluded that multifactorial intervention was less effective in this patient group compared to cognitively intact older people.

- However, as older people with cognitive impairment and dementia are at high risk of falls, it is important that prevention of falls remains a research priority in this patient group.

- Shaw 2007 provides a rationale for a different approach to falls prevention in older people with dementia (MMSE < 20). She suggests that this population have a higher prevalence and severity of risk factors including gait/balance impairment, psychotropic medications plus behavioural risk factors such as wandering.

- Further work is required to determine optimal delivery of interventions and to identify the most important modifiable risk factors.

Fear of falling: techniques for promoting movement

- An older person with fear of falling may be so anxious about moving that they push themselves backwards when trying to stand up from a chair or walk cautiously with short, tentative steps.

- Rank the person's goals in order of difficulty/level of anxiety for the person.

- Practise each step of hierarchy:

- With the physiotherapist assisting (or provide sturdy support and reduce gradually, e.g. parallel bars, plinth in front of the person)

- With the therapist giving verbal prompting

- With therapist near the person

- With therapist standing at a distance

- With therapist out of sight.

- Use praise, support, encouragement and distraction if necessary. Make sure that you 'over consolidate' a stage before moving onto the next stage.

- Never ask a person to practise a task alone or with a carer/relative if they haven't achieved that stage alone or with carer in the presence of the therapist.

- Increase the level of difficulty in very small stages determined by the level of anxiety associated with each stage. Start from where the person is 'at', then increase either a) the distance to walk or b) increase the repetitions or c) increase the complexity of the task. The older person should always succeed.

- Suggested hierarchy for walking across a room despite fear of falling.

- Stand unaided

- Walk on the spot or move in standing, near to something to hold onto

- Walk short distance from chair to chair unaided

- Gradually move the chair further away (person in control)

- Walk across a small room

- Walk across a larger room
- Walk across the room with others walking about too.
- Given that fear of falling can exist in the absence of a history or risk of falls, it is an important clinical problem.
- A systematic review (Rixt Zijlstra et al 2007) found limited but fairly consistent findings of effectiveness in trials of home-based exercises, fall-related multi-factorial programmes and community-based tai chi group sessions.
- Tennstedt et al (1998) conducted a single blind controlled trial to investigate the effectiveness of a community based group programme to reduce fear of falling and associated activity restrictions in activity levels among older people ($n = 434$) (eight sessions over 4 weeks cognitive behavioural intervention). Intervention subjects reported increased levels of activity and greater mobility control immediately after the intervention ($p < 0.05$). A decrease in effects was noted by the 6 month follow up, suggesting that ongoing sessions may be required to maintain improvement.
- An RCT of multi-factorial intervention to reduce the risk of falls in community dwelling older people resulted in significant reductions in fear of falling for intervention subjects compared to the controls (Tinetti et al 1994).
- RCTs considering the effectiveness of Tai Chi; Zhang et al 2006 Wolf et al (1996) and Sattin et al (2005) also found significant reductions in fear of falling.
- In two other trials for falls reduction interventions, one yielded no change in fear of falling Reinsch et al (1992), whereas the other showed an increase in fear of falling among the intervention subjects (Hornbrook et al 1994).

Not achieving goals

- Is the problem identified accurately?
- Is the goal achievable?
- Examine influencing factors:
- Change in social or family circumstances
- Change in physical or mental condition, be on the alert for early signs and symptoms of acute illness, depression, confusion and discuss your concerns with the MDT
- A sudden change in functional ability may be due to a new acute illness
- Has the person been participating?
- Review the case, reassess the person's goals and discuss these with the person, your line manager, peers and the multidisciplinary team. You may need to change your intervention.
- If the person has reached their full potential, the physiotherapist should change the goal to a maintenance goal and teach the individual and/or carers a maintenance programme.

The references for this chapter can be found on www.expertconsult.com.

Strategies taken from Promoting mobility for people with dementia: a problem-solving approach by Rosemary Oddy (Alzheimer's Society 2011) and reproduced by kind permission of Alzheimer's Society and Rosemary Oddy.

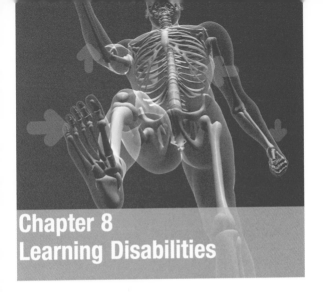

Chapter 8
Learning Disabilities

Introduction

- The basis of any intervention when dealing with a person with learning disabilities (LD) is no different from any other physiotherapy intervention, but a different set of skills will need to be developed so as to make the interventions accessible, appropriate for the needs of the individual and enjoyable.
- Failure to ensure this happens may lead to the individual becoming non-compliant, resulting in a poor outcome to treatment interventions.

Treatment planning based on assessment findings

- The assessment as covered in the assessment volume will define the physiotherapy intervention.
- The interventions must be person-centred to meet the individual's needs.
- As described by Barrell (2007), often the identified therapeutic intervention is not appropriate or not acceptable to the person with a LD, e.g. a client may wish to walk without pain and without a walking aid.
- They may not be happy or are unable to follow a specific exercise programme.
- Alternative options will then have to be devised to involve participation of the individual, in order to ensure that they undertake the necessary exercises.
- These options may include Jabadao, aquatic physiotherapy, or suitable leisure activities adapted to meet the needs of the client.
- In addition Barrell (2007) also highlights that the needs of parent carers, carers and support staff must also be considered.
- People with LD are often semidependent or totally dependent on their carers.

- There may be differing opinions between carers concerning perceived needs of the individual and success in delivering treatment is dependent on good communication and understanding of what is required between all involved.
- Assessment results and intervention plans need to be very clearly identified, discussed and communicated between the multidisciplinary team (MDT), the client and carers.
- Interventions tend to be based on exercise that will enhance movement and the client's functional ability.

Types of interventions

- The type of interventions given by the physiotherapist can be divided into the following categories:
- Advice and signposting
- Moving and handling advice including treatment handling
- Specific treatments/interventions, including aquatic physiotherapy, posture management, rebound therapy, Jabadao
- Management of long-term conditions
- Health and well being
- Teaching carers and support staff to carry out interventions, recognise change and to know when and how to contact the physiotherapist.
- The following will describe interventions that are commonly implemented in LD service, taking into account the specific needs of each person with a LD and providing practical tips.
- It may be that the person with LD needs information about or access to community activities such as appropriate gym classes, swimming clubs, walking groups, riding for the disabled, or wheelchair dancing.

Complex handling assessment

- Manual handling is defined as 'transporting or supporting a load (including lifting, putting down, pushing, pulling, carrying or moving thereof) by hand or bodily force' (HSE 2004).
- To the HSE definition may be added guiding, facilitating, manipulating or providing resistance.
- Thus any treatment where force is applied through any part of the physiotherapist's body to any part of the patient, involves manual handling.
- Physiotherapists are often considered the experts in manual handling and as such are often asked to advise on safer handling for an individual.
- However 'Physiotherapists cannot dictate to another profession how to handle a patient.' (CSP 2008), but as the health care professional with the knowledge of the individual's physical presentation the physiotherapist may be best placed to contribute to the risk assessment and to the development of a handling plan for an individual.
- Manual handling techniques as taught in the majority of training situations and described in most of the literature cover a generic handling approach for care staff. Individuals who present with challenging behaviour either physically or behaviourally are a relatively small population and their handling needs may differ from those of the general population.

- Physical challenges may include:
- Severe spinal deformities and limb contractures, which require the use of specialist slings
- Neurological conditions that present with potentially unpredictable movements, e.g. athetosis or severe spasms that may need specific placing of a carer's hands or require specialist equipment or slings to help minimise the risk of injury to staff or the individual
- Poorly controlled epilepsy, where seizures could occur during a transfer. This can affect the safety of both the individual and carer and the use of any equipment must be considered in respect of this.
- Behavioural challenges may include:
- Communication difficulties that result in individuals not being able to understand any necessary commands or instructions, which make it unclear how much they will be able to co-operate with a transfer. This may be compounded where an individual has more profound difficulties, e.g. no verbal communication
- Physical aggression such as hitting out, kicking, spitting
- Self-injurious behaviour
- Sensory difficulties, where individuals may be unable to tolerate physical touch, or the close proximity of carers or equipment
- Verbal aggression
- Confusion through dementia
- Confusion as a result of medication.
- Many individuals with a learning difficulty present with a combination of both physical and behavioural challenges. Therefore manual handling advisors, physiotherapists and carers may find themselves with a conundrum to solve, i.e. as the handling needs will generally not be met through a conventional approach, in order to meet the individual's needs appropriately and maintain the safe involvement of all parties involved, there will need to be careful planning of the processes and use of equipment.

Consent

- In relation to any physical intervention, which includes manual handling, individuals have the right to be consulted and involved in the formulation of any 'treatment' and/or care plans that directly affect them.
- If an individual is unable to give consent regarding their handling plans, as in any other situation, a solution must be in their best interests and documented as such, following a multiprofessional discussion.
- A physiotherapist is often called upon in these situations for their advice and recommendations.

Risk assessment

- The law is clear on the duty of employers to fully assess all risks to their employees in relation to manual handling, where there is the risk of injury; and where there is the possibility of violence or aggression directed towards staff, other clients or any other persons.

- Many individuals who present challenges resulting in complex manual handling situations may also present risks of injury through violence or aggression. Therefore, these clients require greater in-depth risk assessment and detailed management plans in order to reduce the risks to the lowest reasonably practicable level.

- Balanced risk assessment and management plans need to take the human rights of the individual as well as the safety and human rights of the health care staff or carers into account. It is not always possible to have one handling solution that will meet all of the individual's transfer needs. Each transfer situation must be assessed separately with all relevant risk factors taken into account.

- The individual should be involved, where possible, in the devising of safer handling management plans.

- In addition any plans should be devised on a multiprofessional basis, including the care staff who often have the best knowledge of the individual and their behaviours in specific circumstances.

- The risk assessment process should follow the guidelines defined in the Manual Handling Operations Regulations 1992 and subsequent Health and Safety Executive Guidance (HSE 2004). The risk assessment will need to consider risk factors in relation to: the task, the individual capability of the carer(s) carrying out the handling task, the load (individual) and all environmental factors.

- With individuals who present with challenging behaviours, there may be triggers in the environment which could affect their behaviour and influence the handling situation. These must be incorporated into the assessment of the environment along with the other factors such as the height of surfaces or lighting of the area.

Additional risk situations associated with complex handling

- There are often situations where an individual may have to be moved in what would be considered emergency situations in other contexts.

- Plans need to be considered and put into place to manage such foreseeable risks as they often occur in unforeseen circumstances.

- Such situations may include:

- Emergency removal from adapted wheelchairs for rescue medication

- An individual taking themselves to the floor while being removed from an environment

- Moving an individual to a place of safety when they have placed themselves at floor level and are unwilling to assist themselves from the floor, thus placing themselves and others at risk.

- These examples are not exhaustive, but merely serve as examples to emphasise where so-called 'general safer handling guidelines' cannot be applied.

- With complex handling situations, it may not always be possible to reduce environmental or handling risks with the provision of suitable equipment. By introducing equipment other situational risks may be presented. Therefore, alternative methods for managing the situation in the safest manner have to be found.

- The ideal posture and position for performing a particular task may not be possible to achieve, as this could place the carer in a position where they could be the recipient of physical aggression. Therefore, alternative postures and positions may have to be adopted in order to maintain carer safety.

- In such situations, the risk assessor needs to have an in-depth understanding of the presenting behaviours (both physical and behavioural) of the individual, the 'culture' of the organisation and carers undertaking the day-to-day care of the individual and a range of possible solutions to the presenting problems.

- Where individuals pose an additional risk to handlers through challenging behaviours, the behaviours of concern need to be highlighted, including who might be at risk and how. Additionally a record must be made of the details of triggers and situations that are likely to lead to such behaviours being displayed, the probability of such an occurrence, followed by the stages of intervention in the event of such an episode.

- Complex handling plans should only be put in place having been devised around specific individuals in specific situations.

- They should never be used as generic plans to cover all individuals in any situation. It is essential that any carers that are likely to be involved in carrying out the plan are individually assessed for their suitability in carrying out the plan and receive specific training in the techniques required with regular updates.

Recording complex handling plans

- Any safer handling management plan must be documented and be available for all parties involved to read and understand. It is also important that the process through which the decision was arrived at is documented, so that all carers reading the plan are aware of the potential risks involved.

- Recording personal information regarding the ability of carers to carry out the handling task needs to be recorded in individual staff files. This information is confidential and as such should not be recorded on a client's management plan. It is important that staff make their line manager aware of any physical condition that could affect their ability to carry out a safer handling plan.

- A complex manual handling risk management plan must include additional information over and above that which is usually recorded in a handling plan, for example:

- Basic client details including height and weight where possible and it may also be useful to record the physical stature of the client.

- The date on which the plan was devised needs to be clear on the front page, so that carers can see that it is the most recent and up-to-date plan that they are following.

- Details of the specific handling strategies to manage the situation including the minimum number of people to carry out the plan in the safest possible manner.

- The level of individual involvement in the management plan, i.e. whether or not they are able to give consent and where not, the consultation that has taken place with any significant others involved such as family members and the line managers of carers who will be carrying out the plan.

- Any individual or carer needs, such as any specific equipment required, including where it is stored.

- Any specific training requirements for carers.

- The clinical reasoning process that was undertaken to support the handling decision.

- The risks associated with the technique including both risks to the carers and individual.

- Any consequences that may impinge on an individual's human rights should the plan not be carried out.
- The frequency and likelihood of the risk occurring.
- Any action that should be taken following an incident, such as any documentation requiring completion. This may include informing the plan co-ordinators once the plan has been carried out to enable the plan to be reviewed immediately to ensure that all risks were kept to a minimum.
- The signatures of the risk plan co-ordinators.
- The signatures of any significant others who have been involved in the decision-making process.
- There also needs to be an agreement form designed to be signed by all carers to show they have read the management plan, understand the handling strategies and have received any necessary training specific to the handling strategy.
- Any handling plan needs to be reviewed regularly or in the event of any change to the individual's physical presentation or any changes in their behaviour that would affect the handling strategy. A review sheet should form part of the handling plan.
- It is important that if a specific number of carers have been identified in order to carry out the handing plan in the safest manner, that the required number of staff are available at all times in the event of the plan needing to be executed.
- As part of the review process of the handling plan, regular training is essential to ensure that staff remain familiar with the management plan and the required techniques, particularly where they may only be performed occasionally.
- This may involve the compilation of a resource in the form of detailed photographs showing stages of releasing wheelchair straps, footplates or use of other pieces of equipment or where the staff are required to specifically place their hands during implementation of the plan.

Therapeutic handling risk assessments

- Physiotherapists are subject to the manual handling regulations with regard to risk assessments and have a duty to reduce any risks involved to the lowest reasonably practicable level (HSE 2004). Many physiotherapists carry out risk assessments as part of their ongoing assessment process, but it is important that this information is written in the individual's clinical notes and does not remain as a series of thoughts in the therapist's head. Implicit in the legislation is the requirement to record the risk assessment and any planned risk-reducing methods. If this information is not written down, it is considered never to have been carried out, and in the event of a handling incident occurring, a physiotherapist's memory of what was assessed and what was planned would not be considered robust evidence in a court of law should an individual seek to establish negligence and gain compensation for any harm incurred during the handling process.
- The handling risks that physiotherapists are exposed to differ from those of general care staff, as they are involved in the re-education and rehabilitation of individuals and without any intervention, many people may never progress and regain function.
- Due to the complex physical presentation combined with challenging behaviour, physiotherapy programmes may present additional challenges. Added to this,

certain treatment modalities used may inherently introduce an added risk of an incident occurring, for example during rebound therapy there is added risk from the unstable surface and the poor postures required to position individuals on the bed of the trampoline.

- There are many examples of different ways to record treatment handling risk assessments. An example of this designed and developed by the All Wales Treatment Handling Group is available to physiotherapists as an appendix to the guidelines on manual handling produced by the Chartered Society of Physiotherapy (CSP 2008).

- It is important to examine treatment goals and the methods decided upon to reach those goals. The question should be asked, 'Is hazardous handling involved?' If the answer is in the affirmative, it may be necessary to consider alternative treatment methods, or introduce equipment to reduce risks or even to reconsider treatment goals in conjunction with the individual explaining any reasons why.

- Clinical reasoning must be documented to explain why a particular intervention has been decided upon. The physiotherapist must consider their own health in relation to the ability to implement the treatment safely and also the safety of any person assisting them. For example, can the physiotherapist or any assistants, safely achieve prolonged knee flexion should it be required?

- Any particular risks associated with the individual being treated must be recorded. With adults with a LD this could include any behavioural challenges, uncooperative behaviour, unstable epilepsy, as well as poor sitting ability, tendency to drop to the floor or involvement of particularly heavy individuals or their limbs that require handling.

- Environmental risks must be recorded, such as height of bed may be an issue if working in an individual's home, a potentially noisy or busy environment if treatment is taking place in a day centre.

- It is important to record any risk-reducing measures, such as an increase in staff, the introduction of equipment, a third person following behind with a wheelchair if assisting an individual to mobilise.

Delegation and advice

- Within the field of LD, physiotherapists may frequently find themselves delegating all or part of a physiotherapy programme to carers.

- It is important to be clear whether advice is being given or a specific task is being delegated to another.

- Recording must always be made of the names of individuals the task has been delegated to and any advice given.

- A task should be observed on more than one occasion having been delegated to a carer to ensure the carer is clear on the reasons for the intervention, any risks involved, any reasons why the programme should not be carried out and that the physiotherapist is confident that the carer can carry the intervention out safely.

- Clear written instructions should be issued making sure that they are understood. It is important to remember that no assumptions should be made about people's level of comprehension or ability to read written instructions. These instructions can be complemented with the addition of photographs.

- It must be remembered that if the physiotherapist asks employed carers to carry out part of a physiotherapy programme, it may not be their priority to carry out that task. They are employed as carers and therefore their priority will often be to ensure the individual has assistance with personal care if required, participates in activities of daily living and accessing their local community. They may not make time to carry out a programme of physiotherapy. Where possible, programmes should be incorporated into activities of daily living, such as active assisted movements that can be incorporated into washing and dressing; balance work in sitting or standing can take part during mealtimes or while washing up.

Aquatic physiotherapy

- Aquatic physiotherapy is a frequently used modality of treatment for adults with a LD and it is a welcome medium for interventions providing freedom of movement for individuals with PMLD with the warmth of the water allowing the relaxation of muscles that are affected by increased tone.

- Refer to the aquatic physiotherapy assessment and treatment chapters for details on the principles of treating people in water.

- Many clients with a LD experience epileptic seizures, are PEG fed and doubly incontinent, all of which in some pools may be considered a contraindication to aquatic physiotherapy.

- A thorough risk assessment is necessary as these risks need not exclude an individual from accessing a pool.

Rebound therapy

- Rebound therapy is the therapeutic use of a trampoline and it is widely used as a treatment modality within LD.

- It can be used for any manner of ability/disability. For example:

- It can be used as a stepping stone for the more physically able to access the sport of trampolining.

- For those that will not progress to integrated sports, it can be a valuable weight-reducing activity that is fun.

- It may also help with balance, co-ordination and concentration levels.

- This use of a trampoline may not require the skills of a physiotherapist and may be led by a special needs trampoline coach.

- It can be used to reduce the energy levels of some individuals. Some of these may have challenging behaviour so any participation in rebound must be fully risk assessed for its outcome and the potential risk to individuals and coaches.

- Floor access trampolines may present less of a risk in mounting and dismounting for these individuals.

- It can be used therapeutically for mobile individuals who have some neurological impairment. The trampoline can aid with improving someone's balance, core stability and co-ordination while giving them a challenging and unstable base to work from.

- For individuals with PMLD it is a vital mode of delivering physiotherapy. It is especially beneficial if individuals are tactile defensive or their tone is so high that it is difficult to carry out passive movements in a pain-free manner.

- In this instance rebound therapy is much like an aquatic therapy pool in that the bounce of the trampoline will give the benefits in the same way as the warmth of the water will without the need for hands-on physiotherapy intervention.

- Rebound, like many physiotherapy modalities, does not lend itself well to quantitative forms of research. Therefore, much of the research available is of a qualitative nature where physiotherapists have highlighted some of the benefits observed clinically when using Rebound.
- These include:
- The reduction or recruitment of muscle tone depending on the need of the individual and the depth of the bounce produced on the trampoline.
- Stimulation of bladder and bowel function.
- Stimulation of the respiratory system – for those individuals who have a propensity to chest infections and who cannot produce an effective cough on demand, the trampoline can be an effective way of stimulating a cough. This is by either the general movement or by using bigger bounces which can force air into the lungs and thereby stimulate a cough.
- Sensory stimulation.
- Rebound has an important function to play in postural management when gravity can be used to improve posture rather than be destructive.

Restrictions and contraindications

- Manual handling is the main limitation for rebound due to the unstable and moving base the physiotherapist is working on.
- The physiotherapist must ensure that staff can safely assist the individual on and off the trampoline. This may be independently or with assistance. The latter may be just verbal and/or physical prompts or may refer to hoist transfers.
- Contra indications do exist and must be observed.
- The Chartered Society of Physiotherapy (CSP) has produced a guidance paper for physiotherapists using rebound in practice which encompasses the contraindications (CSP 2007). In addition the interactive forum of the CSP (iCSP) is a useful discussion forum where physiotherapists can share practice issues and good practice with other physiotherapists already using this mode of treatment.
- Rebound therapy can be an invaluable tool in any physiotherapist's repertoire and it may be used widely within learning disabilities.
- Rebound should not be limited to the LD patient group, as the benefits can be applicable for patients with a variety of neurological conditions.
- Rebound also makes therapy 'fun' and provides an alternative to the physiotherapy gym, which can ensure that there is something additional to maintain the interest of the individual in their treatment, when it can be difficult to maintain the incentive in long-term rehabilitation.

Splinting in LD

- Splinting may be seen by many physiotherapists as the domain of the occupational therapists, but for long-standing neurological conditions, such as those that are associated with individuals with LD, cross therapy working is essential.
- The use of splinting is contentious and many neurological physiotherapists argue against the use of splinting for patients with acute neurological conditions.

- However, where the neurological damage is long-standing, splinting may have a part to play in preventing further deterioration of asymmetrical postures or small joint contractures and deformities.

- Adult PMLD individuals may not have volitional movement in their upper limbs and as such LD physiotherapists work with a number of individuals who have developed contractures, particularly of the hands.

- The cause of the contractures may be attributed to increased muscle tone in combination with the effects of gravity.

- The effect of this can lead to anatomical structures tending to 'slip and slide' and can result in deformities similar to those seen in rheumatoid arthritis, such as 'swan neck' and 'Boutonniere' although the mechanism by which they develop is very different.

- Due to the way that physiotherapy intervenes in LD the physiotherapist may become aware of the need for intervention in order to maintain joints in a neutral position as far as is possible.

- Resting splints, functional splints and serial splinting are all possible interventions that can be utilised.

- However, in advanced neurological conditions splinting may have to accommodate any deformity that may already present.

- Splints may be used in an attempt to alter long-term deformity or they may be just as importantly arresting the deformity from deteriorating further.

- The provision of a splint may seem to be for cosmetic reasons, for example in the case of finger flexion contractures. However the tendency for an individual's nails to dig into their palm may lead to the breakdown of the skin and a resulting infection. The use of palm protectors is a simple but effective way of preventing unnecessary complications due to contractures.

- For the provision of splints there may be joint working between a neurologist, occupational therapist, orthotist and physiotherapist. Many neurologists will only administer Botox injections when splints are in place to maintain any increase in joint range of movement that may be achieved as a result of the treatment.

- Therefore, splinting may not be a modality that every physiotherapist participates in, but for student and junior physiotherapists, every opportunity should be taken to gain an insight into this area of work.

- Knowledge of the principles of splinting and how splints can be provided for an individual will ensure that outcomes from intervention will be improved.

Postural management

- Postural management is the maintenance of optimal physical position.

- Ideally posture management should occur over a 24-hour period.

- The majority of individuals with PMLD experience the constant fight between gravity and the opposing up-thrust from their supporting surface.

- Humans with normal postural tone are able to support themselves against these forces to maintain an anatomically correct posture. Within these parameters, individuals can move effectively and efficiently without conscious thought of these opposing forces.

- Individuals with altered muscle tone are unable to maintain a stable, energy-efficient and functional posture and this can lead to damage of anatomical structures.

- As a result of the abnormal tone contractures and deformities often develop.

- Secondary complications that can occur in association with tone abnormalities can include:
- Spinal deformities
- Respiratory incompetence
- Gastrointestinal compromise
- Swallowing issues and dysphagia
- Pressure areas
- Contractures
- Pain/discomfort
- Poor maintenance of weight.
- Conventional positioning, such as most chairs, requires an individual to sit with their hips at a right angle or close to it.
- If an individual has decreased range of movement at the hip joint that prevents them from achieving 90° flexion and the seating provided expects them to do so; their body will accommodate to allow them to be seated. With the example mentioned of reduced hip flexion, this will lead to rotation and/or deviation of the pelvis and development of a scoliosis.
- Therefore, a thorough assessment of the range of movement available at critical joints is essential. This then provides a framework to liaise with seating engineers to provide a suitable wheelchair insert.
- The seating design needs to accommodate an individual's limitation of movement and must allow them to be seated with a stable base, without expending energy to maintain their position and without causing tissue damage.
- Pauline Pope has written a book and produced additional material that provides a comprehensive yet readable narrative regarding posture and its management (Pope 2006).
- Noreen Hare developed resources for evaluating and managing postural deformities and these can be accessed via http://hafpa.info/.
- The responsibility of a physiotherapist does not only involve providing advice around the types of wheelchair seating available, it extends to every aspect of an individual's life, for example, their position at night time and alternative comfortable seating and for any time that they spend out of their supporting wheelchair.
- The physiotherapist will need to liaise with different providers of specialised equipment and be able to co-ordinate the assessment and provision of equipment and its funding.
- The physiotherapist's role also includes the education of carers, family members and care staff in the different environments that an individual accesses on a regular basis. This is important as the maintenance of optimum posture involves everybody that is involved in supporting the individual over a 24-hour period.

Clinical case example A

Background

- CJ is a 40-year-old lady with a diagnosis of cerebral palsy.
- She weighs approximately 9 ½ stone and spends much of her time in a wheelchair which has a moulded insert.

- CJ also has the use of a specialist armchair both at home and in day services.

- CJ lives at home with her parents where she has an adapted en-suite bedroom. There is overhead tracking through to the bathroom where there is an adapted bath and in the bedroom she has an electric profiling bed.

- Physically she presents with a gross kyphoscoliosis with the curvature convex to her left side.

- She had generally increased muscle tone and flexor contractures were present in her upper limbs.

- She had a marked windswept deformity of her hips to the left with a resultant reduced range of hip movement.

- Both of CJ's knees were fixed in knee extension.

- Harrington rods had been inserted into her back in an attempt to control the scoliosis in her late teens and these had gradually been bent due to the force generated through the muscle spasms she experienced.

- The spine is monitored on a regular basis in the local orthopaedic department and regular X-rays are taken in order to rule out breakage of the rods due to metal fatigue.

- CJ experiences regular myoclonic jerks and frequent absences as well as occasional tonic-clonic seizures.

- She has no verbal communication, but is able to demonstrate pain and discomfort although it is not always easy to differentiate between seizure activity and discomfort.

Historical handling practice

- Since she was a child CJ's father has lifted her for all transfers.

- Over the years it has been the role of the physiotherapists supported by other team members to educate the father about the hazards of manually lifting his daughter in the way that he had been used to.

- It took a great deal of persuasion before he would accept the provision of the handling equipment to make it safer and easier to manage CJ.

- In day services a hoist and full sling was used for all transfers, but a modified draglift was used to place and remove the sling.

- The modified drag lift presented a risk to the carers because of the postures required to undertake the task, i.e. bending into flexion with a twisted spine and having to support CJ's body weight.

- This position effectively meant that CJ was being handled away from the carer's base of support adding to the increased risk.

- Handling CJ from under her armpits and pulling her weight forward by this method also placed repeated stresses and strain on her shoulder joints leading to undoubted pain, discomfort and potential damage to the joint structures. CJ was unable to verbally express this.

Solution

- CJ was assessed for and provided with a specialist all-day sling, which accommodated her spinal deformity.

- This was designed so that it could be left in situ behind her in her wheelchair and armchair.

- The previous manual handling that was involved in inserting and removing the sling was eliminated.
- Subsequently the sling could be placed in position in the morning by her father with CJ lying on the bed by rolling her onto the sling.
- The sling could be repositioned in the same way when necessary following personal care by the carers.
- Carers that were carrying out unsafe practice by using a drag lift were given some education on the risk that this manoeuvre posed to their health and the potential for damaging CJ's shoulders (Carayon 2007, Hignett et al 2003).

Clinical case example B

Background

- A is a 46-year-old male who lives in 24-hour staffed accommodation.
- He has cerebral palsy and severe LD.
- A has verbal speech, but this tends to be in the form of 'catch' phrases that he has learnt over the years.
- Despite his speech limitations A is able to hold quite a sociable conversation.
- A's only purposeful movement is of his head and some of his upper limbs.
- He can exhibit a startle reflex, but this same movement can be set off when he is unsure or anxious.
- A is wheelchair-dependent and requires hoisting at all times.
- He has a moulded wheelchair, which has a tilt in space base.
- He uses a leave under sling at all times to reduce the manual handling for both A and the staff, but also as part of his 24-hour postural management plan.
- He has a specialised postural armchair and a profiling bed.
- On his bed he uses parts of two different postural management sleep systems.
- The posture management systems are in place when he is resting on the bed and also at night when he goes to sleep.
- His LD physiotherapist has provided him with a variety of splints.
- These mainly consist of hard thermoplastic hand splints and also soft palm protectors for both hands.
- The different splints have been provided in order to try to accommodate the asymmetric posture of both of his hands.
- A is able to carry out some functional tasks with his right hand, but there is no functional ability in the left hand.
- The position of both hands is one of flexion and ulnar drift with flexion at the metacarpophalangeal joints (MCPs).
- The fingers have a lax feel and tend to exhibit both swan neck and boutonnières deformities.
- His current physiotherapy input is weekly for passive movements and rebound therapy.
- Hydrotherapy would be advantageous, but no facilities are currently available within a practical distance of his living accommodation.
- His splints and wheelchair are reviewed as required.
- Staff training is also carried out in regards to the passive movements he requires and his 24-hour postural management needs.

Challenges

- Staff were carrying out unsafe practice by using a drag lift (Carayon 2007, Hignett et al 2003).

- A is able to verbalise his thoughts and needs, but it is difficult to ascertain his capacity to consent.

- A is a very dominant character and likes to think of himself as being 'kingpin' in his own house and as such is in charge of everyone's whereabouts, including his co-tenants. In order to enable him to feel that he is in control of the house A likes to stay within the kitchen.

- If this doesn't occur he can become verbally aggressive and use very abusive language.

- The volume and intensity of this will increase and he will threaten to report staff for neglecting to observe his wishes.

- This behaviour has arisen when staff have taken him to lie on his bed to have a change of position or to change the splints on his hands.

- This situation has been improved somewhat by the purchase of the postural armchair, but there remained an issue with the fitting of the hard splints.

- Staff were initially prepared to persevere with the fitting of these as the physiotherapist had requested them to be applied.

- However, the staff felt that the abuse was unacceptable and after discussions between the physiotherapist and the whole staff team it was decided to stop the use of the hard splints for the time being and to continue with the soft splints.

- This was quite a compromise as A's hand shape had been improving with the daily use of the hard splints.

- It is hoped that they can be reintroduced at another time; however, in the interim the soft splints are being tolerated and are also maintaining his hand function and position, if not to the same degree as the hard splints.

- A will regularly tell staff that his physiotherapy sessions are cancelled; although when he attends he appears happy to be there.

- The other main challenge to his LD physiotherapist is that despite A having all the postural equipment that he should have in place his posture continues to deteriorate. His weight is more than it should be, but this has been stabilised at the moment with the care staff following a healthy eating menu and in addition they have reduced his portion size.

- However, his trunk is still following a more flexed pattern, but more troubling is that his trunk has also started to take on a rotational deformity.

- His head has begun falling forward and to the side, which he is becoming less able to correct. This not only affects his communication, but it also results in his saliva pooling on his cheek and causing a skin irritation and sometimes dental abscesses.

- The trunk rotation force is the hardest deformity to correct and even though the tilt facility is used to position him in his wheelchair and postural armchair the amount of rotational deformity is becoming worse.

The future

- For the LD physiotherapist this will involve working closely with the wheelchair engineers that are responsible for the production of A's wheelchair to try to build a corrective mechanism into the chair design.

- The concerns of the physiotherapist need to be discussed with the neurologist responsible for A's medication.
- The care staff need to be provided with support to help them to deal with A's changing physical presentation and this includes manual handling and positioning advice.

The references for this chapter can be found on www.expertconsult.com.

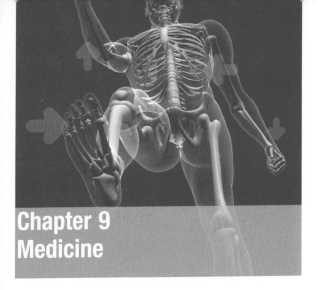

Chapter 9
Medicine

Introduction

- For the student or novice physiotherapist commencing work on a medicine ward they may be wondering 'what conditions will I see?' and 'what is the treatment approach I will be expected to follow?'

- There is no 'recipe' book of treatments that covers every diagnosis or presentation encountered on an acute medical ward and the specific treatment interventions. The aim of this chapter is to indicate the types of assessment approaches that may be used and how these enable the therapist to choose the appropriate interventions.

- The authors anticipate providing the reader with an insight into the role of the physiotherapist in the medical management of patients, the hospital multidisciplinary team (MDT), professional documentation, discharge planning and on-going referral.

- By understanding the role of physiotherapy within acute medicine the reader will be able to make their own conclusions about what working in medicine as a physiotherapist entails.

Admission to an acute medicine ward

- The reasons for admission to a medical ward are varied with each patient's presentation having associated medical issues. Each patient seen by a physiotherapist on a medical ward will be different and will need to be approached as an individual.

- Even a similar diagnosis will not guarantee that a patient will present in the same way and this will mean that they will require a different approach from the MDT and the physiotherapist.

- The diagnosis may not necessarily directly influence or dictate physiotherapy intervention; however, it is important in relation to an individual's prognosis in terms of the course of the condition, life expectancy, possible fatigue, impact cognition, physical ability. All these factors could then influence the decisions to be made regarding the rehabilitation potential or discharge destination, e.g. home, residential or nursing home.

- The variation of presentations/diagnoses to be encountered should not be viewed as a daunting or intimidating prospect, if the physiotherapist has confidence in the assessment findings and reasoning associated with this.

Assessment and goal planning

- The most fundamental thing to remember above everything else is that the assessment should, and needs to, identify the problems that physiotherapy treatment intervention can where possible, work towards resolving or reducing them.

- Equally important is ensuring that the assessment findings and subsequent treatment intervention are defined as a result of patient-related goal planning, which includes inclusion within an MDT framework.

- Talking to some patients about goal planning and it may be difficult to engage them. However, talking about what they feel they need to achieve in order to return home may stimulate a different and far more enthusiastic response.

- It may seem obvious, but it is worth emphasising that both the physiotherapy and the overall MDT intervention goals should be focused on the patients' needs as defined by them, rather than what 'we' as professionals consider should be the outcomes.

Patient demographics

- The type of patient being admitted to an acute medical ward has changed significantly over the years, not surprising if the changes in population demographics are considered.

- The UK has a population that has been aging over the last 25 years, with the percentage of the population aged 65 and over increasing from 15% in 1984 to 16% in 2009, an increase of 1.7 million people.

- The most potentially influential statistic is that the fastest population increase has been in the number of people aged 85 and over, the 'oldest old'.

- In 1984, there were around 660 000 people in the UK aged 85 and over. The total number has more than doubled, reaching 1.4 million in 2009.

- By 2034 it is projected that the number of people aged 85 and over will be 2.5 times larger than in 2009, reaching an estimated 3.5 million and accounting for 5 per cent of the total population (ONS 2010).

- Considering these significant demographic changes it is suggested that more services will be required within the local health community to manage the associated health needs of this population.

- The way in which these services are delivered will continue to change as more patients are managed in primary care settings rather than the secondary care that is commonplace in present day service delivery.

Profile of patients on medicine wards

- Physiotherapists working on a medical ward are likely to encounter patients with complex medical, physical, social and emotional needs that can no longer be managed safely and effectively within the community resources.
- Patients admitted to hospital from the community require a co-ordinated MDT assessment in order to ensure that they and their family/carers have a realistic plan for the future.

Preadmission status

- Ascertaining the pre-admission status and function of patients is essential for the physiotherapist in order to formulate appropriate, meaningful and realistic problem lists, treatment plans and goals with the patient (where possible).
- Above all else this information is fundamental to safe and successful discharge planning.
- The patient's preadmission functional status can be acquired from a variety of sources, e.g. medical and nursing notes (if separate) may have some information regarding an individual's social history.
- The physiotherapist and OT will require a greater depth of information than that provided by the medical and nursing records. This information must be obtained either directly from the patient, or next of kin/family or carers.
- If the patient has been admitted from a residential or nursing home it is useful to contact the establishment as they can provide valuable information.
- This may be particularly important as some residential/nursing homes may not accept the patient back as a resident unless they have regained their pre-admission status.
- The specific areas of preadmission function that need to be ascertained are:
- Mobility
a How did they mobilise prior to admission?
b Any aids used?
c Level of independence or assistance required
d Distance mobilised on a regular basis
- Stairs
a Were they able to negotiate stairs?
b Any aids required?
- Transfers
a Bed to chair
b Sit to stand
c Level of assistance required
d Level of independence
- Bed mobility
a Level of independence
b Assistance required.
- Along with the gathering the previous information it is also essential to record if there are any concerns or difficulties with any of the activities and establishing why these difficulties are occurring.

- One of the most important pieces of information to substantiate is whether the patient has experienced any falls and what the circumstances were.

- Wherever possible a ward physiotherapist would be aiming to assist a patient back to their preadmission levels of function, as in some cases independence is solely compromised by an acute illness.

- A number of NHS hospitals have developed acute medical wards and rehabilitation ward/beds where patients who no longer require acute medical care may be transferred. Physiotherapy and MDT colleagues will require a handover including a copy of the professional documentation completed up to this stage of the patient's admission.

- It is important to identify if a patient is having a decline in their functional ability which may become evident during the subjective assessment or from information gathered during previous admissions.

- It is then the role of the MDT to identify why this decline may be taking place. Is it the result of a pre-existing condition or some other factor such as poor levels of support in the community? When planning a patient's discharge these are factors to consider and appropriate and additional support on discharge can make the difference between the patient remaining in their own home and being readmitted within a short timeframe.

Treatment interventions relating to speciality assessments

- In this chapter commonly encountered conditions are covered along with a range of ideas for treatment that may be used.

- Hopefully, whilst working under supervision the student will realise that the most effective plans for intervention are generated from a combination of knowledge of anatomy, physiology, pathologies, the effects of treatment interventions and the assessment findings. Senior clinicians will draw on clinical experience in addition to these factors to ensure that the patient receives the most appropriate management.

- As mentioned previously, there is no specific 'recipe' to follow when treating patients in an acute medicine setting, students and novice physiotherapists will need to develop their theoretical knowledge base and integrate their experiences into the clinical reasoning process that underpins the choice of interventions.

- Patients often present with a complex medical history and the student/novice will be expected to discuss the complexities with their supervisor or senior clinician in order to develop their ability to reassess and progress treatments appropriately.

- It is important to gather feedback from other members of the MDT, e.g. nursing, OT or care support workers. The knowledge of the MDT assessment findings can assist the physiotherapist in planning the patient's treatment programme.

- As an example a patient who is standing well in a standing hoist with other members of the team may progress quicker if the physiotherapist informs the team that the patient is initiating the stand. The MDT discussion may lead to the patient being assessed for their suitability to use a rotastand or Zimmer frame in order to progress the independent function during transfers with other MDT members.

- Sometimes successive treatments will be a combination of assessment and treatment to determine the most effective approach for a patient. This tends to be the case with patients who have conditions such as Parkinson's disease (PD) where it may be necessary to trial what cues work best for them. When treating patients with varying degrees of cognitive impairment it may require the use of a number of different approaches before the optimum method of communication is identified that will ensure the patient engages with their therapy.
- Assessment should have identified a list of problems that are affecting the function of the patient:
- Reduced muscle strength
- Reduced balance (static and dynamic)
- Reduced range of movement (ROM)
- Poor gait pattern
- Decreased exercise tolerance
- Deterioration of functional ability, e.g. sit to stand and bed transfers.
- When considering the treatment of patients in medicine it is important to remember that there is no specific 'medical' approach as such, the management requires a combination of knowledge and skills from the 'core' areas of musculoskeletal, neurology and respiratory practice. To be effective the physiotherapist will need to incorporate all their skills in order to treat their patients effectively.
- Providing walking aids and walking patients does not address the fundamental problems that have brought the patient into hospital. If walking aids are provided include an exercise sheet for the patient to enable them to progress their mobility following your instructions.
- The assessment will have identified specific issues that need specific interventions, e.g. it is more effective to spend 10–15 minutes working on balance and ROM than just walking someone. Set goals and ensure that these are incorporated into the patient's routine to enable them to achieve the best outcomes during their time on the ward.

Communication

- There are three main ways of communicating:
- Verbal
- Non-verbal
- Written.
- It is essential that patients are addressed by the name of their choice and they should be asked this question on initial contact. Do not assume that patients like to be addressed by their forename. It is not appropriate to refer to patients as 'dear', 'babe', 'love', 'duck', ' pet', 'honey', or any similar term. These terms are unprofessional and can be viewed as being derogatory and patronising.
- Remember that the hospital admission of a family member is an anxious time for relatives. They will often feel out of control of the situation and be keen to acquire as much information and reassurance as possible. It is imperative that communication channels with relatives and carers are established (it is essential to remember that consent is required from the patient before the disclosure of any patient-related information to a third party).

- It is essential to be able to adapt methods of communication with patients.
- Consider the following:
- The environment the patient is in, e.g. busy medical wards can be distracting for many patients
- Cognitive impairment either long-standing or acute
- Patient's ability to hear
- Visual impairment.
- Some patients may respond better to instructions that are given in short sentences, have pauses between sentences and use positive language, e.g. 'move your bottom nearer the edge of the chair' (pause), 'put your hands on the arms of the chair' (pause), 'slide your feet back' (pause), 'on the count of three stand up' (pause), '1, 2, 3, stand up'.
- Provide further instructions such as 'keep standing' rather than 'don't sit down'.
- Using the word 'don't' – your patient will invariably end with the patient doing what you don't want them to do.
- The ability to adapt your voice when giving instructions will also help to influence the outcome.
- If you are working with another member of staff (PT, PTA or OT) ensure you are both aware of who is leading the session, so the patient doesn't become confused about who they should be following.
- Written communication can be effective for patients with hearing problems and also for those patients who themselves are unable to speak, e.g. cerebrovascular accident (CVA) patients, motor neuron disease, multiple sclerosis (MS).
- Non-verbal communication, such as your body posture and body language, eye contact, can help to develop a rapport with the patient to get them to engage in their treatment.
- This is a useful skill to use with patients who have cognitive impairment, when demonstrating what you want them to do.

Musculoskeletal and orthopaedic problems: treatment options

- The following list highlights the common musculoskeletal presentations/past medical histories frequently seen in a medical environment:
- Rheumatoid arthritis (RA)
- Osteoarthritis (OA)
- Back pain, both specific and non-specific in origin
- Previous joint replacements, either recent or old
- Osteoporosis
- Simple spinal fractures
- Pubic rami fractures
- Upper limb fractures, either post fall, mechanical or other causes
- Muscle atrophy and sarcopenia.
- Commonly, musculoskeletal problems tend to be part of the past medical history (PMH) and they usually contribute to a patient's loss of function when they are admitted, e.g. a patient admitted due to heart failure may have OA in their knees that affects their ability to mobilise.

- Patients may also be admitted for elective or trauma surgery and postoperatively may develop a deep vein thrombosis (DVT) or pulmonary embolus (PE). It is important to be familiar with postoperative precautions, contraindications and complications when attempting to increase a patient's independent mobility.

- It may be part of the role of the physiotherapist to inform nursing staff about any precautions as they may not be familiar with them. What may be obvious to one member of the MDT may not be obvious to other members and therefore the ability to communicate and educate other MDT members is an important skill to develop.

- For a number of patients it is important that they have pain relief prior to any intervention in order to maximise the outcomes from the treatment sessions.

- Time treatment sessions to coincide with medication, in order to maximise therapy and patient outcomes. If pain relief is not adequate, then liaise with the medical teams and/or pain management clinical nurse specialists; this may be beneficial in ensuring the patient has adequate pain relief to get the most benefit from physiotherapy intervention.

- For patients with musculoskeletal problems it is important for them to be given exercise programmes to do whilst they are in hospital and to continue following discharge.

- After their assessment, tailor the programme around their problems, e.g. reduced ROM, decreased muscle strength. Use skills that may have been developed in outpatients and or trauma/orthopaedics in order to treat the patient holistically, e.g. if a patient also has an OA knee provide an exercise programme incorporating strengthening exercises and ROM and provide advice about positioning, ice packs and pain relief.

- It is important to document accurately the exercise programme in the notes in addition to giving patients a copy of the exercise programme or you may wish to photocopy the sheet given to the patient. Also stress the importance of the patient taking responsibility for their own management of the problem as you would in outpatients. For patients who have cognitive decline, you may need to discuss this with the patient's relatives or carers. You may also want to refer to community-based services or to a Day Hospital for further rehabilitation if you feel this is appropriate. Discharge planning is discussed in more detail later in the chapter.

Walking aids

- There are a number of walking aids that can be used to assist with a patient's rehabilitation to promote independence and safety, e.g.:

- Zimmer frame:

  Improves a patient's ability to weight bear as they provide a wide base of support. However, when mobilising any distance the patient has to lift the frame for every step, which is unhelpful for patients who fatigue or who have difficulty initiating movement, e.g. PD.

- Wheeled Zimmer frame:

  These avoid the need to lift the frame at each step and provide more fluidity of movement, enabling patients to weight bear with an enhanced base of support. It is wise to consider a patient's home environment and if there are stairs then it will be helpful to issue the patient with two frames, one for upstairs and one for down stairs.

- Gutter frames:

  Useful for patients where their hands have been affected by RA/OA or if they have sustained a wrist/or hand fracture and are allowed to weight bear through the forearm. These are beneficial for patients that rely on upper limb support and can be a good progression from a standing hoist.

- Elbow crutches:

  Useful for patients with good co-ordination and where they need upper limb support when weight bearing. These are standard walking aids given to patients post-elective orthopaedic surgery.

- Gutter crutches:

  Again useful for patients requiring elbow crutches where they are unable to use the hand grips. Ensure that your patient has good co-ordination and good cognitive abilities.

- Walking sticks and quad sticks:

  Useful aids for patients requiring some additional support when mobilising and can be provided as single items or as a pair. It is important to consider a patient's cognitive abilities and their safety as it is not uncommon to see sticks being carried, rather than being used as walking aids.

- Fischer sticks and crutches:

  These have moulded handles and are very useful for those patients with disruption of the joints in the hand, e.g. RA.

- Delta frames and four-wheeled walkers

  Useful for patients with balance issues. Good for outdoor walking. Important to ascertain whether the patient understands the safety precautions and that they are able to operate the brakes safely. In some organisations delta frames are no longer issued due to concerns about the frame folding up unexpectedly. Therefore ensure that the organisation you are working in supports the use of these aids.

- It is always essential to consider different types of gait pattern and weight bearing when providing mobility aids as well as a patient's ability to follow instructions and their cognitive abilities.

- Zimmer frames can also be adapted by OTs with a Buckingham caddy to assist patients with transporting meals and drinks and to carry belongings.

Muscle atrophy and sarcopenia

- Muscle atrophy is a decrease in the mass of a muscle which can be partial or complete. Atrophy results in weakness as the overall muscle is unable to exert the force in relation to its mass. Conditions which can result in atrophy include cancer, congestive heart failure, COPD, renal failure and burns, liver disease and starvation, which are all conditions commonly seen in patients on the medical wards.

- Atrophy results in a decrease in the quality of life for the individual as performing tasks such as standing and walking become more difficult and become associated with an increased risk of falls. Causes of atrophy include exercise, hormones, nutrition, denervation and motor neurone death.

- Sarcopenia is the loss of muscle tissue that occurs over a lifetime and is also commonly used to describe its clinical manifestations (Lang et al 2010). Age-related loss of muscle mass results from loss of slow and fast motor units with an accelerated loss of fast motor units (Lang et al 2010). Clinical manifestations of sarcopenia include loss of mobility and independence and increased risk of injury secondary to denervation, changes in hormonal and inflammatory environment, mitochondrial dysfunction combining to produce losses in the bulk properties of muscle tissue such as muscle mass and strength (Lang et al 2010). Maintenance of muscle mass and strength is critical for preservation of physical activity in older age and important in decreasing the risk of falls and skeletal fractures (Lang et al 2010).

Neurological problems: treatment options

- Common presentations encountered on medical wards include:
- Parkinson's Disease (PD)
- Multiple Sclerosis (MS)
- Cerebro Vascular Accident (CVA)
- Neurology is a 'core' topic area that is not intended to be covered in any depth by this book. The reader is advised to consult a core neurology textbook (e.g. Edwards 2002). However, ideas and treatment suggestions are provided for the three conditions commonly seen on medical wards.

Parkinson's Disease (PD)

- Patients commonly present with problems associated with the initiation of tasks, e.g. sit to stand, gait, bed mobility; especially rolling.
- They may also present with a simian posture, i.e. a stiff thoracic spine, decreased ROM in shoulders.
- The physiotherapist should be thinking about function at home, e.g. reaching into cupboards, washing and dressing.
- Always check medication prescribed and discuss with the patient if they find it effective. In more severe cases treatment may be more effective if timed to coincide with the effects of medication.
- It may be necessary to liaise with the medical team about medications as the patient may benefit from a medication review.
- These patients respond well to different types of cuing:
- Visual cuing, involving the use of markers on the floor for patients to step towards
- Verbal cuing, where the physiotherapist counts or repeats right, left
- Cuing is often more effective if the patient can cue themselves (Morris 2000)
- Proprioceptive cuing where the patient rocks during a sit to stand movement.
- Alternatively it is possible to use a combination of the above, e.g. counting as well as rocking during the move from sitting to standing.
- Patients may need work on their functional abilities, e.g. rolling, lie to sit, sit to stand and this needs to be incorporated during treatment sessions.
- Consider what sort of walking aid the patient has and any need to change it. High-level patients find delta or four-wheeled walkers beneficial, as they enable more fluid movement. For patients whose balance is not adequate for these aids a wheeled Zimmer frame (WZF) can be beneficial as these also provide some fluidity for movement with additional balance support. Standard Zimmer frames (ZFs) are unhelpful as the patient has to lift them for each step and if there is a problem initiating movement, then this is compounded.

- The paper by Morris (2000) is an excellent text in providing a problem-solving approach and advice to problems commonly seen in PD along with advice on what should be worked in the different stages as per the Hohn and Yahr scale (Goetz et al 2004).
- A useful outcome measure for treatment of PD is the Lindop Parkinson's Scale (Pearson et al 2009).

Multiple Sclerosis (MS)

- Patients who are admitted to a medical ward are generally admitted for reasons other than their MS.
- Generally if they have a true relapse, in their MS, they will be admitted to the regional neurological unit for their initial treatment.
- Presenting complaints such as a urinary tract infection, respiratory tract infection or pneumonia can result in their symptoms worsening. This is due to the increase in body temperature which tends to impair their neural transmission.
- As any infection subsides with treatment then the patient's impairments, activities and function will improve.
- This is not to say that the patient will not require physiotherapy. For many patients the infection will subside relatively quickly, however the physical recovery will take longer to recover.
- Points to consider include:
- What sort of MS do they have, e.g. relapsing/remitting, primary progressive or secondary progressive?
- When they have had relapses, how have they tended to progress in their rehabilitation and recovery?
- Level of function prior to admission.
- Any community-based physiotherapy services they may have been accessing. (If so, it is important to liaise with these teams to find out whether there are any problems in particular that need to be considered or addressed.)
- How mobile were they and were any walking aids used?
- This information should be combined with objective neurological assessment findings to formulate a treatment plan.
- The treatment plan will need to consider the following:
- Bed mobility; any physical assistance required?
- Bed to chair/commode transfers. Is any equipment required, e.g. a full sling hoist, standing hoist, rotastand or walking aid?
- Seating, do they have sitting balance? If not it will be necessary to liaise with the occupational therapists to obtain suitable seating and pressure-relief care.
- Mobilising requiring any assistance? If so how much? Walking aid required?
- Strengthening exercises, balance exercises.
- Any tonal problems that need addressing? If so splinting or equipment such as a T-roll may be needed.
- You may need to consider positioning charts for patients with progressive MS if they have had long-term problems prior to admission.

- There are now standardised national guidelines regarding rehabilitation with stroke patients (NICE 2008). There is also a 2-yearly national Sentinel audit which all trusts with acute stroke units take part in (Royal College of Physicians 2008). Further details can be found on the CSP website (www.csp.org.uk).

- Recommendations for the implementation of stroke management are outlined in the NICE standards document as follows 'Patients with stroke are assessed and managed by stroke nursing staff and at least one member of the specialist rehabilitation team within 24 hours of admission to hospital, and by all relevant members of the specialist rehabilitation team within 72 hours, with documented multidisciplinary goals agreed within 5 days' (NICE 2008).

- The standards also state that patients with stroke are 'offered a minimum of 45 minutes of each active therapy that is required, for a minimum of 5 days a week, at a level that enables them to meet their rehabilitation goals for as long as they are continuing to benefit from therapy and are able to tolerate it' (NICE 2008).

- It may be helpful to undertake the initial assessment with the occupational therapists as they will be able to assess the patient for seating needs.

- Depending on the assessment findings and the resulting problem list it may be necessary to address the following:

- Altered tone, consider neural and non-neural components

- Upper limb:

  Shoulder: beware of low tone shoulder which will be vulnerable to subluxation as a result of the loss of supportive muscle tone around the joint. Preventative measures need to be implemented, e.g. an arm rest on the wheelchair when sitting out. Support the upper limb with pillows when in bed

- Owing to the patterning that can occur in the upper limb in the high tone patient, movements to maintain range must be combined with methods of reducing tone

- Elbow: stretching/mobilising/massage can help to reduce flexor hypertonus in the elbow

- Splinting to maintain range can also be helpful, be aware of pressure areas

- Wrist and fingers: passive movements, positioning and liaising with the occupational therapists regarding splinting to maintain the hand's resting position and enable skin care to be carried out by the nursing staff.

- Low tone is generally easier to manage in the lower limbs than high tone (Edwards 2002).

- For patients with high tone the use of T-rolls or wedges is useful in maintaining alignment and preventing contractures and this is used in conjunction with seating.

- The seating needs should be determined in the early stages of rehabilitation with the main aim being to establish the method of transfers that can be reinforced by all members of the MDT on a daily basis.

- Lower limbs

- Hips and knees: if there is high tone a T-roll can help break patterning

- Casting may need to be considered for the ankle in order to maintain ROM

- Massage and mobilisation of the foot and ankle muscles and joints will help to maintain the ROM that will be needed when a patient undergoes gait re-education

MEDICINE

9

– Positioning is particularly beneficial particularly for patients with severe hypertonus to prevent the asymmetry that can lead to the development of contractures.

Positioning in bed

• Depending on the firmness of the bed, side-lying can be useful to increase the extensibility of the trunk by providing a stretch to the supported side. Alternatively a pillow placed under the lower side will provide a stretch to the upper side.

• Side lying may also be a useful position to treat the upper limb if a patient lacks independent sitting balance.

• Supine lying can be useful to provide a secure base of support for patients with high or low tone to ensure that the optimal alignment of muscles and joints is possible.

• Half-lying can be achieved by elevating the head of the bed, rather than using extra pillows to align the head/neck/trunk. The physiotherapist needs to be aware of the risk of contractures, by placing the hips in flexion.

• Prone lying can be useful for maintaining or correcting range into extension at the hips and knees.

• It is important to consider any associated medical issues, e.g. respiratory compromise that the patient may have when lying flat and take these into account when planning treatment.

• The use of a T-roll or pillows can help to break up hypertonic patterning in the lower limbs and provide more symmetrical alignment.

Sitting balance

• In the early stages of rehabilitation taking the patient to a therapy gym is important for regaining sitting balance and is easier to achieve than attempting this on an air-pressure mattress.

• Attempting to rehabilitate sitting with a patient on an air-pressure mattress on the ward is more difficult and more tiring than using a treatment plinth in the gym.

• Ensure the patient is supported appropriately, this includes the feet being part of the base of support.

• Consider the amount of upper limb support when working on static sitting balance.

• For dynamic sitting balance and reaching outside of the base of support, make the treatment purposeful and goal-orientated, e.g. reaching for a bottle of water.

• Ensure that there is support for the patient if they cannot maintain their balance, e.g. someone sitting at their side to stop them falling or mats/pillows positioned to cushion their fall.

Transfers

• There are a range of methods to transfer a patient, dependent on their ability:

– Full sling hoist for patients in the early stages of rehabilitation who do not have sitting balance or sufficient lower limb strength for weight bearing

– Standing hoist can be useful to encourage weight bearing and this method of transfer is often used by the nursing staff when transferring patients from bed to a chair or commode

- Rotastands can be used with patients who have the ability to stand but are unable to step safely or effectively. Consider the ability of the upper limb to be able to grip the rotastand
- Sliding board transfers can be used to transfer patients from bed to a chair or commode, if they have sitting balance, but are unable to stand effectively. Consider level of function in the affected side and any inattention problems
- Stand and step transfers can be used for patients with the ability to stand safely. Consider the use of a walking aid if necessary and the number of staff required to reduce the risk associated with the patient falling.

Seating

- Seating needs to be supportive, maintain alignment of muscles and joints and key segments, e.g. position of hips, pelvis and trunk. Seating can be useful for assisting patients to become orientated to midline balance.
- It is also an effective method in reducing respiratory complications, particularly in those at risk, e.g. patients with dysphagia.
- Effective MDT communication is required to ensure correct positioning, awareness of skin integrity and the patient's sitting tolerance.
- Tilt in Space wheelchairs, e.g. a Cirrus chair, may need to be used for patients requiring maximal support for maintaining sitting balance, with additional support being required on the affected side.
- Standard wheelchairs can be provided for patients who have good sitting balance (may require minimal support).
- Lateral supports can be placed in the chair to support the low tone trunk and achieve good postural alignment.
- Upper limb supports can be provided if there are concerns around the positioning of the hemiplegic upper limb.
- Wheelchair trays can assist the awareness of midline and support of the trunk and upper limb.

Standing balance

- Being able to stand (with or without assistance) or be placed into a standing position is beneficial in maintaining joint ROM in the lower limbs and stimulating antigravity muscles. For patients with hypertonus who require total support to stand, a tilt table can be used in the early stages of treatment.
- Treatment can also be performed in the parallel bars with a mirror being used for those patients struggling to regain midline balance or who have sensory deficits.
- Standing can be undertaken at a high/low table with knee block, which can enable upper limb function to be treated at the same time. Planning is required to ensure the appropriate number of staff are available to facilitate this safely.
- Static and dynamic standing balance can also be treated with the patient in the upright posture.

Gait

- Consider cognitive and inattention problems, use of walking aids if necessary and the level of support required in the early stages of gait re-education.

Respiratory problems: treatment options

- Common respiratory conditions seen in medicine include:
- Chronic obstructive pulmonary disease (COPD) exacerbations (infective and non-infective)
- Pneumonia
- Lower respiratory tract infection (LRTI).
- It is not uncommon to encounter these patients if called into hospital during an on-call situation, especially if they are experiencing high fraction of inspired oxygen (FiO_2), decreased oxygen saturation (SaO_2), increased work of breathing (WOB) and poor airway clearance.
- It is also important to ascertain if the problem is appropriate for physiotherapy, e.g. a consolidated pneumonia is not, treatment consists of oxygen therapy and positioning to optimise ventilation/perfusion (V/Q).
- One of the most challenging decision for a physiotherapist to make, in an on-call situation, is when to decide not to carry out treatment interventions.
- The decision is based on assessment and subsequent clinical reasoning and this is essential when justifying whether to intervene or not.
- In treating the respiratory patient, in particular the acutely ill, it is helpful to establish the problems by using a multisystem approach (refer to Chapter 9 in Volume 1). By doing this you can then establish the main respiratory problems which may involve any of the following:
- Decreased lung volumes
- Increased work of breathing
- Ineffective airway clearance.
- Poor gas exchange and increasing FiO_2 requirements are usually as a result of one or a combination of the above.
- For decreased lung volumes the following treatment intervention can be effective:
- Deep breathing exercises
- Positioning
- Mobilising
- Intermittent positive pressure breathing (IPPB)
- Cough assist.
- For increased work of breathing:
- Positioning
- Relaxation and breathing re-education
- Pacing
- IPPB.
- For ineffective airway clearance:
- Positioning
- Mobilising
- Manual techniques
- Humidification and hydration
- IPPB
- Cough assist
- Suction, either oropharyngeal (OP) or nasopharyngeal (NP).

- When treating a respiratory patient it is advisable to start with 'simple' treatments and then progress.
- For more complex patients seek support and always be aware of your own competence.
- Mobilising a patient is one of the simplest and most effective ways to increase lung volumes and assist the clearance of secretions.
- Consider if the patient requires supplementary oxygen if the plan is to mobilise them over any great distance.
- *Positioning* is a useful adjunct to treatment.
- Upright sitting is the best position to increase lung volumes and improve V/Q mismatch, therefore wherever possible sit your patient out of bed (Hough 2001)
- It is not always possible as a patient may be too unwell to sit out
- Alternative positions such as side lying work well and may be a better option than high sitting, as this can rapidly turn into slumped sitting which will compromise airway expansion
- Combine positioning with other treatments such as IPPB, manual techniques and airway clearance exercises. Manual techniques are particularly useful when a patient is unable to follow commands
- It is important to educate and advise nursing staff about the most effective positioning for a patient and how often this should be implemented.
- *Airway clearance exercises*: either Active Cycle of Breathing Techniques (ACBT) or autogenic drainage (AD). Patients need to be alert enough to follow undertake this.
- If they struggle to grasp FET, simplifying the exercise to deep breaths with inspiratory hold and cough can work well
- Treating a patient in side lying may be effective if they have, for example, a lower lobe infection.
- *IPPB and cough assist* are similar, both provide positive pressure and therefore increase lung volumes, reduce work of breathing and aid secretion clearance. Cough assist can provide negative pressure, thereby stimulating a cough.
- The cough assist is particularly good for those patients who have a very weak cough. For patients that are drowsy a face mask can be used for both adjuncts
- Some patients do not tolerate the treatment as they can find the sensation of positive pressure uncomfortable. Reconsider the treatment choice and opt for positioning, airway clearance exercises and manual techniques.
- *Suctioning* can be daunting for students and less experienced physiotherapists. It is an effective treatment for those patients where treatment options are limited because the patient is too drowsy to comply with instructions and can be used in conjunction with positioning.
- For patients needing repeated nasopharyngeal (NP) suction a NP airway should be inserted, as repeated blind suctioning can cause trauma to the nasal passages, resulting in swelling that can make it more difficult to insert a catheter
- To choose the appropriate size, in clinical practice this has been estimated on the basis of the distance from the nostril to the earlobe or the diameter of a patient's little finger. However, studies have shown these to be less accurate than an estimation based on an individual's height (Table 9.1)

Table 9.1 Guide to the choice of size of nasopharyngeal cannula (based on Roberts et al 2005)

Subject height	NP cannula (PortexTM) size
Short female (less than 163 cm)	6 with pin 1 cm from flange
Average female (163 cm), short male (less than 178 cm)	6
Tall female (163 cm+), average male (178 cm)	7
Tall male (178 cm+)	8

- The most important factor is that the airway is the correct length in order to ensure that it separates the soft palate from the pharynx and not too long so that it aggravates the cough or gag reflex
- Ensure that there is adequate gel on the airway during insertion and once inserted, place a sterile safety pin on the end to prevent the airway from becoming drawn down the nasal passage
- To decide what size catheter to use in conjunction with an airway calculate the following. Multiply the NP airway size by 3 and divide this by 2. If you get an answer such as 10.5, use a size 10 catheter
- Ensure the catheter is lubricated prior to insertion; difficulty passing the catheter can be helped by pulling the airway out a little
- If you are not confident or competent to do this procedure speak to a more experienced physiotherapist or alternatively a member of nursing staff or an anaesthetist who is competent to insert the airway
- The advantage of NP airways is that once in situ the nursing staff can suction as well, thereby reducing the need for frequent physiotherapy, especially at night
- Nursing staff may need to be shown how to do this
- For agitated patients airways are not appropriate, they may pull them out if they find them uncomfortable
- For OP suction a Guedel airway should be used when the patient is unlikely to have a gag reflex present, e.g. unconscious patient
- If a patient has a gag reflex they may vomit and obstruct their airways
- If the airway is too large the glottis may be closed occluding the airways
- These can be sized by aligning the flange with the centre of the patient's lips and the tip to the angle of the mandible.

Oxygen therapy

- This is prescribed by a doctor and should be written in the drug chart along with the appropriate target saturation.
- It is important to know the appropriate saturation for different conditions, e.g. in chronic conditions, lower oxygen saturations are required.
- The aims of oxygen therapy are to:
- Correct hypoxaemia
- Decrease the symptoms associated with chronic hypoxaemia
- Decrease the workload hypoxaemia imposes on the cardiopulmonary system.

- The absolute indication for O_2 therapy is inadequate tissue oxygenation:
  - $PaO_2 < 8$ kPa or $SaO_2 < 90\%$
  - Acute care situations which increase O_2 requirements or risk of hypoxia, e.g. cardiac arrest, shock (BTS 2008).
- Beware of:
  - Hypoventilation in CO_2 retainers
  - Oxygen toxicity
  - Drying of mucosal membranes
  - Discomfort.
- Oxygen can be delivered by:
  - Low-flow/variable-performance devices
  - Simple facemask, inaccurate indication of oxygen being delivered to the patient
  - High-flow/fixed-performance devices
  - Venturi system which provides an accurate FiO_2
  - High-concentration reservoir mask
  - Nasal cannula
  - Used for long-term therapy patients who require low amounts of oxygen (1–4 l/min)
  - Humidification
  - Important for those patients where high flow rates are required for more than 24 hours
  - Patients have excessive thick secretions
  - NB For all trachea patients – O_2 should be warmed
  - Warmed humidification is far more effective than cold as cold humidified O_2 can aggravate bronchospasm (Williams et al 1996).
- Long-term O_2 therapy (LTOT) is sometimes necessary for patients that have severe hypoxaemia. It has the benefits of:
  - Reducing cor pulmonale
  - Increased quality of life
  - Increased sleep
  - Reduced exacerbations and hospital admissions (Hough 2001).
- Patients requiring LTOT will normally be reviewed and assessed by respiratory nurse specialists approximately 1 month after they have been discharged once blood gases have stabilised.
- Patients must have stopped smoking before being considered for oxygen.
- Patients must also be educated as to why they have it.
- Aim to achieve PaO_2 of at least 8.7 kPa without a rise in PCO_2 of greater than 1.3 kPa (www.patient.co.uk).

Pulmonary rehabilitation (PR)

- Pulmonary rehabilitation is a multidisciplinary programme of care for patients with chronic respiratory impairment that is tailored and designed to optimise each patient's physical and social performance and autonomy (General Practice Airways Group 2008).

- Patients with COPD who suffer with breathlessness are inclined to avoid exercise, subsequently becoming unfit and demotivated.
- This patient group can become depressed, anxious and socially isolated.
- Pulmonary rehabilitation can assist in addressing all these issues. It is also effective in improving quality of life, exercise capacity and dyspnoea (GIAG 2008).

  On an acute medical rotation you will probably not be involved in delivering PR as increasingly it is being delivered in the community. However, it is important that you are familiar with the concept and are aware of its role in the multidimensional management of COPD, and where appropriate, when to refer on to this service.

Alternative reasons for admission to an acute medical ward

- There are numerous different reasons and conditions as to why a patient may be admitted which do not fall under the previous categories.
- Conditions include:
- Cardiac conditions, e.g. cardiac failure, arrhythmias, problems with pacemaker, ischaemic heart disease (IHD)
- Renal failure either acute or chronic
- Dehydration
- Urinary tract infection
- Diarrhoea and vomiting
- Falls
- Not coping at home (NB the word acopia is no longer used)
- Confusional states either due to a long-term condition, e.g. dementia or Alzheimer's disease, or acute conditions such as infection or altered blood chemistry
- Psychological reasons, e.g. overdose
- Uncontrolled diabetes
- Oncology.

Cardiac conditions

- These are frequently reasons for admission to an acute medical ward.
- Symptoms commonly include shortness of breath (SOB), decreased exercise tolerance, shortness of breath on exertion (SOBOE), fatigue/lethargy, syncope, chest pain. Patients with cardiac failure may also have oedema, which in extreme cases can be visible from an individual's waist downwards.
- Treatment will consist of coping strategies when experiencing SOB, pacing techniques and building exercise tolerance.
- It is important when treating these patients to give consideration that many cardiac conditions will progressively worsen, so treatments and goals need to be realistic.
- Patients that have experienced chest pain may need a stair assessment.
- This can be useful to teach pacing techniques as patients find it reassuring if they have experienced chest pain in the past how they can exert themselves.

Renal failure, dehydration, diarrhoea and vomiting

- These are other common reasons for admission to hospital.
- Symptoms can include: decreased urine production, oedema, problems concentrating, confusion, fatigue, lethargy, abdominal pain.
- These symptoms can be as a result of altered blood chemistry, e.g. electrolyte imbalance and increased renal function markers.
- Medical treatment will concentrate on rebalancing these and as levels return to normal the symptoms and function will improve.
- However, patients will commonly have difficulties transferring, mobilising and will have general weakness.
- Physiotherapy intervention can include strengthening exercises, balance retraining, mobility practice and gait re-education, but assessment findings will be the most important indicator of what specifically needs to be included in treatment.

Falls

- Falls rehabilitation is also covered in chapters 2, 6 and 7 in this volume.
- In the acute setting, it is important to establish if the cause is mechanical or if it is due to another cause such as postural hypotension, as some causes for falls are not amenable to physiotherapy.
- It is well documented that specific exercise or rehabilitation programmes working around the patient's individual problems are more effective than group work.
- However, as part of your discharge planning you may decide that it is appropriate to refer the patient to a balance and safety group, where their problems can be explored and overcome in more detail.
- Consider the following factors when dealing with falls; age-related changes in sensorimotor function, vision, peripheral sensation and neuropathies, vestibular sense, muscle strength, reaction time as well as other medical risk factors including polypharmacy, residual stroke, PD, postural hypotension, syncope, arthritis, foot problems, psychological and cognitive factors (Darowski 2008).
- For higher-level patients a validated exercise programme such as the Otago scheme can be effective (Thomas et al 2010).

Dementia and Alzheimer's disease

- Consideration needs to be given to the stage of the disease process as patients in the earlier stages will be able to undertake exercise programmes with guidance. Patients are not admitted just because they have dementia, but because of another reason such as a fall or an infection, e.g. urinary tract.
- The medical wards are busy and highly stimulating environments, which for patients who have advanced disease can be confusing and ultimately distressing.
- The medical team will want to treat the underlying cause for admission and then discharge the patient home as quickly as possible to minimise the disruption to their routines.
- Communication is very important, with very confused patients.

- These patients are unable to process protracted pieces of information, so giving short instructions is preferable.
- Make treatments purposeful, containing activities that the patient is familiar with such as sit to stand and mobilising.
- Give them realistic goals to work towards, e.g. 'let's walk towards the nurses' desk.'
- For patients who are fearful of falling, treatments used for falls patients can be used with great effect.
- With patients who have cognitive impairment or psychological problems it can be difficult to ascertain if they are progressing.
- It is essential to establish a rapport with these patients.
- This may take some time to build, however, by seeing the patient regularly and keeping treatments simple and purposeful, patients will be able to benefit from physiotherapy intervention.
- For those patients who have been admitted due to an infection, the level of confusion will reduce.
- It is necessary to find out pre admission levels of impairment from family members or carers.

Oncology management

- The reader is referred to chapter 12 for more information about oncology management.
- Patients can be admitted to the ward as a result of suspicious symptoms that require further investigation and are therefore provisionally diagnosed with cancer or they have been previously diagnosed with it.
- Diagnosis may be of a primary or secondary cancer and symptoms can be varied requiring the physiotherapist to draw on a wide range of clinical skills.
- Discharge planning can be complex, especially for those patients who have a poor prognosis, as there have been changes to funding for continuing care.
- Effective and sensitive communication is required along with effective MDT working.
- Discussion of plans with the patient and family should include other professions such as the palliative care nursing services in the patient's home locality.

Establishing rehabilitation potential

- There are many factors contributing to successful rehabilitation outcomes and in many cases this can be based around the personal preferences of the therapists involved in a patient's management.
- The inter-relating factors that are acknowledged in the literature include compliance, motivation and efficacy (Haynes et al 1979, Maclean and Pound 2000, Maclean et al 2002, Resnick 1996, 2002).
- Haynes et al (1979) defined compliance as 'the extent to which the patient's behaviour (with regards taking medications or lifestyle changes) coincides with medical or health advice'.
- Within rehabilitation motivation is viewed as an important component, but remains vulnerable to subjective judgement and a challenge to objectively measure (Siegert and Taylor 2004).

- Maclean and Pound (2000) propose that the literature relating to the concept of patient motivation within physical rehabilitation falls into three broad approaches:
- Motivation is an internal personality trait of an individual
- Motivation is a product of social factors
- Motivation is influenced by a combination of personality and social factors.
- Brillhart and Johnson (1997) identified five domains associated with motivation and coping ability:
- Independence
- Education
- Socialisation
- Self-esteem
- Realisation.
- If a patient demonstrates deterioration in their communication, function and continence, it is proposed that they may be experiencing deprivation, anxiety and/or decreased confidence in all 5 domains; all of which may be compromising the individual's motivation to engage.
- Maclean et al (2002) highlighted that health professionals' behaviour can enhance or diminish patient motivation. If a patient is labelled non-compliant, difficult or uncooperative by a MDT, communication channels may break down.
- Labelling over time can lead to a self-fulfilling prophecy where a client's behaviour is anticipated by staff. This expectation alters staffs' verbal and non-verbal interactions with the client and can result in the anticipated behaviour being demonstrated.

Prioritisation of caseload

As discussed in Volume 1, Chapter 9 frequent prioritisation of a clinical caseload is essential. There are many different tools that may be used in the workplace, an example of this can be seen in Appendix 9.1.
- As a guide, patients who are a priority for any particular day are those:
- Where discharge will be delayed if not seen
- Where respiratory status will deteriorate if not seen
- New patient referrals that link into the above categories
- New patients referred into the service – requiring assessment in order to prioritise their therapy needs.
- If experiencing difficulties with prioritisation communicate this to your supervisor or a more senior member of the physiotherapy team without delay.
- Use all available staff resources, for example physiotherapy assistants and optimise team working with joint therapy sessions with occupational therapists and nursing staff.

Aims of treatment and goal setting

- The aims of physiotherapy interventions in the acute setting are to maintain and restore functional decline. Goals may depend on individual characteristics such as age, psycho-social factors, health conditions and environmental factors (Mittrach et al 2008).

- Physiotherapy goals should be specific, measurable, achievable, realistic and timed (SMART).

- Physiotherapy interventions are amalgamated into an ongoing and cyclic process. This process involves the identification of an individual's problems and needs, the relationship between the problems and the relevant factors of the person, definition of goals, the planning of interventions and finally the assessment of the effects (Stucki et al 1997, cited in Mittrach et al 2008).

- Goal setting and re-evaluation allows the measurement of the result of any intervention (Mittrach et al 2008), with therapists needing to get to know their clients as a person before it is possible to assist them in setting meaningful goals (Siegart and Taylor 2004).

- Motivation and the formulation of goals are inextricably linked (Siegart and Taylor 2004).

- When a client participates in goal-formulation, planning and decision making, the potential for active participation in the rehabilitation process has been shown to increase (Pollock 1993, cited in Wressle et al 2002).

Discharge planning

- The practice of initiating discharge planning when a patient is first admitted can be a challenging concept to grasp, but there can be generalised pressures to move patients through the hospital system as efficiently and safely as possible therefore this must be considered.

- There may be occasions that physiotherapists are under pressure to agree that a patient can be discharged when physiotherapy assessment or intervention has not been completed. If following the assessment of risk you are not happy that a patient is being discharged do not feel under pressure to say otherwise. Similarly, if a patient is discharged against physiotherapy advice or prior to a physiotherapy assessment ensure this is documented in physiotherapy documentation.

- If a patient's mobility is a specific concern it may be appropriate for physiotherapists to attend a home visit with the occupational therapists and the patient concerned. These visits can provide insight into how an individual functions within their home environment.

- The assessment of the element of risk on discharge can be a difficult dilemma for any physiotherapist. If a patient can mobilise safely and independently on the ward with a rollator frame, but you are aware that their flat is too small to accommodate a frame and would actually be a falls risk if used at home what would you do? This is the type of dilemma you could be faced with.

Onward referral

- Intermediate care teams were formed on the back of the National Service Framework for Older People in 2001.

- The purpose of intermediate care is to prevent unnecessary hospital admissions, but also to expedite discharge from secondary care by providing support to the patient on discharge.

- Intermediate care services tend to be organised geographically with strict boundaries, therefore refer to local arrangements regarding the name of local services and referral criteria. Some services require multidisciplinary involvement to accept a referral.

- Alternatively community physiotherapy services are normally available in most geographical areas to accept physiotherapy referrals, however the demand for these services is high and the service often limited as a result.

- Referral to specialist teams such as respiratory outreach teams (for COPD, asthma). Multiple sclerosis and PD specialist nurses need to be contacted as appropriate. If there is a specific physiotherapy issue, e.g. mobility, function, chest management, it may be beneficial to discuss and advise this with the team in person, on the telephone or through a written discharge report.

- In the absence of discharge co-ordinator nursing staff generally tend to take responsibility for co-ordinating the re-starting of care packages. However, physiotherapists may need to be involved in helping to identify discharge timescales or justification for increases in packages of care or types of community care.

Documentation/CSP standards

- The importance of maintaining a high standard of professional documentation cannot be stressed enough. Fundamentally your professional documentation is crucial for your protection in the event that you are faced with an informal or formal complaint. Members have a legal responsibility to keep an adequate record of their patient interventions to demonstrate to a third party what they did, why they did it and when they did it. The CSP standards describe the components of the written record that will satisfy this legal requirement (CSP 2005).

- The Ombudsman Office received nearly 9000 properly made complaints about the NHS in the last year, 18 per cent were about the care of older people (Parliamentary and Health Service Ombudsman 2011). The total number of complaints made to Hospital/PCT Chief Executives across the NHS is significantly higher.

- Remember: if it isn't written down in the professional documentation – it never happened. If patient-related and/or physiotherapy information is handed over to another MDT colleague it is necessary to document this 'handover' of information and to whom it was handed over in the PT documentation. If MDT notes are in operation this may not be necessary.

- It is advisable to complete patient documentation after the treatment intervention is completed. This is to ensure that the documentation is accurate and reflective of intervention. If 15 plus sets of notes are left to the end of the day, all with perhaps similar types of intervention, important detail may be lost.

- It is recommended to write any information (that is being verbally handed over) into the relevant MDT colleagues' documentation, e.g. medical notes.

- If advice is given to the patient it is necessary to document what was advised.

- Along with adhering to documentation standards it is appropriate that as a professional you have awareness of, and abide by, the CSP professional code of conduct.

Conclusion

The conditions, medical presentations and their combinations that will be seen during a rotation within acute medical rotation are endless. The impact that physiotherapy intervention can have on this client group is significant and overwhelmingly professionally rewarding.

The references for this chapter can be found on www.expertconsult.com.

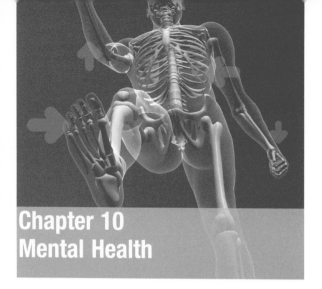

Chapter 10
Mental Health

Introduction

- As a student or newly qualified physiotherapist you may be expected to treat adults of working age or older adults in acute mental health wards, community mental health teams or outpatient settings such as gyms.

- Although it is possible that you will also work with adolescent patients or service users in eating disorder or forensic units, in these areas it is much more likely that you would be working under the immediate direction of a senior practitioner.

- For this reason the treatment plans considered in this chapter relate to referrals for assessment and consequent treatment of an adult with poor general well-being, an older adult with mobility problems and an inpatient in an acute stage of anxiety and depression experiencing musculoskeletal disorder.

- As with all specialities the holistic nature of treatment demands that it be part of a multidisciplinary approach which includes the patient/service user and where appropriate the carer/s.

- All aspects of the service user's life may affect outcomes, including social, environmental factors, alongside the psychomotor signs and symptoms, and so all aspects should therefore inform the approach and delivery of treatment.

- Treatment plans will be based on assessment and driven by goals chosen, or at very least agreed, by the service user (in the case of later-stage dementia the carer may be the person leading the goal setting).

- Goals may be long or short term and should mirror or dovetail with the psychological and social goals, which may already have been set between the service user and others in the team.

Mental Health Act and sectioning

- Patients may be in hospital voluntarily or they may be detained under a section of the Mental Health Act for their own or other people's safety. Detention is often referred to as 'Sectioning' which refers to a particular section of the Mental Health Act (HM Government 2007). A very specific process must be adhered to in sectioning someone and there are reviews and processes which must be followed including the right of appeal for the person.

- Whilst in hospital a patient may be cared for at a specific level of observation related to the assessed risk. Risks may be of absconding, self-harm, harm to others, lack of self care. The level of observation 1–3 refers to the frequency of observation and also the proximity of the observer, for instance level 3, 15-minute observations mean that a member of staff would know where a patient was and what they were doing every 15 minutes but they could view this from a distance, 'level 1 observation constant observations' would mean a member of staff would be within arm's length constantly.

- Consider what this might feel like, especially if one already feels paranoid. The status of the patient will affect the treatment options you have. For instance if a walk is part of your treatment plan then a sectioned patient will have to have ground leave agreed by the responsible medical officer. In forensic settings it is likely that the majority of patients will be on section and will need ground leave which may have to be very specific, e.g. 30 minutes, within the grounds with two escorts between the hours of 10.00 and 12.00; or one hour to walk to and from shops with one escort. For some patients who are under a forensic section of the Mental Health Act permission has to be agreed by the Home Office.

Promotion of well-being

- It falls within the remit of the physiotherapist in mental health to promote well-being, which may encompass weight management plus advice concerning diet, smoking, use of alcohol and physical activity.

- Much will depend upon the resources available to you and the awareness of the team.

- Thus referral to the dietician, smoking cessation adviser or GP for review of medication, may happen via other members of the Community Mental Health team but if referral to the physiotherapist is the first action taken then the physiotherapist needs the knowledge and skills to refer on or to signpost to the most appropriate service.

- A referral is likely to come from the care co-ordinator or possibly self referral from the service user and to be for increase in fitness and reduction of weight.

- Following musculoskeletal assessment and treatment of any specific disorders the goals for general well-being should be set.

Adults with enduring mental health disorder

- For patients with long-term and enduring mental disorder lack of motivation will be, and will have been, a major barrier to fitness. If the service user has been on psychotropic medication for many years then weight gain will have occurred but the lack of activity and diet are likely to be key factors in lack of well-being.

- Patients with long-term and enduring mental disorder are four times more likely to die of cardiorespiratory diseases than are the general population (Phelan et al 2001).
- The body of evidence linking diet with mental health is growing at a rapid pace. As well as its impact on feelings of mood and general well-being, the evidence demonstrates diet contributes to the development, prevention and management of specific mental health problems (Mental Health Foundation 2007).
- Musculoskeletal assessment should have included checking joint range, muscle power, reported pain but should focus on function.
- Questions about what the service user can and can't do physically and what if anything he wants to do about it should be the basis for intervention.
- Specific measurement of body mass index (BMI) and waist circumference may be appropriate on initial assessment or may cause distress and need to be addressed at subsequent appointments.
- The expertise of the physiotherapist should be initially employed to assess and treat any musculoskeletal disorders such as painful joints or injured muscles in preparation for a physical activity programme.
- In many mental health settings technical instructors (TIs), with a background in sport and physical fitness, work with the physiotherapists and can be very effective in delivering the activity plan when it has been devised.
- In some mental health gyms the TIs have a lead role and physiotherapists are involved only if there is a specific need due to injury or physical disorder.
- For patients with low motivation self-reporting questionnaires do not always provide full histories or clear progression lines. An interview screening tool with review will be more useful and can be administered by either the physiotherapist or the technical instructor.
- In this case the physiotherapy student or novice physiotherapist may learn from the experienced non qualified staff member the best way to approach a service user.
- Reviews rating to the baseline screening should take place at regular intervals being sure to involve the service user in a way which is meaningful to them.

Suggested treatment goals

- Long-term goals
- Increased fitness level
- Reduced weight
- Improved motivation/mood/confidence
- Increased level of general activity
- Reduced joint pain on activity.
- Short-term goals
- Attendance at sessions
- Treatment of musculoskeletal disorder
- Improved diet
- Maintenance of weight
- Acknowledgement of need.

- The short-term goals for a person with low motivation and possible fatigue due to lack of activity must initially be about identifying need and encouraging regular attendance.

- This can be facilitated by the use of treatment contracts where the service user agrees both goals and ways of achieving the goals. Contracts provide a structure to describe the methods to be used and this can help the physiotherapist devise relevant and interesting programmes for the service user.

- Motivational interviewing (MI) skills are a useful technique in these circumstances as they encourage the service user to direct the change. Originally used for counselling 'problem drinkers' the interviewing technique produces a relationship which reflects partnership rather than following an expert–recipient model (Rollnick and Miller, 1995).

The question of weight

- A service user may be morbidly obese to the point where even the effort of rising to standing is exhausting.

- Alternatively the service user may have been neglecting to eat regularly and have a low BMI which may cause concern in terms of sufficient calorific intake to support exercise.

- If the decision is to provide a physical activity programme then weight must be considered. Each person's needs should be considered individually but a BMI below about 18.5 would militate against anything other than very gentle exercise and stretching.

- All multigym machines will have a specific weight limit and the service user's weight may exceed this. Always check before suggesting use of exercise machines.

- For extremes of weight levels some useful forms of exercise are:
- Seated gentle exercise with progression to aerobic seated exercise
- Simple sit to stand repetition
- Walking routes which include seated stops
- Stretches.

- A slow start, mild to moderate level exercise should be planned first and explained carefully to the service user as part of their treatment plan and goals.

- Progression from individual forms of exercise should happen at a pace which encourages the service user to continue with activity and /or exercise, until it becomes part of that person's habit.

- Examples of progression:
- Use of a multigym (Figure 10.1)
- Semi-competitive games
- Swimming
- Dancing
- Or even fishing (there is a lot of walking and carrying involved before and after sitting quietly next to a lake or river)
- Any other activity of daily living which the service user sees as important.

- At this point in the treatment new musculoskeletal disorders may become apparent and they should be assessed and treated as part of the total treatment pathway.

Gym Referral		
1st Appointment Health Questionnaire Equipment Induction Taster Gym Programme		
Regular attendance Establish goals of gym attendance and begin		
1st 4 week Review of Goals ? Achieving goals ? Change in programme/equipment used		
Report sent to referrer re: progress Discuss Progression to local leisure facilities (as appropriate)		
Continue Regular Attendance Continue with monthly reviews		
	Some drop out e.g. returned to work, going to local gym, discharged	
Escorted visit to Local Gym		
No	Yes	
Clear Clinical Decision why not	Repeated visits as required	
Continue with Physio. Gym	unhappy	happy
- Clear goals set - 6 months max at this stage - May attend local gym in future	**Return to Physio. Gym**	**Continue on Own**
	- Education of leisure centre - Offer support to Centre - Discharge report	
At any time if no attendance for 6 weeks, a new referral is required and the pathway starts again		

Figure 10.1 Example of a multigym patient pathway.

- However the physiotherapist should be ready for intermittent attendance, relapse in illness or poor concordance with diet regimens all of which will interfere with goal time lines.
- Patience and innovation in treatment intervention can make a long process more successful.

Specific outcomes

- Measurement such as BMI, waist circumference can be used to show weight reduction.
- To evaluate endurance the measures could include
- Distance walked with ease
- Timed measured walk
- Levels of repetitions in multigym programme

Table 10.1 The Borg CR10 exertion scale

0	Nothing at all	'Number 1'
0.3		
0.5	Extremely weak	Just noticeable
0.7		
1	Very weak	
1.5		
2	Weak	Light
2.5		
3	Moderate	
4		
5	Strong	
6		
7		
8		
9		
10	Extremely strong	'Strongest 1'
11		
	Absolute maximum	Highest possible

- Patient self reporting measures can be really useful to demonstrate changes in confidence and motivation but also in physical activity

- The BORG Perceived Rate of Exertion Scale (Borg and Borg 2001) (Table 10.1).

- A subjective measure fulfils the basis of our treatment to give back to the patient some feeling of control over their body and what they are capable of doing with it.

- The service user is invested with the means of regulating how hard they are working whilst at the same time the therapist has some means to demonstrate improvement.

- A regular visual analogue scale with fearful or unhappy at level one and very confident or happy at level 6 can be applied to any of the activities agreed as ways to reach goals or functions which were identified as difficult.

- It cannot be emphasised enough that the baseline for all of the strength and stamina measures is likely to be very low compared to expected norms, so improvement no matter how small will be a health gain.

- The gain in fitness from completely sedentary lifestyle to a moderately active lifestyle occurs at a much faster rate than gains in moderately active to a very active lifestyle.

- Completion of treatment should take the service user to independent (or support worker aided), use of community facilities in leisure centres, swimming pools, walking groups. The student or novice physiotherapist may not be with the service user long enough to reach this point, but they will have put them on that path.

- Although we may be the physical expert it is well to remember that in reducing pain, increasing activity and supporting personal achievement will affect the patient's mental well-being and contribute to raising mood, structuring the day and giving an improved sense of mastery.

- In this way the physiotherapist is truly working holistically.

Older adult mobility in dementia

- For the older adult patient mobility is the most frequent cause of referral to physiotherapy.
- Physiotherapists in many specialties including the 'core' areas of musculoskeletal, neurological and cardiorespiratory will encounter patients with dementia and with an aging population this will become more common.
- The following treatment suggestions are focussed on the approach and possible treatment goals for a patient with moderate dementing changes.
- The classic work of Rosemary Oddy initially written for carers and relatives is a useful resource when treating patients with dementia (Oddy 1998).
- In early stages of dementia the difficulty may be poor mobility, however in later stages the referral to physiotherapy may be to advise on lowering the level of activity.

Treatment goals

- Following assessment the treatment plan will always include achieving safe movement in functional situations, thus, moving in bed, getting in and out of bed, sitting to standing and reverse, stabilising base to allow reaching.
- The other essential is to provide advice to the team and relatives or carers regarding safe management of mobility for the patient.
- Specific goals may be to:
- Increase core strength
- Increase confidence
- Support management of mobility by the multidisciplinary team (MDT) and carers
- Reduce excess mobility.

Aspects of dementia which will affect treatment

- All the impairments which may accompany dementia will not necessarily be seen in one person, but there are a number of symptoms which will affect both the approach to and the success of treatment.

Memory

- Patients with early-stage dementia may find mobility difficult because they begin to go somewhere and then forget why and where they are walking, or they forget that they have difficulty moving which produces a severe falls risk.
- In later stages memory may be so poor that instructions are forgotten almost immediately after they are heard.

Cognition (thought processing)

- Processing instructions becomes difficult and can prove impossible if too complicated.
- Usually when an instruction is given the response is fairly immediate and for functional activities the movement almost automatic.
- For the dementing patient a simple instruction such as stand up may not happen automatically and in trying to think about it the patient can become frustrated.

Perception

- Spatial perception is often affected along with processing of visual input.
- So a space between chairs may be perceived as a chair.
- Changes in flooring from carpet to hard floor or from pattern to plain may be perceived as a step.

Orientation

- The ability to recognise time and place may be lost and a person may be convinced that they are somewhere and in some age other than where they are.
- Very often patients will have a clear reason why they cannot come with you or get out of bed or why they must leave the ward, e.g. 'I am waiting for my son' or 'I have to get home to feed the dog and the bus leaves in 10 minutes'.
- It is therefore important to know something of their history and consider the likelihood of the statement.
- Positional orientation may also be affected and a patient may become distressed if moved too quickly from one position to another so allowing adequate time as discussed previously is of the essence.

Emotional affect

- Depression often precedes or appears alongside dementia and this will have an affect on motivation which may already be low due to the cerebral change associated with dementia.
- Anxiety and fear are common symptoms.
- The anxiety may be specific or global resting on any thought which appears.
- Fear due to reduction in ability to make sense of the environment or to persecutory thoughts may be compounded by a specific fear of falling.

Dual tasking

- Often dementia rids the person of the ability to concentrate on two things at once.
- This is most clearly seen in walking with instruction.
- Instruction should always happen first and if adjustment is needed then walking should be paused, to allow processing of the instructions to take place.

Treatment approach

- The approach is derived first from the attitude of the student or novice physiotherapist who should have a positive attitude and be well motivated; be sympathetic to the individual's difficulties recognising that dementia will affect different people in different ways and ensure that the patient is treated with dignity and respect.
- The key is to plan for success whilst using your skills to make movement enjoyable and including the team, carer and relatives in the plan.

Specific strategies

- Effective communication is essential to influence the different aspects of a patient presenting with dementia.
- Communication techniques comprise of verbal and non-verbal strategies including:

- Single clear instruction
- Repetition or rephrasing
- Calm tone of voice
- Visual and auditory cues, e.g. pat the seat or the pillow to show where you want the person to move to
- Suggest a purpose, e.g. 'let's go to look at the garden'.
- Physical techniques
- Use hand gestures to show the direction of movement
- Rather than pointing take your hand from in front of the patient's chest and move it with an open hand gesture which invites the patient to move forward
- Walk in unison
- Walk beside the patient, supporting if necessary with the open palm hand support and one hand on the back
- Use your body to give close support if necessary
- Use motor memory to aim for automatic movement, e.g. for movement on the side of the bed try invading the person's space slightly by sitting very close to them. Usually they will move automatically up the bed
- To reduce fear:
- Try to discover what is frightening to the patient about moving
- Use reassurance and tone of voice
- Fill the gap as people with dementia who have a fear of falling will find this exaggerated when there is a large space in front of them and therefore will probably refuse to stand up
- Use a person or a chair in front of them to reduce the sense of space
- A walking frame often does not help because the patient is able to see through it and does not discern it as being something which can be leant upon
- Ensure the environment is safe and if possible familiar.
- In all cases allow enough time for the patient to receive the request, process the request and then carry out the actual response.

Treatment techniques

- To increase mobility and core strength and reduce fear of falling exercise can be provided in many ways.

Individual intervention

- The Otago falls prevention system is clear and can easily be adapted for use with people in early stages of dementia.
- It consists of a series of leg-strengthening and balance-retraining exercises and a walking plan that gets progressively more difficult as the patient gets stronger.
- The repetitious nature of the programme uses the motor memory and therefore has more chance of success (Campbell and Robertson 2003).

General activity

- Simple guided walks, supervised swimming may be possible in the early stages.
- Use of equipment such as weights, multigym, balls can be difficult due to the need to process multiple movements; however, experience shows us that automatic movement can be elicited by use of balloons, scarves and particularly music.

Group exercise

- Groups give an extra dimension to exercise and can be useful in early-stage dementia for motivation.

- If the group is co-facilitated for example, an occupational therapist and a psychologist the opportunity to encourage memory by reminiscence, cognition by interaction and challenge alongside physical activities can be provided.

- A wonderful example of this is dance, as provided by a team of dancers, musicians and film-makers who create opportunities for people to indulge in movement play that aims to improve life (http://www.jabadao.org).

- Historically, ballroom dancing has been used with amazing results, for patients who have no motivation to move and may be seen as immobile. They will often rise from their chair and begin to dance if the music and environment are appropriately stimulating for them.

- As most demented patients vary in age from 65 to 100 appropriate dance music should be used from the 1920s to 1950s and 1960s, with rock and roll possibly becoming more popular and taking over from ballroom.

- Tai Chi has been used very successfully as a joint mobility and strengthening exercise.

- One of the elements of Tai Chi is that the movements can be performed just by following the group leader without verbal instruction and this can be very calming for patients with dementia as it avoids dual tasking.

- For some, community walking groups can be a great way of including relatives who value doing something 'normal' with their spouse or parent.

Managing excess mobility or continuous walking

- As the disease progresses, lack of motivation and changed perceptions, which earlier had reduced mobility can be superseded by behaviours that suggest a deep need to move.

- The driving force for the patient may be the desire to get somewhere which is important to them, for instance their childhood home or workplace.

- The physiotherapist can work with the patient and team/carers/relatives to find triggers to help the patient to stop and to sit.

- Triggers could include arranging chairs on the favoured walking route, offering the person a drink or food or noting which member of staff or relative has the best connection with the person and with whom they might sit for even a short time.

- Identifying what interests the patient has and using these to generate a focus with the potential for producing some rest time.

- A care plan should include rest times during the day which follow an agreed pattern, e.g. if the person sits to eat a meal then that is followed by the opportunity to lie down for an hour.

Collusion

- There is debate around the use of collusion to link to ideas that a patient has that are part of the delusional aspects of dementia.

- A patient may wish to phone his or her mother who has been dead for 20 years or is very anxious that he is not at home to feed his children who are now parents themselves.

- Alternatively someone may have memories of being incarcerated, perhaps in a prisoner of war camp and may perceive a locked door as proof that he is still incarcerated and must try to escape.
- To achieve mobility collusion is sometimes considered.
- Saying 'let's go and see where your mother is?' might produce the required motivation and may achieve the goal of increased mobility, but for the patient frustration will be heightened.
- Care must be used and honesty is important if any understanding is to continue. Thus the real situation should be kindly and clearly explained and this should be and will have to be repeated as if it is the first time it has been said.

Advice to carers and relatives

- The skills you have used to encourage mobility and retain strength in the patient need to be translated into useful tips for the carers and relatives who have to maintain safe mobility in the home.
- A crib sheet with scenarios relevant to the patient and suggested management can be very useful.
- For some relatives seeing and trying techniques are more effective than written information alone.

Outcome measures

- Timed up and go.
- EMS Elderly Mobility Scale.
- Falls assessment (FRat).
- Smiling faces.
- General increase in manageability.
- Whatever methods are used remember always plan for success, use a wide range of verbal and non-verbal communication skills and always allow sufficient time for response
- This may lead to mobility in the demented patient being maintained or even improved.

Adults with anxiety disorder

- Physiotherapy skills can be used directly to affect mental health disorders.
- In a referral where a musculoskeletal problem has been diagnosed it may be clear on examination that without addressing the high levels of anxiety a clear indication of the underlying problems associated with neck or lower back pain cannot be seen.
- In some areas liaison between mental health and outpatient physiotherapy services is such that patients initially referred to outpatients are re-referred to the mental health specialist to assess and reduce physical manifestations of anxiety before the musculoskeletal specialist treats the spine.
- In other cases the mental health physiotherapist will use specific skills in anxiety management before using the usual musculoskeletal techniques.

- Physical symptoms of anxiety include muscle tension, raised heart rate, shallow and fast breathing, sensations of heat, paraesthesia, blushing/flushing, aching muscles, fatigue, migraine, difficulty swallowing.
- As physiotherapists we have techniques which can reduce these symptoms and working with the MDT we can cofacilitate reduction in anxiety-provoking triggers.
- Anxiety disorders comprise of a number of distinct illnesses which are defined by the Diagnostic and Statistics Manual of Mental Disorders (American Psychiatric Association 2000), or the International Classification of Diseases ICD 10 (World Health Organisation 2011).
- Specific anxiety disorders include panic disorder, panic disorder with agoraphobia and obsessive–compulsive disorder.
- It is important to note that anxiety and depression occur together more often than they occur alone, where depression is present it will be treated by medication and can be positively affected by some of the physiotherapy treatments directed towards anxiety.

Goals

- Reduction of physical signs of anxiety.
- Patient confidence in self-help techniques.
- Reduction of pain.
- Increase in independence.
- Increase in physical function.

Treatment techniques

- Initially musculoskeletal assessment may be possible but may be compromised by the level of anxiety both in terms of thoughts and physical signs of anxiety.
- Presuming that the physiotherapist or student will have gained basic musculoskeletal skills elsewhere then the focus here will be on how anxiety might be addressed by physical and within the team, psychological means.

Massage

- Massage is a core physiotherapy technique which can prove very effective in treating muscle tension and anxiety (Diego et al 1998).
- In a mental health setting it is most usual to provide massage for hands, feet or head and neck. Centring treatment on distal areas reduces the need for removal of clothing, allows treatment to be offered without the need to find a specific treatment room, reduces the need for specific chaperones (although each case should be risk assessed on an individual basis).
- Whole body massage is rarely appropriate, but as a treatment for a patient with long-term recurring anxiety it can be used.
- The agreement of the patient is essential and explanation to the patient may include demonstration of the process on a colleague.
- Techniques that produce muscle relaxation should be used and may include the Western system of effleurage, gentle kneading, picking up for larger muscles, plus methods which the physiotherapist has trained in, for instance, reflexology, Indian head massage, aromatherapy massage (Fritz 2008).

- For all non-core massage techniques the physiotherapist must have evidence of training and must comply with their organisation's policy on complimentary therapies (CSP 2001).
- Evidence collected by the Chartered Society of Physiotherapy for the Mental Health NHS Framework notes that 'numerous studies have been published related to the effects of massage and lowered levels of anxiety (Field et al 1996). These studies have utilised a wide range of study designs including randomised controlled trials (RCTs). The outcome measures used within these studies have included saliva cortisol levels and self-report measures for anxiety such as the State-Trait Anxiety Inventory (Spielberger 1980). However, these studies have not considered people with diagnoses of anxiety or long-term mental health disorders, but rather groups of the general population. The major limitation of these studies is that the population samples are primarily groups of healthy individuals who do not have a recognised history of clinical anxiety.

Relaxation training

- The physiotherapist may have some training in relaxation techniques from other areas and these skills will be useful for use with patients in the mental health setting.
- In mental health relaxation is vital to enable effective treatment to be implemented in the many subspecialty areas of mental health physiotherapy practice.
- There are numerous techniques that the physiotherapist can use and the choice of technique will depend upon the need of the service user, the level of anxiety, demeanour of the service user and the skills of the physiotherapist.
- Relation training may be given individually or in a group.
- Relaxation techniques are practised by many people in the mental health team, including occupational therapists, psychologists, nurses and psychiatrists as well as physiotherapists.
- The physiotherapist may be expected to provide a physical-based relaxation technique only, but there is no need to be confined to this. The physical relaxation measures include fostering and establishing body awareness of looseness in one's joints, biofeedback, focussing one's mind and thoughts on letting the muscles relax, and developing body awareness of the tension on one's muscles.
- Physical techniques include Jacobsen also called progressive muscle relaxation, Mitchell, hold/relax and diaphragmatic breathing.
- Alongside physical methods we may use guided imagery, visualisation, covert rehearsal, autogenic and more (Donaghy and Payne 2010).
- Jacobsen's technique is essentially a two-step process, which involves relaxing and tensing various muscles.
- Practice is essential for the service user to understand which muscles are usually tense for them and to feel the link with relaxation. It is generally recommended to begin from the feet and move upwards. Starting with the right foot, then proceed to the left, and then to the calves, thighs and so on. Tensing and relaxing each muscle in turn, this process should be repeated on each muscle working right up the body to scalp. To gain the most out of this exercise, breathing techniques should be added and taught carefully, e.g. diaphragmatic breathing.

- The Mitchell method was developed by Laura Mitchell in the 1960s, her reasoning was based around the concept that many muscles work in opposing pairs, for example the 'biceps' and 'triceps' muscles. When one contracts the other must relax. So when you flex the elbow, the 'biceps' muscle contracts, to enable it to do so, the 'triceps' muscle must relax. Thus the Mitchell relaxation method is based on the simple principle of contracting certain muscles to encourage their opposites to relax (Appendix 10.1).

- Each physiotherapist will have a method or methods which they prefer, experience will be the best teacher as evidence for specific techniques is limited. For the treatment method with the best evidence base available the Jacobsen method should be considered.

- Awareness of tension is the first step to being able to reduce abnormal muscle tension. Many service users who have held tension in their muscle for years cannot recognise it as such because for them it is 'normal'.

- A useful method for demonstrating tension is to use the half body or awareness method (it has many names and is adapted in many ways).

- The method consists of using a script which allows the person to focus on one side of the body first and then getting them to compare the more relaxed side with the 'normal' side.

- With the person in lying or reclined sitting the instructions may begin as follows:

- 'Focus just on your right foot

- Be aware of how your foot feels

- Notice what is touching your foot ... the floor ... the mat ... your sock

- Be aware of the position of your toes

- Feel the heaviness of your foot resting on the floor'.

- The script would then continue up the right side of the body bringing the person to awareness of the right knee, thigh, right side of back as it touches the supporting surface, right hand, arm, right side of neck, face and scalp.

- Then the physiotherapist would ask the person to notice any difference in feel comparing the right to the left side.

- Following that the script would be repeated for the left side to bring the body back to balance.

Breathing techniques

- Breathing techniques can be taught in isolation, but usually work better alongside physical or psychological relaxation.

- The use of diaphragmatic breathing may be well known to novice physiotherapist from their work elsewhere. As the name suggests it is the engagement of the diaphragm to produce deep controlled breathing which should give the most effective opportunity for perfusion of oxygen to the bloodstream.

- In the anxious patient, especially one who has a long-term anxiety disorder shallow breathing may be the norm and requesting that the person take a deep breath may in fact be frightening initially.

- Allow the service user to go at their own pace and just to start with slowing the rate of breathing.

- A simple technique is to ask the patient/service user to count how long an in breath takes and then allow the out breath to last one count longer. This can then be progressed to extending the in breath too.

- Care should be taken in relation to teaching breathing methods.

- Risk of unleashing prior memories needs to be monitored. Always note what reaction a service user has when asked to lower the level of breathing, i.e. to take a deep breath and feel it in the lower belly, abdomen.

- If the service user appears to become much more anxious or places their hands protectively over their lower abdomen it may be that a memory of abuse has been elicited. Although not common, if this behaviour is seen the physiotherapist should find a different way to change breathing habits and should discuss this with the team.

- It is not the physiotherapist's place to ask the question or counsel the service user.

- If the service user discloses abuse the physiotherapist must make it clear that they have a duty to discuss this with the care co-ordinator.

- One easy rule to give a person who is breathing quickly and possibly beginning to panic is 'Just breathe out' although this seems oversimplistic it works well and is very effective in catching the first symptoms of panic before they escalate to a panic attack.

- Other methods including 'Yoga' breathing, huffing and 'laughter therapy' can be effective in changing anxiety-based breathing habits.

- For some patients focussing on breathing can make their anxiety worse and may aggravate any symptoms related to swallowing difficulties. If this occurs try to find another method of reducing tension which may act as an adjunct to reduce poor breathing habits.

Guided journey

- An imaginative or guided journey is a verbal relaxation system, which taps into the cognitive art of relaxation.

- The script should include visualisation of a pleasant environment and movement from one place to another. For instance a beautiful garden, focussing on colour, shape, sound, smell. Take the patient for a walk around the garden in their imagination.

- It is better to create a place for the patient rather than ask them to remember a real place as the emotions attached to real memories can evoke both happiness and sadness and not necessarily relaxation.

- Take care not to use scenes which frighten the patient, e.g. high mountains, deep water, all this should be addressed in the assessment but if working in a group you may not have individual assessments, so be aware of the possible negatives in scene setting.

- In addition to taking the guided journey, positive thoughts may be added and physical triggers given to allow the patient to return to the setting described or the physical relaxation achieved quickly in other environments.

- The additional techniques are best taught practically and although outlined here the advice to novice physiotherapists would be to observe an experienced therapist before attempting positive thought addition.

- Triggers that can be added to both physical and cognitive techniques include the use of trigger words which might describe the physical feelings of relaxation, e.g. loose, heavy, floating. Alternatively triggers which relate to emotions or cognitions, e.g. calm, chilled, restful.

- Physical triggers or cues should be very simple such as pressing together the index finger and thumb and again this can be done alongside the word cues and provide a way of relaxing in public situations and for treatment purposes when coming to the physiotherapist for treatment of pain or dysfunction.

Acupuncture

- The physiotherapist may be trained to use acupuncture for pain reduction but it has been shown to be effective in both general relaxation and well-being and is used specifically in reduction of withdrawal symptoms for service users on opiates and alcohol detoxification programmes (Tyndall 2003).

- The technique used is called the 'five point protocol' and this protocol can be used prescriptively and therefore can be taught independently of a whole acupuncture qualification.

- Although used in detoxification programmes using this protocol, physiotherapists should only apply the technique following accredited training and within the CSP scope of practice and also adhere to the policy structure within their employer organisation.

Joint working for cognitive behavioural therapy (CBT)

- The physiotherapist may treat the patient with musculoskeletal disorder alongside anxiety as part of a cognitive behavioural approach which is led by another member of the multidisciplinary team.

- This approach may acknowledge that the patient's perception of pain is related to anxiety itself or to the triggers, which stimulate both anxiety and pain.

- CBT is a type of therapy that aims to help the service user to manage their problems by changing how they think and act.

- It is an approach which physiotherapists are using more often in the treatment of chronic pain and long-term conditions.

- CBT encourages the patient to talk about:
- how they think about themselves, the world and other people
- how their actions affect their thoughts and feelings.

- By talking about these things, CBT can help to change how the patient thinks about pain or anxiety and enables them to recognise the triggers for either or both (Beck 1985, Bourne 1995).

- Unlike other talking treatments, such as psychotherapy, CBT focuses on the problems and difficulties which are current, rather than issues from the past.

- Focus is on practical ways to improve the patient's state of mind and manage anxiety on a daily basis. An ethos which can be reflected in the physiotherapist's approach to pain management.

- In the treatment of generalised anxiety disorder CBT has been found to be more effective than psychoanalysis and other forms of non-directive counselling or behavioural interventions including relaxation training used in isolation.

Anxiety management programmes

- The physiotherapist may facilitate an anxiety management programme with other members of the MDT.

- The level of input will vary and often depends upon the structure of the team and the skills within the team.

- The physiotherapist's input may be to provide relaxation training and to give a teaching session on the effects of exercise and activity, or they may be much more involved and provide sessions relating to the panic cycle (Figure 10.2), fixed thoughts, cognitive errors, symptoms of panic both physical and psychological, goal planning, distraction, reframing and other anxiety management techniques.

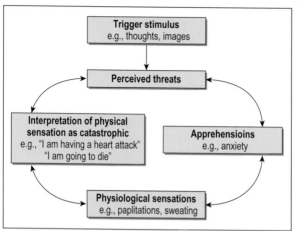

Figure 10.2 The panic cycle.

Table 10.2 The component symptoms of panic disorder	
Component	**Prominent features**
Emotion	Severe and incapacitating anxiety
Cognition	Thoughts of dying, going mad, or losing control
Behaviour	Escape, avoidance, safety seeking
Somatic symptoms	Sympathetic arousal, e.g. sweating, palpitations, hyperventilation
Associations	Depression, agoraphobia, substance misuse

- As part of an anxiety management programme panic disorder and panic attacks may be successfully addressed.
- Panic disorder is an extreme form of anxiety disorder usually triggered by stress or by environmental or emotional factors (Table 10.2).
- Recurrent panic attacks are a feature of panic disorder and are very disabling leading to people being housebound for years in some cases (http://www.nhs.uk/Conditions/Panic-disorder/Pages/Symptoms.aspx).
- A panic attack may occur when you are treating a patient.
- Their body will experience a rush of intense psychological and physical symptoms.
- They may feel an overwhelming sense of fear, apprehension and anxiety.
- As well as these feelings, they may also experience physical symptoms such as:
- Nausea
- Sweating
- Trembling
- Palpitations or irregular heart rate.

- The patient needs to be supported and led to understand that although it can be very frightening and intense, a panic attack is not dangerous and will not cause any physical harm.
- Just being with the patient and helping them to see the panic through to resolution and return to normal function is important.
- Relaxation may help in lowering the threshold of anxiety level and therefore reduces the likelihood of a panic attack.
- Breathing techniques can help, as can the use of a trigger and cues for relaxation.
- All of these will go hand in hand with cognitive work done by the team.
- If it is the environment which has triggered the attack then planning and graded exposure can help and should be part of a patient's programme.

Exercise and activity and the influence on anxiety

- The effects of exercise on anxiety have been discussed in the NICE guidelines on depression and described in many studies which provide consistent findings of a link between exercise and anxiety reduction (Scully et al 1998, Biddle and Mutrie 2007).
- The literature suggests that the beneficial effects of exercise in alleviating anxiety seem to be stronger for those reporting greater initial stress.
- As stated by Donaghy and Durward (2000) in the CSP evidence for the Mental Health NHS Framework, 'although there is no consensus of opinion on the level of exercise intensity or its duration, the greatest trait anxiety reducing effects appear after 20 minutes and when training occurs over a minimum period of 10 weeks (Petruzzello et al 1991).'
- The input a physiotherapist might be able to give in an inpatient environment may not reach the levels suggested in the evidence, but the use of group walks, multigym programmes, competitive games may all be used as part of an anxiety-reducing treatment plan.
- The anxiolytic (anxiety-reducing) effects can only be said to relate to generalised anxiety. Some studies have included clinical populations with increased generalised anxiety; however, many of the studies have been undertaken with student and normal populations and a very small number of studies have included inpatient psychiatric clinical populations with specific anxiety disorders.
- Some experimental studies indicate that exercise has a low-to-moderate anxiety reduction effect, with positive evidence that single sessions of moderate exercise can reduce reactivity to, and enhance recovery from, psychosocial stressors.
- Exercise has similar outcomes to other non-pharmaceutical interventions such as counselling and relaxation.
- This information may be something that the physiotherapist has to promote in the therapeutic environment.

Outcomes

- Self-reporting measures can be used for stress reduction, but the ease with which an assessment of the musculoskeletal disorder accompanying anxiety can be made compared to the difficulty with reaching a diagnosis initially is a clear outcome measure.
- Reduction in pain scored on a visual analogue scale.

- Easing of activities of daily living, and social interaction are also good subjective measures.
- Thus physiotherapy can provide a range of treatment options to treat anxiety alongside or independently of musculoskeletal disorder.

Conversion disorder

- The final focus of treatment in mental health is one which will be experienced less frequently for most physiotherapists, but for those in specialist units may be seen on a daily basis, is conversion disorder, which is sometimes referred to as somatisation.
- Signs and symptoms of conversion disorder typically affect movement or senses, such as the ability to walk, swallow, see or hear.
- Conversion disorder symptoms can be severe, but for most people, they get better within a few weeks.
- Conversion disorder symptoms may occur because of emotional distress or psychological problems.
- Symptoms usually begin suddenly after a stressful experience.
- People are more at risk for a conversion disorder if they also have a medical illness, dissociative disorder, or personality disorder.
- Some doctors falsely believe that conversion disorder and similar disorders are not real conditions, and may tell patients that the problem is 'all in your head'.
- However, these conditions are real and they cause real distress and cannot be turned on and off at will.
- Research on the mind–body connection may eventually increase understanding of these disorders.
- They are classified using the ICD-10 tool as dissociative (conversion) disorders, which suggest the symptoms arise through a process of dissociation.
- Patients are likely to be seen in specialised units, but may also be encountered in acute mental health wards, neurological wards and in the community.

Treatment

- There are different conditions under the label of conversion disorder which may support the choice of one of several models of treatment available to the physiotherapist.
- A patient's condition may be described as somatising, which means that for them the symptoms are real, despite no medical evidence being found.
- Some patients may know that the symptoms are not real and be using the symptoms for some sort of gain, either financial or personal in terms of attention or importance.
- A physiotherapist may be involved in coming to a decision as to which type of disorder it is, but it is not the role of the novice physiotherapist to make that decision independently.
- The appropriate model of approach is adopted by the whole team and there has to be a strong liaison within the team.
- The importance of case reviews to discuss progress and to set short-term goals for the following week is vital, in most units the client will attend and be part of the goal setting.

- Inclusion of all relevant individuals ensures that both the therapy team and the patient know the focus of the programme and to avoid what is termed in mental health 'splitting'.
- Splitting describes a technique of playing one person against another or suggesting to one professional that another professional is not doing their job properly.
- If a patient suggests this or makes a complaint or suggestion about the physiotherapist then best practice is to share this with all the team and to make a clear and detailed record of the comment or complaint.
- In this way the patient understands that there are no 'secrets' in the team and that they are part of that team.
- Always know what the route is for the patient to make a formal complaint.
- In most cases hospital will have a leaflet explaining this from their PALS team.

Goals

Short-term

- Bring the patient to some understanding and acceptance of their condition.
- Identify any physical causes of dysfunction.
- Strengthen weak muscles.
- Treat causes of pain.
- Achieve personal self-care activities.

Long-term

- Bring patient to full understanding and acceptance of their condition.
- Restore the person to the highest functioning level without the props of wheelchairs, sticks and dark glasses.

Methods

- Positive reinforcement of activities that they can partake in.
- Demonstrate evidence of musculoskeletal restriction and highlight areas where restriction cannot be evidenced.
- Recondition muscles.
- Provide a way of beginning to move.
- Initially this may be an easier option than recognising the psychological components of their illness, but the success is for the patient to be able to accept both parts of the disorder.

Reconditioning

- Sometimes when disability has been around for 20 years or more then there are more specific deconditoning factors that need physical approaches to correct.
- Strengthening regimes, activity programmes may be useful and the treatment is therefore a combined physical and psychological approach.
- The role of the occupational therapist is interwoven with that of the physiotherapist and is vital in transferring any gains in physical activities into more functional behaviours, regimes and returning the patient's skills to a premorbid level.

- A period of admission removes the individual from the environment and background that may have been a contributing cause or the catalyst for their difficulties.
- The following section provides a vignette of a patient with conversion disorder and the treatment that was given.
- Each patient will be different, but the general principles outlined can be followed for any patient.

The patient

Background

- A middle-aged lady who has been using a wheelchair for the last 10 years.
- She had had previously held a high-powered job, but her life was 'shattered' when she became aware that her husband might be having an affair.
- She had an episode of disability that was diagnosed inconclusively as a possible left-sided stroke.
- The relationship with her husband improved and she started to regain her previous level of mobility.
- One year later the husband admitted to an affair and he left to live with his new girlfriend.
- The lady suffered another episode of much greater severity and although having periods of therapy has remained in a wheelchair for the last 10 years.
- She has a supportive daughter who was 23 when the partners split.

The physiotherapy assessment findings

- Poor neck posture with evidence of a neck injury following a road traffic accident, which she reported to have happened 20 years ago.
- Weak gluteal musculature bilaterally, no neurological cause, possibly due to disuse.
- Disuse weakness of the whole of left side lower limbs and varied weakness of upper limb, with associated posturing on movement of the left arm.
- Poor rotator cuff stability bilaterally.
- Mobility was limited to a couple of steps when necessary in order to transfer.
- Able to independently self care.

Treatment plan

- Work initially on bed exercises to regain strength in core stability muscles.
- Address posture in all planes in lying, sitting and standing.
- Use of positioning in crook lying for stability, ensuring neck alignment and leg positioning. Pillows may be needed to allow leg to remain in good position initially.
- Use verbal and physical cues to encourage active movement in the left leg.
- Progression to gym work in lying, sitting and standing.
- Improve mobility of neck and upper thoracic area by application of mobilisations and connective tissue massage.
- Strengthening exercises in all positions for both sides of the body.
- Focus on establishing symmetry.
- Weight transference concentrating on good symmetrical alignment.

- Transferring into normal chairs.
- Talking when standing.
- Gradually increase walking distances.
- Talking when walking.
- Transfer core stability exercise to the standing position.

Summary

- Treatment was designed to enable the patient to take small steps and concentrate on developing a pattern of gradual increase in resistance and activity.
- The next steps involved the team working towards independence in society for the patient.
- The physiotherapist will be part of setting goals that involve the patient going out to the shops without her wheelchair and getting on public transport, or being part of a group of other people.
- The fear associated with being in public without the wheelchair, which has been a prop for years cannot be overestimated.
- The whole team will be part of the rehabilitation needed to achieve full return to her pre-morbid life.
- Ongoing interventions may include CBT, assertiveness training, anxiety management.
- The physiotherapist will be central to the provision of a home exercise programme and introducing the patient to the use of community gyms which will provide her with extra confidence in maintaining the physical gains that she has achieved during her period of treatment.

The references for this chapter can be found on www.expertconsult.com.

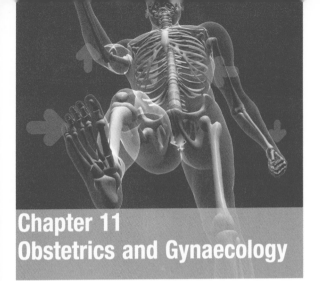

Chapter 11
Obstetrics and Gynaecology

Postoperative major surgery – treatment

Respiratory care

- Upper abdominal surgery is known to cause severe and prolonged alterations in pulmonary mechanics.
- Opiates and sedatives can also affect the natural 'sigh' mechanism (Richardson and Sabanathan 1997).
- Respiratory physiotherapy is essential to prevent the development of atelectasis and chest infections.
- Active cycle of breathing techniques with supported huff/cough should be taught, and incentive spirometry provided for those at most risk.
- Active treatment should be undertaken when pain relief is most effective and independent work encouraged.
- For patients who develop respiratory complications, oxygen therapy, humidification and nebulisers may be necessary.
- Positive pressure devices, such as CPAP, can aid lung expansion (Cook 2004).

Initial bed activity exercises

- When an epidural is in situ, the presence of equal, bilateral lower limb sensation and general mobility must be assessed.
- Simple active ankle and knee exercises should be encouraged; gentle pelvic rocking/knee rolling may help relieve flatulence (Cook 2004).

Initial transfers

- Patients should be taught how to move in bed, e.g. from lying to sitting via side-lying to minimise intra-abdominal pressure; moving up the bed by bending their knees and using their thigh muscles, digging in with their heels, pushing up with their hands and straightening their knees so that the hips lift up off the bed and back towards the pillow (Cook 2004).
- The occupational therapist (OT) may need to assess regarding any assistive equipment and techniques, e.g. a bed-lever may be supplied to aid general bed mobility.

Positioning

- Supported resting positions such as half lying with a pillow under their thighs and side lying with pillows between the knees and under the lower abdomen may be beneficial.

Posture

- Good posture in standing and supported positions in sitting, using appropriately placed pillows or lumbar rolls, may also help to reduce backache in the postoperative period.
- Patients may benefit from a recliner chair or specialist pressure relief; a graded sitting tolerance programme should be instigated for the most severely debilitated (Reed and Sanderson 1992).

Mobility

- Early ambulation should be encouraged.
- On day one, the patient should be assessed regarding ability to transfer out to a chair, including the potential use of a hoist.
- Standing should be encouraged and the need for a walking aid assessed.
- By day two most patients should be able to walk, with the assistance of two, for a short distance and progressed to independent mobilisation as able (Cook 2004).
- Less extensive or laparoscopic surgery would require similar multidisciplinary team (MDT) input, although progress is usually quicker.

Postoperative complications

- Tumour-related complications can include:
- Renal failure due to bilateral ureteric obstruction
- Acute haemorrhage from tumour occasionally resulting in hypoglycaemic shock
- Fistulae between vagina and bladder or rectum
- Pyometra (pus in the urine cavity) due to obstruction of cervical canal by tumour (Hatch and Berek 2005).
- Immediate postoperative complications can include:
- Bleeding (internal), deep venous thrombosis, respiratory problems, paralytic ileus, urinary tract and wound infection (O'Connor 1998, Sharpe 1998, Cook 2004)

- Lower limb, lower abdominal or groin lymphoedema may also develop in those who have had pelvic or groin node dissection
- Bladder and bowel dysfunction are common in the immediate postoperative period; suprapubic or urethral catheterisation and laxatives are therefore desirable in the first week
- It is essential to monitor the patient's ability to void after removal of the catheter, a functional assessment may be required regarding access to and transfers on/ off the toilet, rearranging clothing and cleaning of the perianal area and hands (Reed and Sanderson 1992) alongside adequate control of bladder and bowel.

Physiotherapy management in the convalescent/ post-acute phase

Counselling/information provision

- This may be an anxious time for the patient as they await pathology results.
- Gynaecological cancers have profound psychosocial implications in addition to the obvious physical manifestations. Women are confronted with cancer and its related treatments, which may impact adversely on body image, sexuality and relationships, including the possibility of imposed infertility and/or menopause.
- Altered body image is an important factor and becomes problematic when it affects the individual's quality of life (Shearsmith-Farthing 2001).
- It is important that appropriate, timely and confidential information is provided.
- Literature and websites sponsored by cancer charities are useful; some details are supplied at the end of the chapter.
- Eighty per cent of centres now offer aromatherapy for the relief of stress and anxiety (Kohn 2003).
- Menopausal symptoms may begin quite quickly after Bilateral salpingoophrectomy (BSO); advice on the control of symptoms should be provided by the consultant surgeon/oncologist; HRT can be contraindicated in some cancers (Biglia et al 2006).

Rehabilitation (including pelvic muscle floor retraining)

- Pelvic tilting, knee rolling, abdominal bracing and knee bends may be taught as exercises for the lower abdominal muscles and lower back.
- Expert opinion also suggests that pelvic floor muscle training after gynaecological surgery may mitigate problems such as urinary incontinence both in the short and long term (Cook 2004).
- Many physiotherapists delay instruction until the catheter is removed, although there is no evidence of harmful effects resulting from undertaking pelvic floor exercises whilst a urinary catheter is in situ (Haslam and Pomfret 2002).
- Ideally these exercises should have been taught preoperatively, however in both scenarios a vaginal assessment is unlikely to be possible.
- Therefore, the use of diagrams and models to verbally describe the anatomy and function of these muscles is essential as many women find it difficult to achieve correct pelvic floor contraction on verbal instruction alone (Bø et al 1988, Bump et al 1991).
- A combination of fast, slow and anticipatory pelvic floor muscle contraction should be taught to prevent leakage and control urgency.

- Patients may present with bladder problems ranging from hesitancy and poor flow, to incontinence, frequency and urgency, which may or may not have been present before surgery and/or related to the underlying malignancy.
- Individualised advice is required as this can be difficult to manage.
- Cranberry juice may be recommended to help prevent urinary tract infections, although this is contraindicated for patients on warfarin (Jepson et al 2004, Aston et al 2006).

Constipation management

- Some patients may also develop constipation, therefore education regarding correct diet and defecation position and technique should be taught.
- This includes sitting with the knees apart and higher than the hip joints; this may require the feet to be on a support.
- The trunk should be flexed forward at the hips supported on the forearms, and with the neutral spinal curves maintained.
- A bracing technique should be adopted which means to make the waist wide and to let the abdominals bulge anteriorly (Chiarelli and Markwell 1992, Markwell and Sapsford 1995).
- Straining should be avoided.
- The use of a pad to support the perineal area may be useful.

Diet

- Dietary advice can be helpful including information on supplementary feeding for those with depressed appetite and for those with stomas.

Ascites

- Ascites (the presence of fluid in the abdomen) may sometimes be present before surgery or in the later stages of the disease.
- This makes deep breathing and expansion of the bases of the lung difficult; patients should be encouraged to breathe as deeply as possible, and provided with oxygen therapy if appropriate.
- Ascites can also affect functional activities because range of movement can be restricted and tolerance reduced.
- Some relief may be gained from paracentesis (Krishnan et al 2001).

Activities of daily living (ADL)

- Following assessment and advice, the provision of ADL equipment can promote independence in personal care, toileting, bathing, transfers, seating and pressure relief.
- Written and verbal advice on a graded return to domestic, social and work activities are also essential.

Discharge preparation

- Before discharge, patients with stairs at home should have a supervised trial.
- If required ADL reports should be completed and adequate home-care provision organised by liaison between the hospital and community or social services.

- District nursing services to assist with the management of continence/wound/stoma and input from the community MDT to assess, facilitate and encourage mobility and independent activities are often required.
- For some, nursing home or respite care is needed, and input from voluntary sectors, such as a hospice, Marie Curie or Macmillan, can also be essential for palliative support.

Minor surgery

- Examples of minor surgery are laparoscopic hysterectomy, vaginal hysterectomy, prolapse repair, Trans vaginal tape (TVT).
- Following such surgery advice on pelvic floor muscle exercises and return to ADL should be provided.
- Additional information for those returning to high-impact sport can also be provided.
- Sources of information: Association of Chartered Physiotherapists in Women's Health (ACPWH) leaflet Fit for Life, Royal College of Gynaecologists (RCOG).

Prostate surgery

- In some settings the WH physiotherapist may visit men who are going to have or have recently undergone either a radical prostatectomy or a transurethral resection of prostate (TURP).
- There is some evidence that suggests that pelvic floor muscle training helps prevent or restore continence.
- To undertake a pelvic floor muscle (PFM) contraction the men should be advised to contract around the back passage, bring this feeling to the front with a scrotal lift and should be held for as long as possible (Dorey 2006).

Pelvic floor dysfunction (outpatients)

- Pelvic floor dysfunction encompasses the problems of genital prolapse, urinary and faecal incontinence, voiding dysfunction, and discoordination spasm of the muscles of the PF.
- These conditions may occur alone or in combination with one another.

Continence

- Continence problems occur in many patients especially as they get older, although it is not an inevitable part of ageing, or can be associated with conditions such as stroke, multiple sclerosis, diabetes or post-partum.
- When undertaking general rehabilitation, either as an inpatient or as an outpatient, it is often good practice to remember that patients may need to go to the toilet more often and quickly than usual.
- Multidisciplinary input is invaluable for such patients as functional problems of access, appropriate clothing and recognition of toilet area often helps.
- During a rotation in Women's Health, patients with pelvic floor dysfunction are assessed and advised as outpatients and can be referred by a GP, gynaecologist, urogynaecologist, obstetrician, midwife, urologist, neurologist, allied health professionals and in some areas by self-referral.

Pelvic pain

- Explain the rationale for proposed treatment modalities.
- Interventions that may be applied may include cognitive–behavioural therapy, PFM relaxation and re-education exercises, manual therapy, adjunctive therapies and pain management.
- Direct treatment to the presenting symptoms and address objective findings.
- If there is no response to treatment within a reasonable timeframe (allow 3–4 months) refer the patient for either psychosocial evaluation or pain management.
- This is a complex specialist area of treatment (Frawley and Bower 2007, Knight and Shelly 2008).

Urinary incontinence

- Following assessment it is important to teach the patient about the PFM and lower urinary tract function using diagrams, drawings and models.
- Explain a correct PFM contraction and if the woman consents vaginally assess PFM contraction.
- If active contraction is possible agree an individual training programme to be conducted at home.
- If strengthening is the main goal then the main factors to be considered are the same as for any muscle, i.e. overload, specificity, maintenance and reversibility.
- For patients with SUI recommendations are for women to exercise performing a minimum of 8 contractions 3 times a day, with training lasting for 3 months (NICE 2006).
- Ask the patient to suggest where and when exercises should be performed.
- Supply an exercise diary or 'biofeedback back' with computerised adherence registration.
- If the patient is unable to contract the muscles, try manual techniques such as touch, tapping, massage, fast stretch or using biofeedback, e.g. electromyography biofeedback, perineometry, ultrasound or electrical stimulation.
- In addition to a strength training regimen ask the patient to precontract and hold the contraction before and during coughing, laughing, sneezing and lifting (conscious precontraction, the 'knack').
- Follow-up with supervised training, weekly or more often.

Electrical stimulation (ES)

- Transcutaneous electrical stimulation (ES) is most frequently administrated using vaginal or anal plug electrodes, or percutaneous electrical stimulation, e.g. posterior tibial nerve stimulation.
- ES for Stress urinary incontinence (SUI) is focussed on improvement of the urethral closure pressure and sphincter activation, or as a kind of feedback procedure in patients who are unaware of how to contract the PFM and are unable to do so voluntarily.
- Office-based equipment as well as portable electrical stimulation devices have been developed.

- There is a lack of consistency in the ES protocols used in practice.
- The most common protocol uses a frequency of 10 Hz, pulse duration of 250 ms, and duty cycle of 1 : 2, although frequency and duration of application tend to be varied.

Biofeedback

- Biofeedback is defined as 'the technique by which information about a normally unconscious physiological process is presented to the patient and/or therapist as visual, auditory or tactile signal'.
- By using biofeedback it raises awareness of PFM activity and improves compliance to exercise.
- The main biofeedback tools are:
- Digital vaginal palpation, the therapist provides 'verbal biofeedback' about PFM contraction
- Digital self palpation
- Hand-held mirror
- Educator™
- Vaginal cones
- Manometry
- Electromography
- Real time ultrasound
- Dynamometry.
- Patients who undergo a vaginal assessment receive verbal feedback on correct technique of PFM contraction and the use of further biofeedback techniques depends on patient, clinician and availability.
- Biofeedback can also be used to teach PFM relaxation.

Advanced manual therapy

- On vaginal examination areas of reduced or nil PFM activity or areas of increased or overactive muscle fibres are often detected during a voluntary contraction.
- Manual therapy techniques such as trigger point release can be used in a patient where such muscle imbalance exists and is indicated for defecation dysfunction, Over active pelvic floor (OAPF) and urinary incontinence.
- Following such treatment in order to maintain the resting length of the muscle the patient must learn how to exercise it and a self-help technique called 'sniff, flop and drop' has been found to be beneficial (Whelan 2008).
- Once this technique has been established the patient can progress to an exercise programme of contracting the transversus abdominis, then the pelvic floor muscles holding these contractions while breathing in and out.
- A home exercise programme can then be developed.

Pelvic floor stability and trunk muscle co-activation

- As with any muscle the PFM do not work in isolation, but there is debate as to the benefit of actively co-contracting transversus abdominis (TrA).

- There is evidence that a co-contraction of the TrA occurs during PFM contraction and that a co-contraction of the PFM during TrA contraction may be lost or weakened in patients with symptoms of pelvic floor dysfunction (Bø et al 2009).

Bladder training and behavioural training

- Components of behavioural treatment can include:
- Introduction of voiding schedules
- Bladder control strategies
- Urge suppression techniques
- Urethral occlusion
- Biofeedback
- Self-monitoring with a bladder diary
- Behavioural lifestyle changes such as weight loss
- Fluid and diet management.
- These strategies are useful both for urge and stress urinary incontinence and can achieve significant improvements in continence in some patients.
- Self efficacy and motivation play a large part in their successful use.

Mixed urinary incontinence

- PFMT is recommended as a first line of treatment for stress and mixed UI in women.

Urge urinary incontinence

- It has been shown that PFMs play a role in overactive bladder and urge incontinence in women as well as men.
- Voluntary contraction of the PFMs not only can occlude the urethra, but also can inhibit or abort detrusor contractions.
- This is a skill that can be accomplished by most patients and provides significant reduction of incontinence.
- The first step in behavioural training is to help patients to identify their PFMs and to contract and relax them selectively without increasing pressure on the bladder or pelvic floor.

Medications

- There are several medications that can be prescribed to the patient with urgency or urge incontinence.
- These are mainly anticholinergic agents which abolish or try to reduce the severity of detrusor muscle contraction.
- Side effects such as dry mouth or eyes or constipation sometimes occur.
- At present there is one medication which may be prescribed for SUI (Duloxetine hydrochloride), and one for nocturia (Desmopressin).
- Intravesical Botulinum toxin A is emerging as a useful alternative in neurogenic detrusor activity.

- It is important to remember that drug treatment should be part of a behavioural package and that fluid management, drill and pelvic floor re-education remain the cornerstones of conservative management.

Bowel dysfunction

Faecal incontinence (FI)

- Principles are to keep the stool formed and keep the rectum empty.
- Stool consistency can be altered either by dietary manipulation or by use of constipation agents or both.
- It is important to recognise that the introduction of a high-fibre diet or fibre supplements in the diet can be used to soften the stool as well as to make it formed.
- This can be achieved by regulating the amount of oral fluids.
- If the stool is already liquid then the introduction of fibre supplements with limited oral fluids makes the stool firm as the fibre draws fluid from the stool itself.
- Constipating agents that work by slowing intestinal and colonic motility are also beneficial.
- The most common agents are codeine phosphate and loperamide.
- These agents increase the residue time for the stool in the colon and therefore provide a better opportunity for absorption of water from the stool.
- Keeping the rectum empty is important, particularly in the elderly patient who often has faecal loading or impaction.
- In these patients FI is secondary to the faecal impaction and often the treatment of the faecal impaction results in complete resolution of the symptom of FI.
- The simplest way of keeping the rectum empty is by regular use of glycerine suppositories and occasionally daily enemas or washouts are necessary.
- Establishing a regular complete rectal evacuation at a predictable time may be beneficial.
- Dietary management of FI or urgency is difficult to control as it is difficult to predict in different patients.
- Clinically a lot of patients derive benefit from moderating their fibre intake.
- Incontinence of flatus is difficult to control, products such as probiotics and aloe vera are reported as helpful in reducing flatus by some patients.
- Quantity and type of fluid is important.
- Alcohol seems to cause the bowels to be loose in some people and some have a bowel that is very sensitive to caffeine (Norton 2007).

Exercise

- There is little evidence to support the use of PFM exercises for FI, except for the early post-partum period following a third-degree tear.

Biofeedback

- This attempts to teach the patient to alter rectal sensitivity and to respond to the normal decrease in anal pressure then the rectum is distended (rectoanal inhibitory reflex) by a voluntary squeeze to avoid incontinence.

Electrical stimulation

- Intra-anal electrical stimulation has been reported to be a useful adjunct to exercises or biofeedback with some suggestion of improved effect.

Constipation

- Conservative measures include dietary manipulation, judicious use of laxatives and specific drug therapy.
- Once a mechanical cause for constipation has been ruled out all patients should be given advice regarding a high-fibre diet, fibre supplementation and increased oral fluid intake prior to rectal and colonic transit studies.
- Increase in exercise in sedentary patient, improving poor toilet facilities, providing privacy can improve the status.
- Defecation techniques can be taught (Chiarelli 2008).

Abdominal massage for constipation

- Abdominal massage for the relief of constipation was taught for many years in physiotherapy schools but its use went out of fashion in the 1960s.
- However, it has regained popularity with some evidence of effectiveness in people with chronic constipation and/or faecal incontinence when used as part of a holistic bowel management strategy.
- The massage is applied in a clockwise direction and has four basic strokes, stroking, effleurage, kneading and vibration.
- Daily massage lasting for approximately 15 minutes is usually recommended and it may take up to 3 weeks to show effect.
- There are no known adverse effects and is thought to have a mechanical and a reflex effect on the gut, thus encouraging peristalsis and may also utilise the mass movement of the gut increasing the strength of the contraction.
- Thus massage may reduce gastrointestinal transit time, soften stool and load the rectum (Emly 2008, McClurg et al 2010).

Laxatives

- Laxatives should not be used as a first line of treatment for constipation and the choice of agent largely depends on presenting symptoms, nature of complaint, patient acceptance and compliance.
- There are four main groups of laxatives:
- Bulking agents
- Stimulants
- Osmotic preparations
- Faecal softeners and rectal preparations (Irwin, 2008).

Obstetrics

Outpatient group work

Back care classes/pelvic girdle pain classes

- Some WH services will provide an 'early-bird' class with the aim of promoting good health in pregnancy.

- Others will provide a back care class or pelvic girdle pain class specifically for people who have developed musculoskeletal problems.
- For some women with early aches and pains, advice and exercise may provide relief or resolution of their problems.
- Women who require 'hands-on' treatment will find all the information given in such a class of benefit too.
- Classes may include some or all of the following:
- An overview of the physiological and musculoskeletal changes in pregnancy
- Posture correction and back care advice
- Comfortable positions to sleep and correct ways to get in and out of bed
- Advice about choosing baby equipment such as prams, baths, baby slings. It is imperative that the physiotherapist has a good understanding of products on the market and can analyse them from an ergonomic perspective and advise appropriately
- Exercise which relieves discomfort in pregnancy should include pelvic tilting in sitting, standing and 4-point kneeling; transversus abdominus exercises in different functional positions; Thoracic spine mobilisation exercises (rotations, extensions and side flexions)
- Information about common ailments such as carpel tunnel syndrome, varicose veins, rectus-abdominus divarication, ankle swelling, etc. and how to relieve them
- Advice on safe exercising in pregnancy (ACOG 2002; www.acog.org)
- Relaxation techniques – the Laura Mitchell method of relaxation is often used by women's health physiotherapists.

Antenatal exercise classes
- Exercise classes may be provided in the antenatal period.
- There are many benefits of exercise in the antenatal period, for example women are thought to sleep better, have improved posture, have increased strength and stamina to cope with the changes of pregnancy and the process of labour.
- It is also logical to think that women who maintain a level of exercise through pregnancy will return to their pre pregnancy weight in the postnatal period.
- Women can be taught safe cardiovascular exercise and core stability or Pilates style exercises in a safe environment by a physiotherapist who understands the increasing musculoskeletal demands on their body.
- Women should be screened prior to entry into a class.
- It is advisable to exclude those with the following:
- Haemodynamically significant heart disease
- Restrictive lung disease
- Incompetent cervix/cerclage
- Multiple gestation at risk of premature labour
- Persistent second or third trimester bleeding
- Placenta praevia after 28 weeks of gestation
- Premature labour during current pregnancy
- Ruptured membranes
- Pre-eclampsia/pregnancy-induced hypertension (ACOG 2002).

- Relative contraindications are:
- Heart problems, high blood pressure/hypertension, or maternal cardio arrhythmia
- Anaemia
- Asthma, chronic bronchitis or lung problems
- Diabetes
- Thyroid problems
- Seizures
- Extremely over- or underweight
- Muscle or joint problems
- History of spontaneous miscarriages
- History of previous premature labours
- Carrying multiples (e.g. twins, triplets)
- A previously sedentary lifestyle
- Smoking (BabyFit recommends immediate cessation of smoking during pregnancy)
- Orthopaedic limitations
- Intrauterine growth restriction in current pregnancy (ACOG 2002).

Aquanatal classes

- Aquanatal classes involve pregnant and sometimes postnatal women exercising in the medium of water.
- The benefits of exercise in water are well documented and include reduced risk of injury to joints, little or no muscle soreness post-exercise and the hydrostatic pressure of water may reduce oedema.
- Pregnant women who have pain when mobilising will see particular benefit from the water as they will feel significantly lighter in the water and walking should be less painful.
- There are particular considerations and contraindications to aquanatal exercise.
- Further information can be found on the ACPWH website and in Chapter 3 in this volume (http://acpwh.csp.org.uk/publications/aquanatal-guidelines-guidance-antenatal-postnatal-exercises-water).

Parent education classes

- It is usual for midwives to lead a set of four to six parent-education classes for pregnant mothers and fathers.
- Physiotherapists may lead one or two or provide standalone classes.
- The aim of parent-education classes is to provide education, thereby improving knowledge and consequently enabling informed decision making.
- Some classes will be designed for specific groups of women and their partners, such as teenage pregnancies.
- The content is very similar irrespective of the dynamics of the classes.
- Women will make a choice about whether to attend an NHS-run group of classes, whilst others will choose to attend privately run classes such as those run by the National Childbirth Trust (www.nct.org.uk) or a Lamaze trained childbirth educator.
- The physiotherapy content of parent-education classes includes:

- Coping strategies for labour, distraction techniques in early labour, which can include mobilising, reading, playing games, etc.
- Advice on early pain relief, such as Transcutaneous electrical nerve stimulation (TENS), massage, keeping mobile, breathing awareness, visualisation and positions of comfort.
- Positions in labour for the second stage, breathing awareness and how to effectively push.
- Discussion about after birth care, positions to care for baby when feeding, bathing and changing, discussion on baby equipment, returning to exercise post-natally.
- Advice given on the increased importance of pelvic floor exercises in the ante and postnatal period, and how to perform effective pelvic floor exercises.
- It is imperative that a full understanding of the birthing process is gained to take such a class and that ideally the physiotherapist has observed a number of deliveries.

Outpatient musculoskeletal care

Pregnancy-related pelvic girdle pain

- Pregnancy-related pelvic girdle pain (PGP) is the general term now used to describe pain, dysfunction and instability in the symphysis pubis joint, sacroiliac joint and/or lumbosacral region.
- The term symphysis pubis dysfunction (SPD) used to be used widely to describe pain and dysfunction in this area and is still used by some GPs, midwives and obstetricians.
- SPD describes a problem with the anterior aspect of the pelvis.
- As the pelvis consists of three bony articulations forming a ring, it is reasonable to presume that disruption at one joint will affect the other two joints in some way.
- This is observed in clinical practice and in line with the European guidelines for PGP the terminology of this dysfunction has been changed.
- PGP can occur at any stage of pregnancy, during delivery or postnatally.
- It is different from diastasis symphysis pubis (DSP) which is confirmed on diagnostic imaging, when it is shown that there is an abnormal pathological, horizontal or vertical displacement of the symphysis pubis (Bjorklund et al 2000). A diastasis of the pubis is classified as a gap of more than 1 cm between the symphysis pubis. Normal gap between these the symphysis is 2–3 cm and it is known to increase to 9 cm in pregnancy with no dysfunction.

Symptoms

- Pain varies between individuals both in severity and location. The common pain distribution areas include:
- Directly over the symphysis pubis
- Radiating into the groin
- Lumbosacral region
- Lumbar spine
- Sacroiliac area
- Anterior and posterior thigh
- Trochanteric area
- Pelvic floor and perineal area.

- Women will have difficulty mobilising, often exhibiting a 'waddling' gait and have difficulty abducting the lower limbs or performing any activities which involve standing on one leg (such as getting in and out of a bath or car, or going up and down stairs).
- ADL such as household chores, turning in bed, caring for other children and work related activities may be challenging.
- They may complain of a clicking or grinding sensation in the SPJ or SIJs.
- They may report that sexual intercourse is painful or difficult.

Diagnosis

- Diagnosis is reached through the subjective and objective assessment after excluding any other possible diagnosis.
- Differential diagnoses include urinary tract or other infections, renal problems, early labour contractions or Braxton Hicks contractions.
- All women with PGP present differently.
- The key message to remember is that this is a treatable condition that can safely be treated with manual therapy.
- All women should have a full assessment of their pelvic joints and be treated according to the assessment findings.

Possible treatment strategies

- Manual therapy – mobilisations, manipulation, muscle energy techniques, etc.
- Exercise therapy.
- Pain relief – discussion with the multidisciplinary team can help optimise analgesic modalities. Acupuncture and TENS may be of use.
- Advice on ADLs – help where possible from family and friends, back care and ergonomic advice particularly regarding looking after other children.
- Provision of a pelvic girdle support belt can reduce pain and aid mobility in severe cases, as do crutches.
- Women who have a lot of internal stairs in their homes may be helped by a commode to reduce the excessive weight-bearing of repeated stair use.
- Education about the condition is of high importance.
- Advice is crucial in order to limit the pain, this includes advice about periods of rest, maintaining activity within pain free limit, accepting help were possible, planning the day effectively through pacing, avoiding one leg standing positions and asymmetrical pelvic alignment, i.e. sitting down to dress, avoiding crossing legs.

Advice for delivery

- It is crucial that all health care professionals are aware of the woman's condition prior to her delivery. This may involve a case conference or documentation in the women's notes regarding her condition and in particular, to note the width of comfortable hip abduction available a guide through delivery.
- Upright positions to deliver should be taught, such as 4-point kneeling or side lying.
- Active delivery should be encouraged other than in extremely severe conditions.

- It is useful if the woman's birthing partner can be an advocate for her condition.
- Women who require perineal stitching ideally should have this in side lying.
- Refer to www.pelvicpartnership.org.uk for more information.

Postnatal care for PGP

- On the wards, women should have a bed near bathroom facilities, ideally a side room with direct access.
- They should have their analgesia optimised with non-steroidal anti-inflammatory drugs and low potency opiates such as codeine, as management of bowels should be considered with women taking medications which are likely to cause constipation.
- Some women with acute pain may well need a short period of bed rest.
- Mobilisation should be attempted with or without a support belt and/or crutches depending on the severity of the pain.
- Early pelvic floor exercises and core stability should increase the functional recovery.
- An assessment should be made about the level of help required at home and community agency referrals made where needed.
- As an outpatient, the postnatal woman with PGP should be referred to an appropriate physiotherapist who has expertise at the treatment and management of PGP.
- Treatment options are based on clinical findings and similar to that in the antenatal period.
- Standing stork X-ray, MRI or ultrasound investigations may prove useful if pain starts immediately postnatally, or pain and function are not improving (http://acpwh.csp.org.uk/publications/pregnancy-related-pelvic-girdle-painfor-mothers-be-new-mothers).

Back pain

- Back pain is very common in pregnancy.
- Despite this it is important not to allow others to consider it a 'normal' ailment of pregnancy.
- There are multiple reasons for back pain in pregnancy which include the change in posture, increased weight gain, and alteration in the muscle activity causing an 'imbalance' of the activity.
- Back pain in pregnancy is a treatable condition which if not treated may well lead to chronic pain. Postnatal back pain is also common due to the increasing demands of caring for a baby whilst recovering from pregnancy and the birth process.

Symptoms

- Generalised low back pain with or without referred pain.
- May have pins and needles or numbness.
- Pain may refer into the perineum.
- May be associated with PGP.

Possible treatment strategies

- Postural correction (Figure 11.1a, b).
- Manual therapy.

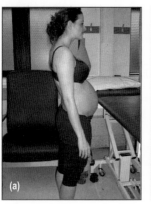 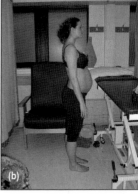

Figure 11.1 (a) Postural changes in pregnancy; (b) posture correction.

- Exercise therapy.
- Hot/cold therapy.
- TENS/acupuncture.
- Analgesia.
- Support belt.
- Advice about ADL.

Rectus abdominus divarication

- This is a very common condition that occurs when the two rectus abdominus muscle bellies separate at the linea alba and an obvious gap appears.
- It will become evident when a woman pulls herself forward out of bed, bath or performs a sit up.
- During pregnancy it is important to avoid movements where an obvious doming of the abdomen occurs.
- Teaching women how to roll to get out of bed and exercise safely may reduce the gap postnatally; however, the size of the baby and the stretch occurring to the abdomen dictates the gap to a larger extent.
- Teaching and maintaining a strong transversus abdominus is likely to help the postnatal recovery of this muscle.
- Postnatally, the gap should be assessed in crook lying and felt just above the umbilicus.
- A head lift will approximate the muscle bellies so that the gap width can be assessed and monitored through treatment.

Treatment

- Pelvic tilting.
- Core stability exercises.
- Advice about getting in and out of bed without causing further divarication.

- Avoiding excessive straining, lifting and constipation.
- Large L-sized Tubigrip may give symptomatic relief.

Rib flare

- Rib flare usually occurs in the third trimester and is characterised by pain over the lower ribs, it may radiate around the ribs, over the thoracic spine and will increase with any movements of the ribs and thoracic spine such as deep breaths, twisting movements, laughing or coughing.
- It occurs due to the changing angle of the ribs as the fetus grows.

Treatment

- Maitland's mobilisations of the thoracic spine or rib angle may provide pain relief.
- Stretches to mobilise the thoracic spine, such as rotations and side flexions.
- Hot/cold therapy.
- Teaching good sitting postures.

Coccydynia

- Coccydynia is classified as pain over the coccyx.
- It may start insidiously or there may be a history of trauma.
- Pain may develop postnatally after delivery when the coccyx has become bruised or displaced.
- Women will generally report pain on sitting and in changing position.
- Both LBP and PGP can refer to the coccyx.

Treatment

- In an acute phase, ice may help reduce any bruising or swelling.
- Sitting in an anterior pelvic tilted position may offload direct pressure on the coccyx. Coccyx sitting rings can be purchased, alternatively rolled up towels can be placed in a ring to relieve pressure.
- Specific Maitland's joint mobilisation techniques may be helpful.

Carpal tunnel syndrome/wrist pain

- Carpal tunnel syndrome (CTS) is the most common nerve compression syndrome in pregnancy, which occurs due to compression of the median nerve where it passes through the carpal tunnel.
- This probably occurs due to excess fluid pooling around the carpal tunnel in pregnancy.
- De Quervain's syndrome is also seen in pregnancy, where tendonitis occurs at the base of the thumb to extensor pollicis brevis and abductor pollicis longus.

Symptoms

- CTS is characterised by pins and needles and numbness in the median nerve distribution which are worse at night and after waking.
- Also may include general stiffness throughout joints.
- Women may complain of dropping things regularly and have poor grip.
- Women with De Quervain's will have specific pain at the base of the thumb.

- Finkelstein's test can be used to diagnose. Ensure differential diagnosis of radial nerve involvement is undertaken.

Treatment

- CTS- ice packs, resting with the hands in elevation, wrist and hand exercises and wrist splinting, especially at night to limit wrist flexion.
- De Quervain's – frictions, soft tissue massage, ice packs and rest.
- As this is a tendonitis, avoidance of aggravating movements will relieve pain.
- Postnatally a proportion of women will have unresolving CTS and De Quervain's.
- Ensure that the symptoms are not due to adverse neural dynamics.
- Steroid injections may be of benefit for a true De Quervain's.
- Referral to an orthopaedic surgeon with an interest in hand therapy should be made in non-resolving women.

Meralgia paraesthesia

- This condition is characterised by slight sensory loss and/or burning over the anterolateral aspect of the thigh.
- It occurs due to compression of the lateral femoral cutaneous nerve probably due to fluid retention.
- There is no motor involvement and the aim of treatment is to reduce and manage the discomfort.
- Treatment can include TENS and massage and stroking of the affected area.
- Full resolution should occur postnatally once fluid levels in the body and weight have returned to prepregnancy levels.

Round ligament pain

- Round ligament pain is relatively common and occurs due to the stretch of the round ligament which runs from the uterus to the vulva.
- Women will classically report a sudden sharp pain in the lower abdomen on movement, coughing or laughing.
- It should resolve within seconds, causes no harm to mother or fetus.
- There is little treatment that is known to be effective; however, women often find comfort in the knowledge of the cause of the pain.
- There are other causes of abdominal pain which should be referred to a doctor urgently, such as appendicitis, ovarian torsion and preterm labour.
- It is the physiotherapist's responsibility to refer if there are any concerns that the symptoms are not indicative of round ligament pain.

Varicose veins

- Varicose veins are common in pregnancy due to smooth muscle changes.
- The varicoses are usually in the calf, are often painful and women complain about the look of them.
- Advice can be given about brisk walking exercise to encourage efficient venous return through increased muscle activity.
- Circulatory exercises, avoidance of excessive periods of sitting or standing with the legs dependent as well as elevating feet when resting may help the symptoms.

Vulval varicoses

- These varicosities in the vulval area are much less common than varicose veins in the legs.
- Treatment includes advice regarding supportive underwear or wearing a sanitary pad in the underwear to create more pressure.
- Pelvic floor exercise, avoiding excessive standing and constipation may help.

Guidance of the use of TENS in pregnancy

- TENS may be beneficial to women in pregnancy for the treatment of back and PGP after other treatment strategies have been exhausted.
- ACPWH (2007) guidance has deemed that without evidence that it is harmful, and with consensus opinion it is safe to use TENS in pregnancy, especially when the alternative is analgesic medication which crosses the placental barrier.
- The usual contraindications to TENS should be adhered to.
- If women have a history of an irritable uterus, preterm deliveries or miscarriages caution should be taken (see information on the ACPWH website www.acpwh.org.uk).

Emotional needs

- Pregnancy itself is a very emotional period.
- There is a huge amount of change that occurs both physically and emotionally.
- To then have to cope with a pain which is quite severely disabling can bring feelings of depression, inability to cope, anxiety about the impending delivery and future motherhood.
- Understanding women's worries and listening to their goals will in part support their emotional needs through this period.
- Physiotherapists working in this field should also have good links with their local women's health counselors and means of referral.
- They should also be in contact with specialist midwives in their local area.
- Most midwifery services will have midwives who specialise in a specific area of expertise, such as human immunodeficiency virus, obesity, teenage pregnancy or safeguarding and will have experience at managing the more complex obstetric patients.

Postnatal (PN) ward care

Aims of PN care

- To provide information on reducing pain through non-pharmacology mechanisms.
- To teach and advise on pelvic floor exercise and abdominal exercises.
- To provide information on back care and health promotion for the future.
- In the PN period and particularly immediately after delivery, women will have feelings of exhalation and complete exhaustion.
- They may have a painful perineum after a vaginal delivery or a painful incision site from a caesarean delivery, or ongoing LBP/PGP.

- Women often ignore these ailments over the immediate need to look after a newborn baby.
- However, at some point they will seek help and they may remember the physiotherapist who saw them just after having their baby, who gave them some helpful information.

Treatment after a vaginal delivery

- Advice on positions of rest and trying to take rest is important.
- Advice should be given on rolling and getting out of bed without putting stress through abdominal muscles or perineal stitches.
- Women may find putting a hand over their perineum and supporting the stitches through the pad reduces any pain when coughing or performing a Valsalva manoeuvre (such as opening bowels).
- Good positions for feeding the baby.
- Advice on ADL's, such as changing and bathing baby.
- Teach pelvic floor exercises.

Treatment after a caesarean delivery

- Advice on positions of rest and trying to take rest is important.
- Encourage regular analgesia in the early stages.
- Advice on not lifting anything heavier than the baby for the first 6 weeks.
- Advice on not driving a car for 4–6 weeks or until an emergency stop can be performed safely.
- Advice should be given on rolling and getting out of bed without putting stress through abdominal muscles or lower abdominal stitches.
- Women will find comfort from placing a folded towel over the incision and applying pressure when getting out of bed, coughing, laughing and other such movements which stretch the incision.
- Good positions for feeding the baby.
- Advice of ADL, such as changing and bathing baby.
- Teach pelvic floor exercises.

Rationale for pelvic floor exercise post-delivery

- The exercises should be started as soon after delivery as possible.
- After a vaginal delivery, performing some gentle pain-free contractions will reduce swelling and increase circulation, therefore encourage healing of any tear or stitches.
- Long-term pelvic floor exercises may reduce the incidence of developing pelvic floor dysfunction.
- Although elective caesarean section is thought to be partly protective towards the pelvic floor muscles, pelvic floor exercises should still be performed by women after a caesarean section.
- The effect of pregnancy is thought to be damaging to the pelvic floor muscles alone and pelvic floor exercises are important for women to perform as a protective mechanism irrespective of mode of delivery.

Perineal tears

- Perineal tears are common in women during labour.
- They are classified dependent on the degree of damage.
- First- and second-degree tears may well not require sutures whilst some second-, and all third- and fourth-degree tears require suturing (Table 11.1).
- It is difficult to predict who will suffer a third- or fourth-degree tear, however risk factors are known to be birth weight over 4 kg, persistent occipitoposterior position, nulliparity, induction of labour, epidural analgesia, second stage longer than 1 hour, shoulder dystocia, midline episiotomy and forceps delivery.
- There is an increased risk of bladder and bowel dysfunction after sustaining a third- or fourth-degree tear, particularly with symptoms of flatal and faecal incontinence.
- The key to managing these tears is to correctly identify them, surgical repair by an appropriately trained registrar or consultant obstetrician and correct postnatal management.
- Postnatal management should initially include antibiotics, laxatives and pelvic floor exercises.
- Women should ideally be seen on the postnatal ward by a physiotherapist who can give advice on defecation techniques, pelvic floor exercises and long-term recovery.
- In some units the physiotherapist will offer them an appointment as an outpatient rather than see them on the ward.
- They should be followed up 6–12 weeks after delivery by a consultant who has a specialist interest in perineal tears.
- Many hospitals have dedicated perineal clinics in which a physiotherapist and specialist consultant will assess and treat this group of patients.
- Women should be asked about any bladder or bowel dysfunction or perineal pain.
- They should have a vaginal examination to assess wound healing, vaginal and anal tone as well as pelvic floor muscle function.
- Symptomatic women and those with poor pelvic floor muscle function should undergo physiotherapy, which would include pelvic floor muscle rehabilitation, treatment of scar pain, advice on defecation techniques and advice on returning to sexual intercourse.

OBSTETRICS AND GYNAECOLOGY

11

Table 11.1 First- to fourth-degree perineal tears.

First degree	Injury to perineal skin only
Second degree	Injury to perineum involving perineal muscles but not involving the anal sphincter
Third degree	Injury to perineum involving the anal sphincter complex: 3a: Less than 50% of external anal sphincter (EAS) thickness torn 3b: More than 50% of EAS thickness torn 3c: Both EAS and internal anal sphincter (IAS) torn
Fourth degree	Injury to perineum involving the anal sphincter complex (EAS and IAS) and anal epithelium

- Symptomatic women may be referred for further tests to assess the integrity of the internal and external anal sphincters and rectal sensitivity.
- Women should be counselled in regards to the previous delivery and questions answered regarding possible future deliveries.

Other postnatal complications

- Post-partum haemorrhage.
- Uterine infection.
- Perineal infection.
- Caesarean section wound infection.
- Urinary tract infection.
- Thrombosis.
- Respiratory complications.
- Mastitis.

Postnatal exercise classes

- The aim of postnatal exercise classes is to provide an environment in which a postnatal mother can come, usually with her baby, to exercise safely after pregnancy and childbirth.
- The anatomical and physiological changes should be considered when planning a programme with particular emphasis on pelvic floor muscle rehabilitation, abdominal muscle recovery and back care.
- Women are usually ready to come to such a class between 6 and 12 weeks after delivery of their baby.
- There should be a screening process prior to entry into the class, which should include questions about previous delivery history, identification of any perineal discomfort or pelvic floor dysfunction, any musculoskeletal problems during or after pregnancy, general wellbeing and measurement of rectus abdominus divarication.
- The classes may vary in content to include any or all of the following usually over a 6-week rolling programme:
- Low-level aerobic exercise, working cardiovascular fitness
- Core-stability-based exercise programme concentrating on pelvic floor muscles and abdominal rehabilitation
- Advice about progressing exercises and other classes available in the local community
- Back care advice.

The references for this chapter can be found on www.expertconsult.com.

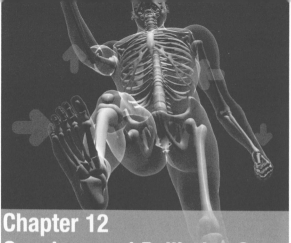

Chapter 12
Oncology and Palliative Care

Introduction

- Cancer rehabilitation, although a relatively new concept, is now recognised as an essential component in the cancer journey (Rankin et al, 2008).
- Rehabilitation in cancer care 'aims to improve quality of life irrespective of aetiology or life expectancy' (Cheville et al 2007).
- Patients can therefore maximise their independence and obtain the best physical, social, psychological, and work-related function during and after their cancer treatment.
- Palliative care rehabilitation is still poorly understood by many professionals, but it is becoming increasingly accepted that patients, regardless of prognosis or diagnosis, can benefit from rehabilitation services at all stages of their disease.
- There are four accepted rehabilitation stages recognised by Dietz (1980) (Box 12.1).

Underlying principles of management

- Before considering treatment it is vital to have an understanding of the assessment required for this group of patients and the reader is referred to Chapter 12 in Volume 1.
- Physiotherapists working in the field of cancer and palliative care are able to offer comprehensive assessment and treatment regarding the management of different symptoms in the acute, primary and tertiary care settings.
- A physiotherapist's primary aim in oncology and palliative care is to maximise independence and reduce the effects that cancer or progressive degenerative illnesses have on an individual's physical, psychosocial and economic functioning.

> **Box 12.1** Cancer rehabilitation stages
>
> - Preventative: reducing the impact of expected disabilities and assistance in learning to cope with any disabilities
> - Restorative: returning the patient to pre-illness level without disability
> - Supportive: in the presence of persistent disease and the continual need for treatment, the goal is to limit functional loss and provide support
> - Palliative: further loss of function, put in place measures which eliminate or reduce complications and to provide support (symptom management)

Dietz 1980.

- Physiotherapeutic objectives will be diverse (Küchler and Wood-Dauphinée 1991), but will be determined by a whole-person approach to assessment (physical, psychological, social and spiritual) followed by appropriate goal setting in partnership with the patient (ACPOPC 1993).
- There are a number of principles which should be applied to cancer and palliative care rehabilitation, the most important of these is co-ordinated care, requiring effective communication with a multidisciplinary team (MDT) working approach (Bliss et al 2000).
- It is particularly important when treating or giving advice to patients to provide written information to reinforce the treatment plan.
- In oncology and palliative care, in many instances the aim is for symptom management and not complete alleviation of the problem.
- This is something that can be challenging for less experienced physiotherapists or those coming from a different environment where the aim is complete resolution of symptoms.

Communication skills in oncology and palliative care

- Communication underpins every aspect of the care provided for patients and their families and is the key to effective team work (Heaven and Maguire 2008).
- Good communication consists of the ability to assess the patient's communication needs and to tailor communication to these needs, while maintaining realistic hope (Lugton et al 2005).
- Good communication skills:
- Facilitate the exploration of the patient's unspoken concerns
- Clarify the patient's priorities and enable them to set their own realistic goals
- Reduce uncertainty and the likelihood of unrealistic expectations while maintaining hope
- Explore treatment options
- Allow the patient to be involved in decision making/planning for the future
- Reduce the possibility of misunderstandings
- Support effective multidisciplinary teamwork
- Enhance the support of families and carers.
- Patients in oncology and palliative care will have many worries and concerns that they find difficult to express.
- During interactions, it is important that the patient is given full attention and is not rushed.

- It is essential to be aware of both verbal and nonverbal communication such as facial expression, tone of voice and body language.
- Open questions should be used to encourage the patient to talk, for example 'How are you feeling today?' rather than 'How is your pain?'
- It is essential to establish what the patient knows about their condition, a useful phrase might be 'Can you tell me about what has been happening to you?'
- Enquire from the patient if they have had any problems since the initial assessment and what the specific nature of the problem is.
- In an outpatient or community setting where the patient has been referred for a specific problem, it is important to give a patient the opportunity to share other problems too.
- As an example the following statements represent the interaction that may occur:

'Following the assessment last week how have you been feeling?'

'Was there anything that you wanted to talk about last time you were here?'

'Is there anything else I can help you with?'

- These questions provide the patient with an opportunity to raise other issues that concern them.
- Following the initial assessment a patient may have had time to reflect on their issues.
- This can happen after specific questions have been asked, which may not always happen as people are often frightened of asking the 'wrong thing'.
- The patient may decide to change the priorities that they decided on a previous attendance, this is an indication that the patient has engaged with the process and not avoiding confronting the problems that need to be dealt with.
- Sometimes this conversation may bring out information that was previously unknown and indicate the underlying anxieties that a patient may have.
- Throughout the treatment, the patient should be encouraged to express feelings. For example, it may be appropriate to ask 'is there anything about the treatment that worries you?'. 'What is it about the treatment that concerns you?'
- The physiotherapist may get a chance to find out about the patient's anxieties. For example:

Patient 'I don't want to die the way my brother did'

Therapist 'What do you mean by that?'

Patient 'Well, he became very different in the end, it was not very dignified and that upset me'

- Sometimes patients have concerns about their quality of life. Reflecting a question back to the patient may allow deeper meanings to be aired, for example:

Patient 'Will I ever get out of this wheelchair and walk again?'

Therapist 'Why do you ask?'

'Well, I really don't want to carry on if I am going to be in a wheelchair forever'

- It may be useful to verify what the patient has just said to avoid any misunderstanding.

Therapist 'When you said you wouldn't want to carry on what do you mean?'

- It is not always possible to provide a direct answer to a direct question from a patient particularly in terms of prognosis.
- It is best to be honest and maintain hope during communication and therefore a vague answer to questions initially will allow their response to be gauged.
- More specific details may be given depending on the reaction of the patient or if they request more information.
- It is not always possible to provide answers to the questions asked by patients as in many cases the answer may not be clear.
- Always give the patient enough time to talk in the way that they want to, encourage them to talk but avoid pressurising them. For example:

Patient 'I feel frightened …' (pause)

Therapist 'Sometimes you feel frightened about …'

Patient 'Sometimes I feel frightened that I will not be in control of what happens to me'

- The physiotherapist should be aware of the patient's need to talk and provide opportunities for this to happen, however there may be times when the conversation begins to uncover issues that are beyond the ability of the physiotherapist to manage.
- In these cases it may not be appropriate for a conversation to be continued and the physiotherapist will need to discuss this with the patient and offer alternative options for issues to be discussed.
- In these cases the physiotherapist should be aware of the appropriate professional to refer the patient to.
- The physiotherapist may not always know the answer to a question. It is important to acknowledge this by saying 'I don't know' or 'I'm not sure about that'.
- Offer to find out the answer to the questions or the most appropriate person to provide the answers.
- It is important to remember that patients may want to know certain things at different times during their illness and the physiotherapist must be sensitive to these changing needs to avoid upsetting the therapist–patient relationship so necessary for achieving treatment outcomes.

Goal setting

- Any additional information disclosed by the patient following the initial assessment may lead to the treatment goals that were set following the initial assessment needing to be re-evaluated and reset.

- The goals will need to be discussed with the patient and jointly agreed as being practical and achievable in the short, medium and long term as necessary.
- The physiotherapist must always try to engender the possibility of the patient achieving success and not allow goals to be unattainable.

Multidisciplinary working

- The key to successful physiotherapy treatment in oncology and palliative care is working closely as part of a MDT.
- This will provide a continuum of care through diagnosis, treatment and survivorship.
- This group of patients can have complex and multifactorial issues that need to be addressed by a team with relevant skills and knowledge.
- The physiotherapist should ensure consideration is given to all aspects of the patient's problems, and involvement of other members of the team is arranged when necessary.
- NICE have described the domains of care in cancer rehabilitation and each assessment of a patient's rehabilitation needs should consider:
- Physical, which includes optimising functional ability and management of symptoms such as breathlessness or fatigue
- Nutritional involves optimising nutritional status to ensure maximum benefit from physical programmes; management of nutrition-related symptoms
- Psychological, involves health care professionals recognising signs of psychological distress or developing knowledge and skills to deal with certain levels of distress
- Informational, material provided for the patient in written, audio and visual format
- Practical, development including activities to enhance daily living or returning to work
- Spiritual, involves finding personal value; identifying personal meaning; seeking, finding and maintaining hope; being able to express emotions
- Social, covers relationships, socialising, hobbies and pastimes
- Financial, concerns such as being able to pay the rent or mortgage, loss of earnings; travel and other types of insurance (NICE 2004).
- If the physiotherapist is unsure if referral to another professional is indicated they should discuss this with a senior colleague or with the other professional directly in order that each individual case is given due consideration.
- Working in a close MDT in oncology or palliative care can be one of the most rewarding aspects of this specialty and is one thing likely to provide maximum benefit to the patient.
- Living with advanced incurable disease can affect all aspects of life, creating psychological, spiritual, and existential challenges as well as demands for symptom control and physical care. It is therefore rarely, if ever, possible for any one professional to meet all the needs of a patient or family (Haugen et al 2009).

'A single profession, like a single model of care, cannot meet the holistic, fluctuating needs of patients and carers. The knowledge and skill of many professions including medical, nursing, pharmacy, social work, physiotherapy, occupational therapy and chaplaincy bound together by communication and teamwork is vital' (Mount et al 2006).

Psychological aspects

- It is vital to consider the psychological aspects of being diagnosed with and living with cancer or a life-limiting illness when considering physiotherapy management.
- The common issues are discussed below.

Anxiety and depression

- Fear and anxiety are normal reactions to stressful situations, such as those undergoing treatment for cancer.
- Depression is when a patient's mood is low most of the time for several weeks or more and the relationship between cancer and depression is complex and multifactorial.
- The physiotherapists should be aware of the issues and be able to identify the patients who may need referral on to a specialist.
- Common presentations can be breathlessness, muscle tension, dizziness, sweating and panic attacks, all of which may be identified by a physiotherapist.
- Depression may also be expressed by a patient with no motivation, or who feels helpless, hopeless or guilty or to blame.
- The most common anxiety and depression assessment scales used in a health setting are the Hospital Anxiety and Depression Scale (HADS) or the Brief Edinburgh Depression Scale (BEDS).
- Both scales are simple and short, providing a pragmatic method of screening for anxiety and depression.
- Mild anxiety and panic attacks may be eased by the physiotherapist teaching simple relaxation techniques or the patient taking part in gentle exercise with support.
- Treatment may consist of active listening and allowing the patient to share their concerns, fears and frustrations.
- If the physiotherapist does not feel able to manage the patient's problems or feels they need further investigation it is essential to refer on to the relevant member of the team, which may be a social worker, counsellor or psychologist.

Breathlessness

- Twycross (2003) defined breathlessness as 'the subjective experience of breathing discomfort'. Breathlessness has been noted to be 'subjective and like pain, it involves both perception of the sensation by the patient and their reaction to the sensation' (Heyse-Moore et al 1991).
- Therefore, the patient's emotional state and other symptoms can and will have a direct impact on the symptom of breathlessness.
- The treatment of breathlessness in oncology and palliative care employs similar techniques to those used in respiratory physiotherapy.
- The evidence shows that non-pharmacological management of breathlessness is effective for both malignant and non-malignant disease (Bausewein et al 2010; Bredin et al 1999, Corner et al 1996).
- Before providing specific advice, it is helpful to provide the patient and family some basic education about the anatomy and physiology and the functions of breathing. This should be done at an appropriate level for each individual and

once a patient has a good understanding of how the lungs are structured and work, often this will lead to an alleviation of anxiety.

- The following are suggestions that may assist the patient, the technique must feel comfortable for the patient or they may increase anxiety:
  - Get in a position to ease shortness of breath, e.g. forward leaning (Appendix 12.7)
  - Try to make the breath out twice as long as the breath in. This requires practice as patients often focus on inspiration
  - Breathe out through pursed lips
  - Time walking to the breathing, e.g. step one – breathe in; step two and three – breathe out. This is a useful technique to use when climbing stairs
  - Give advice in the presence of family and carers, as their behaviour can affect the patient's breathlessness. The physiotherapist should make sure family and carers understand that the patient should not try to converse when short of breath and they should support the patient in whichever way the patient prefers, e.g. holding their hand
  - Use a hand held or table fan to help reduce the shortness of breath and ease anxiety.
- The following are suggestions to manage breathlessness when carrying out daily activities:
  - If bathing, don't have the water too hot or too deep and let the water out first before you get out
  - If showering, don't have the shower head spraying into your face and make sure a window or door is open for ventilation
  - After washing, wrap yourself in a toweling robe and rest until able to continue
  - When dressing, do as much sitting down as possible
  - Avoid bending over at the trunk, try to kneel or sit if working at low level
  - If gardening try to move plants into pots and work at waist height
  - In the kitchen, have frequently used items at worktop level or above to avoid unnecessary bending.

Pacing and planning

- It is important when breathless to plan and pace daily activities and social events allowing periods of rest between activities.

Anxiety and relaxation

- Breathlessness will often cause anxiety and can be a very frightening experience.
- Education and reassurance will often ease some of this distress but simple relaxation techniques may also be useful.
- The most commonly used methods include simple diaphragmatic breathing and progressive muscle relaxation.
- Any relaxation method must be tailored to the patient and their preferences.
- Some patients may also find the calming hand tool useful which was designed to help control panic attacks (Burnett and Blagbrough 2007).
- Good control of breathlessness can alleviate both physical and psychological distress to patients and their families and therefore can have a significant impact on quality of life.

- The physiotherapist does not aim to alleviate the breathlessness, but to help teach the patient how to manage the symptom.
- These techniques are appropriate for anyone suffering from breathlessness, due to cancer or any other condition.
- For further information see the breathlessness rehabilitation pathway (NCAT 2009a) available online.

Body image

- The image we have of ourselves is our own impression of our physical appearance and what sort of person we feel we are.
- This image is built up over time from observing ourselves, the reactions of others, and a complex interaction of attitudes, emotions, memories, fantasies and experiences, only some of which we are aware of (Regnard and Kindlen, 2002).
- Our body image is also affected by social interactions and how we relate to others, our feelings of achievement and self worth, our sexual image of attractiveness and our spirituality and morality.
- Cancer and its treatment can produce various temporary and permanent changes which can have a devastating effect on patients' feelings and their attitude to their own body which can affect their psychological health.
- It is often thought that body image problems should be referred for psychological assessment and treatment but it is the responsibility of all health care professionals to be aware of body image issues in the oncology and palliative care setting.
- The physiotherapist's ability to actively listen to the concerns of the patient are of paramount importance, and often a simple open discussion and acknowledgement can help to bring down barriers, reduce feelings of isolation and fears of rejection.
- The focus of intervention in the body image services generally covers seven domains and it is important that the physiotherapist has an awareness of these areas of treatment as some of them may sit well with standard physiotherapy interventions and planned outcomes (Box 12.2).
- Work in these domains can improve perception of body image by working on self esteem, anxiety and mood, increase coping efficacy in situations that are challenging, increase social activity and improve relationships with others.
- Whilst awareness of body image treatments is essential the physiotherapist must be aware of their own competencies in communication skills and must not hesitate to liaise with other more experienced members of the MDT.

Hope

- Hope has been described as 'a multidimensional dynamic life force characterised by a confident yet uncertain expectation of achieving future good, which, to the hoping person is realistically possible and personally significant' (Dufault and Martocchio 1985).
- The fostering of hope and the prevention of feelings of abandonment are part of the physiotherapeutic intervention (Doyle et al 2005).
- Hope needs a goal and realistic goal-setting is a core physiotherapy skill.

Box 12.2 Management of body image, the seven domains

1. Camouflage and masking

   The use of clothing to cover or shield an area, such as a scarf, jewellery or make-up

2. Functional adaptation – e.g. use of a stick for proprioception in peripheral neuropathy

3. Enhancing self worth through

   a) compassion through touch therapy

   b) competencies and achievements

4. Supportive expressive therapies – disclosure and counselling

5. Desensitisation programme – gradual exposure formally or informally as in repeated consistent reactions of others

6. Enhancing coping strategies by

   a) goal setting – identify desired outcomes

   b) reframing – challenging assumptions and beliefs

7. Compensatory activities with a pleasure focus, i.e. generate positive mood states

Table 12.1 Key factors relating to hope

Factors supporting hope	Factors threatening hope
Attainable goals that help to maintain a sense of control	Physical or emotional loss
Affirmation of worth	Losing the future
Honest information	Loss of healthcare professionals interest
Symptom management	Devaluation of personhood
Trust in care	

Kymla et al 2009.

- Patients need attainable goals to help maintain a sense of control and to reframe a vision for the future.

- Some patients choose to avoid receiving information as a strategy to maintain hope therefore gentle honesty, empathy, optimism and excellent communication skills are required to navigate the patient through the uncertain course ahead.

- Living with incurable progressive disease does not necessarily mean living without hope.

- Kylma et al (2009) conducted a review of 34 articles and identified key factors contributing to and threatening hope in palliative care.

- Some of the key factors that are of particular relevance to physiotherapists are listed in Table 12.1.

- Because hope is inextricably linked with life, health and illness, it has become an essential component of healthcare.

- As well as supporting the patient it is important to give emotional support to the patient's significant others, as they will be jointly involved in fostering hope in the patient.

- Suggested hope-fostering interventions include:
- Affirmation of the patient's worth/being present to the patient
- Working with the patient holistically/taking time to talk/creating a partnership
- Focusing on life while facing a future of a potentially shortened life
- Helping the patient to engage actively in own care
- Keeping an open, positive perspective on the future
- Assisting to devise and revise realistic, meaningful goals
- Supporting the patient's hopes and wishes
- Encouraging the patient to share fears
- Giving information in response to the patient's need for information.
- The wider the gap between the patient's expectations and the reality of the situation, the poorer quality of life will be.
- 'The gap between hopes and realities may be narrowed by improving patients' function by treatment or by reducing their expectations through better understanding of the limitations imposed by their disease' (Calman 1984).
- In curative hope work, the patient is defined as getting better; in palliative hope work, the patient is defined as feeling better.

Preventative advice

- Some problems in oncology and palliative care may be prevented or their impact reduced by implementation of preventative advice.
- In many cases this will be in the form of education for the patient about possible risks of complications or problems that may arise due to their disease process or treatment effects.
- This could be issues such as risk of lymphoedema or range of movement problems or early advice on managing fatigue or breathlessness.
- It is also important to advise on problems that may arise simply from a lack of knowledge or understanding, such as weakness or reduced mobility due to lack of activity.
- It is vital that patients are given such advice early in their physiotherapy management to put the patient in better control of their condition and make them more aware of when to seek further help or support.

Exercise tolerance and deconditioning

- Weakness and deconditioning due to lack of exercise are common problems in cancer sufferers.
- Cancer treatments too by their very nature are toxic to the body and the resulting loss in physical functioning can be severe.
- Within the palliative care setting patients can have significant muscle weakness and mobility issues and the complexity of a combination of symptoms can be a challenge to the physiotherapist.
- Complicated syndromes such as cachexia have a marked effect on muscle mass and exercise tolerance.
- Cachexia is due to a derangement in the body's metabolism due to factors produced either by the tumour or by the body in response to the tumour, e.g. cytokines (Hawkins 2007a).

- In general activity has proven to be beneficial in the cancer patient and the assumption that rest will help increase energy levels and exercise tolerance should be challenged (Hawkins 2007b).
- Another common problem can be the onset of proximal myopathy due to the use of steroids.
- The mechanism of this process is not fully understood, but it is important that patients are aware of this side effect of steroid treatment and are given exercise advice to raise their awareness and help reduce the effect this may have on their function.
- Guidelines for exercise prescription are outlined in Box 12.3. The fundamental principles of exercise such as frequency, intensity and duration are well known to the physiotherapist.
- The progression, adaptation and individuality of exercise prescription apply equally to the cancer patient at all stages of illness and should be as a result of a thorough assessment and with agreed achievable aims and goals.
- Exercise should be monitored using a variety of tools that will provide the information required to gauge the effort expended by a patient, e.g. Borg scale for perceived exertion, pulse oximetry or a timed walk test.
- Be aware special considerations that pertain to cancer rehabilitation patients and use comprehensive assessments to develop appropriate exercise interventions.

Box 12.3 General guidelines on exercise in oncology and palliative care (Courneya and Mackay 2001)

- Patients should be encouraged to maintain normal functioning, mobility and activity
- Exercises should involve large muscle groups
- Frequency should be 3–5 times a week, but daily exercise could be more beneficial
- Duration should be at least 20–30 minutes of continuous exercise, but may have to be in shorter bouts for individuals with poor conditioning
- Progression should increase in frequency and duration first followed by increase in intensity as the patient becomes more fit
- The progression should be gradual, especially for patients with severe side effects of treatment
- Exercise/movement should be tailored to patient needs, ability and disease status
- Appropriate warm up/cool down phase as part of exercise to avoid exacerbation of swelling
- Compression should be worn during exercise

Types of exercise

- Start with low- to moderate-intensity exercise
- Paralysed limbs can be moved passively
- Walking, swimming, cycling and low-impact aerobics are recommended
- Heavy lifting and repetitive motion should be avoided
- Flexibility exercises maintain range of movement

- Continuously monitor the patient's response to exercise and maintain a record of exercise, effects and progression.
- The contraindications to exercise for patients with cancer are similar to other patients with a few additions, e.g. fever, cardiovascular instability, untreated deep vein thrombosis or pulmonary embolism and neutropenia.
- In palliative care the emphasis is on 'little and often' (pacing), the targeting of weakened areas and avoiding exhaustion.
- Exercise prescription should take into account potential sudden variations in symptoms and be able to be adjusted accordingly.
- It is vitally important to agree with the patient and family realistic goals and so minimise demoralising failure.
- It is important to note that patients may be managed in a palliative care environment for a considerable time, sometimes years and therefore they can often tolerate moderate levels of exercise based on their symptoms.

Precautions

- Care must be taken with symptom management and there should be continuous monitoring with certain issues such as bony metastases, poor balance, dehydration, nausea, fatigue, skin reactions, peripheral neuropathy, postural hypotension, body image, pain and thrombocytopenia.

Mobility

- Mobility and function are two common determinants of a patient's quality of life.
- Evidence suggests that there is a positive association between physical activity and quality of life (Helbostad et al 2009, Lowe et al 2009).
- Patients should have access to an appropriate level of rehabilitation to facilitate function at a minimum level of dependency and optimise their quality of life, regardless of life expectancy.
- The challenge increases with disease progression; the physiotherapist can help the patient and carers decide which activities they can realistically perform, within the limits of energy, safety and capabilities and can assist them to devise a strategy for the future.
- The physiotherapist's role is to help the patient adapt to their changing condition and anticipate and prepare for any likely disease progression, while maintaining hope.
- In oncology and palliative care, mobility problems may arise for many reasons. They may be:
- Related to the illness
- Related to the treatment for the illness
- Related to debility
- A concurrent disorder.
- Due to the diversity of the presenting problems, a range of techniques may be employed to address the various aspects of mobility problems which may include:
- Active exercise
- Gait re-education (including the use of orthoses or walking aids)

- Analysis of movement and posture
- Normal movement techniques
- Pain management
- Lymphoedema management
- Balance training
- Activity pacing
- Fatigue management
- Transfer practice
- Wheelchair assessment
- Skin care
- Education of family and carers regarding moving and handling techniques
- Referral on to other agencies as appropriate.

- Where possible it is advisable to liaise closely with an occupational therapist to ensure an optimum outcome for the patient.

- A wide range of mobility aids are available to meet the diverse needs of this client group and the selection of the appropriate device is essential. This should be based on:

- The type of assistance needed, for example, to reduce weight bearing for the relief of pain, or to correct balance
- The overall physical and cognitive abilities
- The care setting in which the device will be used.

- It is important to review the suitability of mobility aids regularly to ensure that they continue to meet the patient's current needs.

- The physiotherapist should plan for likely disease progression and deterioration in order that the necessary equipment is in place in a timely fashion.

- As deterioration occurs, the patient may need greater assistance to maintain their functional ability.

- At some point, the focus on function will diminish and comfort will become the priority.

- For further information see the mobility and loss of function rehabilitation pathway (NCAT 2009b) available online.

Fatigue

- Cancer-related fatigue (CRF) is a complex multifactorial but common symptom of cancer patients in all phases of treatment, recovery, advancing disease and palliative care.

- It has been described as a common persistent and subjective sense of tiredness related to cancer or to treatment for cancer that interferes with usual functioning and 70–100% of cancer patients suffer with CRF (Lundh Hagelin 2006).

- Education and information about cancer-related fatigue should be given to the patient as early as possible, ideally prior to treatment commencing, with the aim of reducing any potential distress and frustration that fatigue may cause.

- It must be remembered that fatigue is often the first sign of ill health and specifically in cancer sufferers a potential indicator of disease status and therefore can induce fear and anxiety.

Fatigue management advice

- It is important for all healthcare professionals to be able to identify cancer-related fatigue and be able to supply basic advice and written material about the condition.
- Macmillan information sheets on cancer-related fatigue are freely available for download or hard copies can be ordered from the website and this is an excellent source of information for patients. *www.macmillan.org.uk*
- The same principles can also be adopted for patients with non-malignant conditions who are suffering fatigue.
- Educate the patient about the importance of food as a fuel.
- If eating is difficult liaise with dietetic colleagues or the MDT about nutritional supplements.
- Consider complex syndromes such as cachexia which can have a marked effect on muscle mass and exercise tolerance and the importance of dietetic input for this condition.
- Teach patients the five P's of energy conservation
- Plan – always try to plan ahead
- Pace – your activities, i.e. do a bit, rest a bit
- Prioritise – what's important
- Posture – think about your position, could you sit and do it
- Permission – should you do it, delay it, delegate it, or dump it.
- Fatigue can be considerable during the first 72 hours post chemotherapy.
- The effects of both chemotherapy and radiotherapy are cumulative, so mild to moderate intensity exercise is appropriate.
- The programme should incorporate a cardiovascular component such as walking in conjunction with targeted strengthening exercises and monitored progress.
- Exercise should be timed so as not to exacerbate symptoms of treatment.

Long-term patients and fatigue

- The patient on long-term follow up who has completed treatment and who is still suffering fatigue often has a poor understanding of the long-term effects of treatment.
- Their aims and expectations of activity are often unrealistic and a negotiated exercise plan with short- and longer-term goals needs to be negotiated.
- This should target weakened areas, include aerobic exercise and a gradual increase in intensity and duration.

Fatigue and palliative care

- Fatigue in palliative care patients is often complex with hourly or daily variations.
- Thus exercise must be safe and relevant to the symptoms, involving close liaison with the MDT.
- The exercises should be aimed at prevention of loss and maintenance of functional ability and will help to give a positive focus for the patient and family.
- For further detail see the fatigue and energy management rehabilitation pathway NCAT (2009c) available online.

Specific conditions and interventions in oncology and palliative care

Bone metastases

- Bone metastases or 'bone mets' are a common finding in certain advanced cancers, particularly breast, prostate, lung and kidney (Cancer Research UK 2008).

- When cancer cells spread to the bone, they commonly lodge in the spine, rib cage, pelvis, limbs and skull. These cells can damage the bone and this may give rise to a number of different symptoms.

- Patients will often have localised pain in the affected area, but this may be referred. Initially, it may come and go and may be worse at night.

- However, it is important to note that not all pain indicates metastasis. In some cases a bone affected by metastasis may become weakened as the process of bone remodelling is destroyed. This is seen particularly in the femur and humerus, which can be at risk of fracture. In some cases this is the first sign of bone metastasis.

- Bone metastases are also common in the spine and can lead to risk of metastatic spinal cord compression (MSCC). Although caution must be taken with a patient diagnosed with, or at high risk of developing bone metastases, physiotherapy intervention is not contraindicated (Crevenna et al 2003).

- Treatment planning must be on an individual basis and aim to design a programme that combines safety and bone protection strategies, i.e. use of bisphosphonates which slow the bone damage caused by metastasis (Ramaswamy and Shapiro 2003). It is important to use mobility and strengthening goals where appropriate. There is very little research on the topic of physiotherapy and bone metastases therefore research on breast and prostate cancer and osteoporosis provide the best evidence (Schwartz et al 2007).

- Maintaining mobility is important for many patients and the risks and benefits must be considered in full consultation with the patient and MDT.

- It is also important to work alongside other treatment regimens such as radiotherapy. This is often a treatment choice which is useful in relieving pain and controlling the growth of the tumour cells in the particular area (Fairchild et al 2010).

Lymphoedema

- Lymphoedema may occur as a result of the treatment of a tumour due to accumulation of fluid and other elements (e.g. protein) in tissue spaces, due to an imbalance between interstitial fluid production and transport (usually a low output failure).

- Lymphoedema may manifest as swelling of one or more limbs and may include the corresponding quadrant of the trunk.

- Swelling may also affect other areas, e.g. head and neck, breast and genitalia.

- Lymphoedema treatment may incorporate several aspects of care and the emphasis is for self management as far as possible.

- These include skin care, exercise, simple lymphatic drainage (SLD) and compression and are termed the four cornerstones of care.

Skin care

- Daily skin care to maintain healthy skin is essential and patients are advised to moisturise 1-2 times daily with appropriate emollients treating any cuts or grazes to prevent infection.

Exercise

- A system of isotonic exercises, working proximally to distally.

SLD

- A gentle specific massage technique to improve lymphatic flow, which the patient can do for themselves or which can be carried out by a carer.

Compression

- Suitable compression garments will be measured by a lymphoedema practitioner if appropriate and should be worn as prescribed.

Specialist intervention

- Specialist intervention may be required for larger or more problematic lymphoedema and may include manual lymphatic drainage (MLD), multi-layer lymphoedema bandaging (MLLB), kinesiotaping and, rarely, intermittent pneumatic compression.
- Kinesiotaping is a taping method that can substantially aid lymphoedema by increasing the body's ability to drain lymphatic fluid to healthy lymph nodes, i.e. specifically aid lymphatic drainage. Please refer to kinesiotaping UK online for further information.

Palliative care

- In palliative care the focus of treatment depends on symptom relief and quality of life and therefore appropriate interventions should be used such as light support bandages rather than compression hosiery.

Role of the physiotherapist

- The physiotherapist should reinforce lymphoedema prevention and can initiate simple treatments to alleviate some of the physical problems associated with lymphoedema supporting the agreed management plan prescribed by the lymphoedema practitioner.
- Basic advice such as good skin care should be promoted, with regular moisturising using gentle upward strokes to help reduce the risk of infection.
- Wearing compression hosiery should be advised if prescribed and especially worn during exercise and regular SLD encouraged.
- The lymphoedema patient, however, often has associated problems such as muscle weakness, joint stiffness, complex scarring, poor posture and pain and is often fearful of exercising.
- The physiotherapist is ideally placed to offer advice and treatment for postural correction, positioning, scar work, range of movement, myofascial release, and to promote normal activity.
- The physiotherapist should be aware of the general guidelines on exercise as recommended by the lymphoedema framework.

- Patients may find the physical symptoms of lymphoedema impact on body image and may raise fears of recurrence.
- They present with confidence issues, anxiety and low mood. Our core physiotherapy skills can have a positive impact on effective self management by improving associated symptoms and by working within the MDT to promote effective self care.

Metastatic spinal cord compression (MSCC)

- MSCC is an oncological emergency, requiring precise assessment of symptoms, urgent investigations and immediate treatment.
- The physiotherapist must have an understanding of cord compression to enable a thorough assessment and to devise an accurate treatment plan.
- Rehabilitation for patients with MSCC improves functional outcomes and patients who achieve high functional gains may have better survival (Tang et al 2007).

Spinal cord compression checklist

- The physiotherapist may use a similar checklist to the one in Table 12.2 to assure a consistent and thorough assessment and treatment plan.

Table 12.2 Example of a treatment checklist
Treatment
Passive/assisted/active exercise
TA stretches
Calf massage
Specific stretches
Respiratory monitoring and management
Assisted cough
Progression of sitting
Advice to patient of symptoms to be aware of
Reporting to nursing staff
Close monitoring with baseline assessment
Rolling
Sitting over edge of bed through rolling
Lying to sitting
Sitting balance assessment and exercise
Sitting to standing as appropriate
Ambulation as appropriate
Provision of walking aids as appropriate
Sliding board transfers as appropriate (straight/downhill/uphill/car)
Wheelchair skills as appropriate
Pressure lifts as appropriate
Upper limb strengthening work

During and post treatment (depending on spinal stability)

- Education, information and support.
- Improve muscle power/strength.
- Facilitate progression from flat bed rest to 60° position.
- Facilitate bed mobility and transfer out of bed.
- Improve sitting/standing balance.
- Facilitate independent transfers where possible with the use of equipment if necessary.
- Assessment of home and provision of equipment.
- Gait re-education.
- Progression of functional activity to maximise independence.
- Educate regarding the use of a wheelchair if necessary.
- Encourage independence in activities of daily living (ADLs).
- Facilitate management of anxiety, relaxation.
- Educate and support regarding fatigue management and pacing of activities.
- Education and support regarding long-term use of collar/brace if required.
- Patients with MSCC require ongoing support and rehabilitation following their initial inpatient programme.
- For those patients who retain or regain mobility they will require follow up to aim to progress this further and to enable physiotherapists in the community setting to be aware of these patients in case of deterioration or recurrence.
- For wheelchair-bound patients they will need monitoring to maintain transfer and bed mobility abilities and to maintain ROM and upper limb strength.
- For patients who are less well and may be transferred to hospice services, they should have access to physiotherapy for rehabilitation to maintain quality of life in whatever way is appropriate for each individual patient.
- It is essential that physiotherapists in the acute setting refer this group of patients on to community teams to ensure continuity of care and maximal opportunity for functional and quality of life improvement or maintenance.
- It is imperative to monitor for signs of deterioration even in the rehabilitation phase as it could be an indicator of compression at another level of spinal instability.
- Therefore, ongoing assessment is an essential part of the intervention stage.
  Please refer to the NICE Malignant spinal cord compression guidelines (2008) for further information. A flowchart for decisions about the timing and safety of mobilisation is shown in Figure 12.1.

Brain and central nervous system tumours

- There are two main types of brain tumour, primary and secondary (metastatic).
- They are not common, accounting for less than 2% of all cancer diagnoses in the UK.
- Primary brain tumours are those which arise in the brain itself and secondary (metastatic) brain tumours are the result of spread of disease from another site.
- Patients can present with a variety of symptoms dependent on the type, location and nature of the tumour. They also have the potential to change very quickly, particularly the high-grade primary brain tumours.

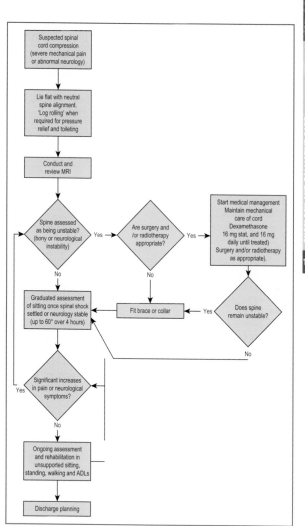

Figure 12.1 Flow chart for decisions about the timing and safety of mobilisation once MSCC suspected.

- Treatment for a patient with a brain or central nervous system tumour will focus on the impairments found during the assessment process, in the same way as for a patient with a CVA or spinal cord injury for example.
- The main difference will be to consider the levels of fatigue or pain that the patient may be experiencing, as well as the psychological impact of the diagnosis.
- Dependent on your assessment findings, the actual treatments will be similar to those used in any neurological condition and may include:
- Proprioceptive rehabilitation
- Sitting and standing balance rehabilitation
- Gait re-education
- Strengthening programmes
- Transfer practice including lying to sitting, sit to stand or alternative transfers
- Wheelchair mobility
- Encouraging independence in functional activities and ADLs
- Assisting the patient in returning to vocational activities and hobbies.

Plexopathy

- Tumour infiltration or as a result of disease progression and radiation injury are the most common causes of plexopathy in oncology and palliative care (Reddy 2006).
- Symptoms include pain, loss of motor control, sensory deficits and an overall deterioration in function.
- Treatments should be based on the findings of the assessment.
- While pain management is usually the most urgent symptom to be addressed, it may be appropriate to use range of movement exercises/stretches, postural correction, advice on skincare and splinting to promote comfort and minimise further deterioration.

Peripheral neuropathy

- In people with cancer, peripheral neuropathy is usually caused by damage to nerves from surgery, radiation treatment, or chemotherapy.
- It can also be caused by a tumour pressing on or penetrating a nerve.
- Chemotherapy-induced peripheral neuropathy as a result of neurotoxicity is a complication most commonly associated with the cytotoxic drugs vinca alkaloids, platinum-based compounds and taxols and the degree of reversibility is variable.
- Treatment should be focused on the relief of pain, strengthening weak muscles, facilitating movement, maximising function and independence and preventing further complications.
- It may be necessary to provide assistive devices and adaptive equipment to support the patient's independence.
- It is important to highlight to the patient the potential safety risks associated with sensory dysfunction.

Progressive neurological conditions

- Many patients with progressive neurological conditions will have palliative care needs, most commonly those diagnosed with more aggressive conditions such as motor neuron disease (MND), multiple systems atrophy (MSA) and progressive supranuclear palsy (PSP).
- However, patients with other conditions such as multiple sclerosis and Parkinson's disease should also access palliative care services towards the end of their disease process or if there are complex symptom management issues.
- Treatment will be based on the findings of the physiotherapy assessment but should be based on goals set with the patient and focus on function.
- It is important to consider fatigue management and pacing with this group of patients and educate them about the balance between activity and rest.
- With many patients with aggressive neurological conditions, the physiotherapist should educate the patient that functional activities can be considered part of their exercise routine and that they should not be doing traditional exercise programmes at the expense of being able to function.
- It is also important to consider liaison with the acute or community sector regarding this group of patients as they will often have been receiving input from these services prior to referral to palliative care.

MND

- MND is a progressive neurodegenerative disease that affects the upper and lower motor neurons leading to weakness and wasting of muscle, loss of mobility and difficulties with speech, swallowing and breathing.
- MND has an incidence of 2 per 100 000.
- It is important for the patient to understand the nature of the disease and that the affected muscles cannot be strengthened.
- This must be balanced by providing positive information regarding using equipment to compensate and simple exercises to maintain remaining strength as much as possible.
- Patients should always be advised on a stretching regime to avoid muscle and joint stiffness.
- Mobility will often be affected at some stage of the disease and walking aids may not be useful if hand function is poor.
- Therefore, the physiotherapist will have to be adaptable and often inventive to maintain a patient's mobility for as long as possible and close liaison with colleagues, particularly the occupational therapist, will be vital.
- Respiratory management will often be key, including teaching deep breathing exercises and assisted cough techniques.
- It may also be appropriate to provide orthotics and splinting, such as orthoses for foot drop and neck collars.

MSA

- MSA is a progressive neurological condition caused by degeneration of neurons in the basal ganglia, cerebellum and brain stem causing problems with movement, balance and autonomic functions.
- MSA has an incidence of 5 per 100 000.

- Patients should be provided with a stretching regime and techniques or equipment to maintain mobility and movement.
- Patients will often have postural hypotension and the physiotherapist can provide education on how to manage this.
- As the condition progresses, respiratory and secretion management may become more important.

PSP

- PSP is a degenerative brain disease affecting eye movement, balance, mobility, speech and swallowing due to degeneration of neurons mainly in the basal ganglia and brainstem.
- PSP has an incidence of 5.3 per 100 000, although many patients are initially misdiagnosed with Parkinson's disease.
- Patients may require advice and equipment to maintain mobility and prevent falls.
- These patients will often have balance problems and a tendency to fall backwards.
- They will require a stretching regime and strength maintenance programme. Respiratory care will also be important.

Problems associated with presenting conditions

Pain

- Pain can be described as 'an unpleasant sensory or emotional experience associated with actual or potential tissue damage, or described in terms of such damage' (IASP 1994).
- It is a complex phenomenon, which is the culmination of several factors, which may be physical or non-physical.
- The aim of treatment is to relieve pain, where possible, and to improve function and quality of life, using evidence-based techniques.
- A patient-centred approach which involves family and carers will facilitate goal setting and treatment planning.
- The physiotherapist can utilise a range of interventions, including therapeutic exercise, positioning, graded and purposeful activity, postural re-education, the use of appropriate moving and handling techniques, massage, soft tissue mobilisation, transcutaneous electrical nerve stimulation (TENS), the use of heat and cold packs, relaxation or coping strategies.
- In addition, cognitive behavioural therapy (CBT) techniques or acupuncture may be useful.
- The education of the patient, family, carers and other professionals is another important role that should not be overlooked.
- The management of pain requires a multidisciplinary approach and the physiotherapist must ensure that other members of the team are involved as necessary to help manage physical, psychological and spiritual aspects of pain.
- The concept of total pain is particularly important in the palliative care setting and emphasises the importance of a team approach, this concept is demonstrated in Figure 12.2.

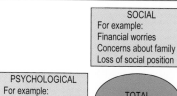

Figure 12.2 Total pain diagram.

Range of movement problems

- Decreased range of movement (ROM) at any joint in the body can occur as a result of surgery, side effects from treatment, deconditioning, the disease itself or a combination of many factors.
- Active ROM exercises can help build up or keep muscles as strong as possible. They can help keep joints flexible.
- Performing ROM exercises will facilitate blood flow to the joint area that is being exercised and may also help prevent blood clots such as DVT, especially if the patient is bed-bound.
- The key principles of exercise prescription include:
- An individualised programme based on comprehensive assessment
- Focusing on maintenance and/or improvement at relevant stages of the pathway
- Concentrating on all aspects of fitness
- Working towards goals identified by the patient
- Regular reviews and reassessment.

Cording

- Lymphatic cording or axillary web syndrome (AWS) can appear after axillary node dissection with breast surgery (Tilley et al 2009).
- Cording refers to a ropelike structure that develops mainly under the axilla but can extend to involve the medial aspect of the ipsilateral arm down to the cubital fossa and even to the base of the thumb.
- These cords often typically reduce range of movement of the shoulder and can be painful for the individual, restricting activities of daily living.

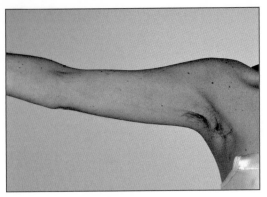

Figure 12.3 Cording in the upper limb.

- There is very little evidence to guide physiotherapists to the correct treatment, however a range of techniques have been suggested in a paper by Fourie and Robb (2009). This involves soft tissue massage with the patient in supine and with the affected arm at the limit of abduction.

- Stretches combined with passive and active exercise regime will also aid recovery. An example of cording is shown in Figure 12.3.

- Seromas can sometimes present following breast surgery and this is a collection of body fluid in the tissues.

- If there is a waterbed-like feature around the scar area the physiotherapists should refer the patient back to the breast care nurse for further assessment. The exercise regime and advice may need to be modified and adapted for the individual patient to avoid increasing pain levels.

- Following surgery connective tissue can often become tight and create a feeling of resistance, this can then reduce shoulder mobility.

- The aim of scar massage is to produce a strong, mobile scar (Rankin et al 2008). Once again, there is little evidence available for the correct treatment of scar massage. Fourie (2006) suggests that tissue mobilisation will encourage the alignment of collagen fibres along the lines of stress, thereby reducing the cross-link bonds responsible for the restriction of gliding planes. Massage is also thought to reduce scar hypersensitivity by stimulating regeneration of nerve endings.

- It is essential that throughout all treatment sessions the physiotherapist fully informs and educates the patient as to the reasons for the specific intervention. This should ensure better patient compliance and speed up the recovery process.

Summary

- Physiotherapy treatment in oncology and palliative care should be conducted on an individual basis and is dependent on a number of factors.

- Treatment approaches from other areas of physiotherapy practice, such as neurology and respiratory care, are often appropriate for this group of patients with the main consideration being the awareness of other factors specific to this specialty such as fatigue, pain and metastases.

- The psychological and spiritual factors of this group of patients also play a significant part in treatment planning and their importance should not be underestimated.

The references for this chapter can be found on www.expertconsult.com.

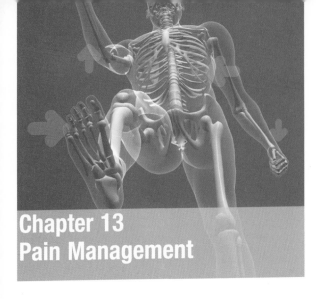

Chapter 13
Pain Management

Once assessment has established the type of pain the patient is experiencing, priorities and interventions can be determined and directed at those factors contributing to pain, distress, disability or reduced quality of life.

Acute pain relief

Despite substantial advances in pain research in recent decades, inadequate acute pain control is still more the rule than the exception. Numerous studies show that fewer than half of postoperative patients receive adequate pain relief ... The 2010–2011 campaign, with its theme of 'Anticipate, Assess, Alleviate', aims to improve acute pain management worldwide.

IASP 2010 Global Year Against Acute Pain.

Drug therapy

Patients who have been injured or undergone surgery will have nociceptive input that requires analgesia. Successfully treating acute pain markedly reduces the likelihood of chronic pain developing. While adequate comparison trials between drug and non-drug methods have been neither supported by drug companies nor performed, experienced therapists know that non-drug methods may be as effective as analgesics, and that *both* should always be used.

Therapeutically effective analgesia should also be given in the form that is most likely to ensure maximum placebo effect. Analgesia must satisfy the brain's desire for an adequate treatment that will allow it to reduce the synaptic strength and connectivity within the CNS supporting the pain state (Wall 1999, Roche 2002).

Many physiotherapists have limited or no prescribing rights but they can support the health care team in ensuring that:

- Prescribing, giving and timing of adequate analgesia facilitates effective physical treatment. Analgesia should be at a level where there is no pain or a level of discomfort that the patient considers manageable.

- Patients with pain on movement following a period of inactivity and tissue stasis receive adequate analgesia prior to initiating the movement. Linking aversive levels of pain to movement can mean anticipation and fear of pain becomes more powerful than the pain itself; preventing patients fully participating in treatment that itself reduces pain.

- Those who regularly take analgesia or other psychoactive drugs like alcohol may require higher doses. If this is suspected during activity, the physiotherapist can discuss this with the patient's prescriber.

- Care is taken that patients do not take doses that put kidney or liver function at risk. Before requesting postoperative non-steroidal anti-inflammatory drugs (NSAIDs) or larger doses of opiates check creatinine levels and look closely at the past medical history (PMH).

- Great care is taken with the elderly. Do not use NSAIDs or larger doses of opiates with the over 70s. Relatively moderate doses of opiates or accumulating levels over time can precipitate acute confusion and permanent deterioration in memory and function, particularly in those who are not accustomed to them.

- Local and epidural anaesthetic blocks are used to help reduce or stop local pain. They enable rehabilitation despite severe pain that is less responsive to analgesics, or when a patient's condition means therapeutic doses cannot be tolerated or are unsafe. New products including improved local anaesthetic patches and creams are becoming available all the time. Experienced staff may be able to advise you on what is available for your patients.

- Patients who don't like taking 'drugs' and normally take as little as possible are encouraged not to let analgesics wear off before the next dose. Remind them: taking medication regularly in the early stages means taking less in the future; simple analgesics, even morphine, do little harm in therapeutic doses.

- If you suspect that patients are taking more than prescribed due to forgetfulness or multiple sources, e.g. over the counter and alcohol as well as prescribed, they must be warned of the risks, non-drug methods promoted, fears (which often encourage analgesia use) addressed, and the physician informed.

- Ensure paracetamol is given as well as opioid-based medication; it is a powerful painkiller. As it is an over-the-counter analgesia, patients often believe it is 'mild', ineffective for more severe problems. This is not the case. Care is needed to ensure the maximum daily dose is not exceeded. Care is also required for patients who take paracetamol and any analgesia on a regular and prolonged basis since these are associated with chronic medication-withdrawal headaches.

Non-drug therapy

For all patients, whether inpatient or at home, the use of non-drug methods to reduce pain and its impact, in addition to medication, should be promoted. See Box 13.1.

Physical activity: our most potent pain reducer and aid to rehabilitation

In addition to acting on the musculoskeletal, cardiovascular, respiratory and endocrine systems, physical activity and function have an impact on the brain. Input and output to the sensory and motor cortex are sustained so that the representation of

---

Box 13.1 Non-drug methods to reduce pain and its impact

- Cold or heat for injuries. Heat can be used for muscle spasm, but not in the presence of a significant healing response or inflammation. Sometimes both heat and cold can be used alternately

- Activities and conversations as distraction

- Friends, neighbours and relatives can offer reminders to limit exertion and to encourage moderate activity. The meaning of 'appropriate rest' must be understood so they don't assume it means doing nothing

- Acupuncture, may provide a powerful placebo effect for many patients. It can be worth exploring for the individual patient as an aid to rehabilitation and to assist night-time sleep

- Keep the 'pain gates' closed as far as possible:

- Avoiding keeping still for long periods including night times (a full bladder has its uses!)

- Use brief, rhythmical, relaxed movement of the muscles and joints of the affected part between short rest periods, e.g.:

  - Rocking in a rocking chair

  - Pendular movements of the arm, leg, hand or foot

  - Shoulder rolling; 'nodding dog' head movement

  - Gentle trunk rotation, hip hitching, stomach pull-ins

- If a part is too painful to move initially, advise on movements of other parts of the body before the most painful area, e.g. move the neck, shoulders and hips before the painful back

- Don't prevent weight-bearing unless there is very good reason to. If paced, it reduces pain and swelling and increases confidence. Encourage smooth, gentle, relaxed walking for legs and spine, as 'limp-free' as possible; gentle pushing movements for arms. Any walking aids should have a clear wean-off programme initiated from the start to reduce future pain and disability (plus minimising loss of confidence and dependence)

---

peripheral parts in the cortices is kept as normal as possible. The CNS production of pain-reducing endorphins and antidepressant monoamines is enhanced and production and impact of glucocorticoid stress hormones reduced (Duclos et al 2003). Exercise may also act as a coping mechanism and help divert patients away from negative thoughts (Box 13.2).

Understanding and accepting or making judgements?

Pain may be unexpectedly more or less than expected for the injury experienced, and can wax and wane over time in ways that may not always be predictable (Cronje and Williamson 2006). Patients can find this disconcerting and concerning, causing them to doubt what the health professional tells them about their condition. Health professionals have a tendency to underestimate or misidentify patients' pain, some assume that if a patient is smiling they can't be in pain (Kappesser and Williams 2002). Is this accurate, fair or reasonable?

Measurement of pain alone does not indicate understanding, belief or empathy. Patients frequently report feeling they have not been believed. To say 'it can't be that bad' demonstrates a complete lack of understanding of:

> **Box 13.2** Physical activity after surgery or injury: advice you can give to your patient
>
> ### Immediately
>
> - Calm the pain down using 'pain gate-closing' activities 'little and often' with frequent short rests for 2 days
> - Reduce overall activity and rest between activities, particularly for the first 2 days, avoiding complete rest
> - Relax muscles when resting and whilst moving
> - Walking is the best pain-reliever, breathing exercise and basic function to support the body in recovery
> - If a part feels strangely painful, weird or numb, keep touching, stroking, pressing and massaging around the area. Watch yourself doing this; it assists the brain to keep 'in touch' with the body
>
> ### After 2 days
>
> Gradually move and do more to:
>
> - Improve the circulation and aid healing
> - Strengthen and stretch healing tissues
> - Don't avoid normal daily activities – do tiny amounts if it's very painful initially
> - Work other parts of the body including heart and lungs as normal; focus on weight bearing
> - Reduce muscle spasm, checking muscles are as relaxed as possible when in use. If muscle tension/spasm builds, take more frequent rest breaks
> - Don't let chronic pain develop: move regularly, use and touch the injured part, building up to normal use, including a graded return to work or simulated work activities
>
> ### From 2 weeks
>
> - Prevent scar tissue tightening: massage external scars; stretch internal scars
> - Continue to build activity. Remodelling processes respond to use: challenge them in the chronic healing stages
> - Keep searching for physical concerns/fears as a result of your injury or its context: face them in a gradual and graded way with guidance

- Pain and its behaviour.
- Other contributing factors such as fear or frustration.

Saying to a patient that 'it can't be that bad' can lead to a downward spiral of the patient trying to demonstrate how strong their pain is, coupled with stronger beliefs by the health professional that they are making a fuss. This results in a breakdown in therapeutic alliance.

A more helpful alternative may be to take the opportunity to consider 'I wonder why this patient is behaving like that; why I find this unexpected?'

Physiotherapists are in a unique position since they treat patients in pain in different contexts to other professionals and may therefore pick up factors about patients' pain that others do not. They are also trained in pain neurophysiology and pain management, so can be a good ally for patients in providing explanations about their pain. They can alert other health professionals when further investigation is required or an exploration of patients' past experiences or home situations are needed.

What should/could I do when the patient has red flags?

These are indicators of serious pathology, and the appropriate medical practitioner should be informed as a matter of urgency. Remember that the patient still has pain and requires management for this. They can still be given advice on pain relief and gentle mobilisation.

Hypersensitivity pain states masquerading as acute pain: have faith!

The difference between acute (nociceptive) pain associated with injury or disease and overuse symptoms can be difficult for patients to understand, particularly in patients experiencing episodic neuropathic pain conditions, e.g. low back pain (LBP) or headaches. The tendency to central hypersensitivity will make unaccustomed use symptoms more painful. The presentation of masquerading conditions can be puzzling to lay people, making them fearful of their tissue strength and of instigating appropriate pain management involving movement.

The way that society has publicly managed pain in the past is partly responsible for the development of these behaviours. While professional practice is improving in this area, patients are all too often given inappropriate walking aids for simple sprains, or supports for the back/neck. When aids are provided patients need to know how and when to wean themselves from these.

Patients need to understand the appropriate management of acute pain and chronic hypersensitivity. With no signs of tissue damage, frequent movements, interspersed with brief rest periods can be instigated immediately. Patients need evidence of the strength of their tissues and to appreciate that pain is not a sign of damage: helping them learn from their own experience is vital.

Preventing chronic pain and disability

Addressing key risk factors: flags

Shaw and colleagues' (2005) early risk factors help focus the treatment plan for yellow flags.

Patients with increased pain affecting sleep despite analgesia

All appropriate methods of attaining pain relief, both drug and non-drug therapies should be discussed with such patients. Benzodiazepines should only be used temporarily: they prevent sleep beyond 2 weeks' use.

Practical advice on managing pain at night may help, e.g. maintenance of through-night analgesia, position changes, and movement in or out of bed. Advice on using pillows to support fractures/injuries can be invaluable. Nerve blocks to help achieve sleep should be supported where needed.

What a patient does or doesn't do in the daytime will influence the night. Daytime naps, particularly beyond lunchtime/early afternoon are disruptive to the body clock and sleep. Equally, being overactive in the daytime can increase pain, so that when the body finally rests, sleep will be prevented. Crawford (http://www.painconcern. org.uk/2011/04/leaflets/a-good-nights-sleep) gives good advice on sleep hygiene.

Belief that pain is harmful or potentially disabling

Beliefs about pain can influence behaviour and inhibit healing and recovery, e.g. the assumption that the severity of pain relates to the severity of injury. This can escalate to avoiding painful movements and reduced function on the assumption that activity will inhibit healing or recovery, when in fact the opposite is usually the case.

Fear of pain is more disabling than the pain itself (Waddell 1998, Crombez et al 1999).

Information and patient experience are important factors for reducing fear. Information that may help patients includes:

- The time limit of inflammation for their particular injury (maximum 7 days) and the expected healing process (maximum 3 months). Don't mistake hypersensitivity for inflammation; pain doesn't mean it hasn't healed.

- An explanation of acute and chronic pain: input about the original damage is altered by central processing; how hypersensitivity develops (http://www.ppip.org.uk/viewdocuments.aspx; Butler and Moseley 2003).

- An explanation of diagnoses such as 'degeneration', 'black or bulging discs' (normal age-related changes) set in the context of pain-free populations with identical findings.

- The fact that epidemiologically the incidence of severe spinal pain and sciatica becomes increasingly less likely beyond the age of 50.

- The body's ability to regenerate and improve the health of its tissues with the right conditions.

Intensive neurophysiology education for LBP patients can produce significant improvements in reported function and self-efficacy and physical performance tasks (SLR and forward bending range) (Moseley et al 2004). Information alone does not change behaviour for all patients (Fordyce 1976, Muncey 2002a). It is important that patients learn to change previous beliefs through actual, disconfirming experience.

Fear-avoidance behaviour from fear of pain or fear of harm/causing damage to tissues

Continuing avoidance of pain-provoking activities is a strong risk factor for chronicity and is best tackled pre-emptively when administering acute treatment and advice (e.g. Fordyce et al 1986).

Vlaeyen and colleagues (1995, 2000) proposed a model of fear-avoidance, finding that exposure (the treatment of choice for phobias) is also effective for fear-avoidance related to pain disability (Figure 13.1).

Each time a situation and associated anxiety is avoided it becomes more likely that avoidance will occur the next time the situation or activity occurs. Avoidance is reinforced by the feeling of anxiety reduction. Therefore avoidance can occur repeatedly in the long term with patients becoming convinced that they cannot cope in such situations.

By avoiding feared movements or feelings patients fail to learn:

- How to cope with difficult situations.

- That anxious feelings do not increase to the point where they lose control or something terrible happens.

If fear-avoidance is present or developing it should be tackled immediately. Beliefs contributing to avoidance are explored and patients guided to try small amounts of the avoided activities, gradually building up in a systematic rather than pain-dependent way. Patients then need to consider all movements or activities they continue to avoid. Some forms of avoidance can be subtle, e.g. continuing to follow doctors' advice rigidly and for longer than necessary when it promotes avoidance; not accepting challenges; talking about activity rather than actually doing it.

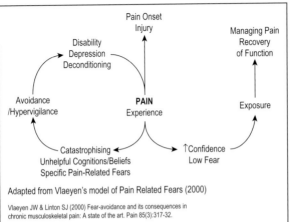

Figure 13.1 Model of fear-avoidance. *Adapted from Vlaeyen J.W.S. and Linton S.J., 2000. Fear-avoidance and its consequences in musculoskeletal pain: a state of the art. Pain 85, 317–322. This figure has been reproduced with permission of the International Association for the Study of Pain® (IASP®). The information may not be reproduced for any other purpose without permission.*

Catastrophising

Catastrophising refers to having a negative view of the pain experience, the situation and the future: fearing the worst. Such preoccupation has been identified as a risk factor for pain-related fear and long-term disability.

Example of catastrophising:
'I can't cope with the bus jolting my back, so I won't be able to go to work. My colleagues will think I'm not pulling my weight and get fed up with me, my supervisor will report me to the management and I'll lose my job'.

Physiotherapy management strategies might include:
- Identify patient's beliefs about the cause of their pain and its treatment.
- Explanation to help patients understand their condition.
- Where needed, challenge what patients think, feel and do about their pain.
- Educating patients about graded return to normal activity, in the presence of pain.
- Setting collaborative goal-focussed targets aimed at return to meaningful and rewarding activities.
- Providing information on pacing activity, relaxation and flare-up management.

Overall management should focus on providing the patient with ways to help them regain control over their life, with active strategies to help them maintain or recover lost function.

Low mood due to the consequences of the injury

Physiotherapists will not directly treat depression, they can still have a powerful effect via:

- Increasing activity levels which directly affect mood.
- Ensuring patients feel believed.
- Ensuring patients realise that others with similar injuries recover even though pain may continue for a while.
- Encouraging patients to work towards specific activities/goals that are rewarding and meaningful to them, particularly where they thought these may be unachievable.
- Helping patients develop hope for their future.

If depression is a problem help patients recognise what strategies have helped them manage mood in the past. Assist them in putting together their own plan for when their mood is low in the future. Follow your department's suicide policy to check for risk.

Expectation that passive treatments rather than active participation in therapy would help

Patients report they attend A&E or their doctor frequently, make frequent requests for medication, treatments and therapies. They seem unwilling to take their medication according to prescription, or comply with self-management strategies, e.g. 'When I get this leg pain I usually see a marvellous physio, the manipulation really fixes it. Can you do it too?' Robson and Gifford (2006) help us think about the actual neurobiological effects of manipulation rather than the folklore, but the psychological consequences also need consideration if it appears patients are not expecting anything other than symptomatic treatment and becoming dependent on interventional treatment (Muncey 2002b).

Patients not making expected improvements after 2–4 weeks of treatment for an acute problem

Whilst you should be aware of red flags, most cases taking longer than normal to recover may be influenced by fear of activity or harm. Patients pick up on a therapist's anxiety too, such as when responding to questions about bladder function, tripping and dizziness.

Both therapists and patients need to remember that injuries such as fractures and ligament sprains take quite a considerable time to return to feeling like they did before the injury. While function can return pretty quickly, pain may still be present first thing in the morning, after inactivity, doing something new, and when stressing the part in more challenging ways. This is not a sign of anything more than remodelling and some secondary hypersensitivity. It merely requires ongoing stressing of the collagenous tissues and challenges to the somatosensory cortex.

Patients who have significant difficulty with activities of daily living (ADL) or work for more than 4 weeks

These will be early signs of blue or black flags for which there is strong evidence for LBP (Waddell et al 2008) and whiplash-associated disorders (Burton et al 2009). Provide a strong message about the importance of being at work, and advice about light duties and a paced return to usual work.

> **Box 13.3** Stepped approach to managing musculoskeletal problems
>
> **<2 weeks: support**
> - Advice
> - Symptom control
>
> **2–6 weeks: intervention**
> - Identify psychosocial obstacles
> - Develop a plan for early return to activity and work
>
> **6–12 weeks: progression**
> - Check for ongoing obstacles
> - Expand vocational rehabilitation
>
> **>12 weeks: multidisciplinary approach**
> - Move to cognitive behavioural approach
> - Maximise return to work/activity
>
> **>26 weeks: social solutions**
> - Community support
> - Provide communication channels
> - Avoid unnecessary medical intervention

From www.kendallburton.com

Supporting work maintenance: developing a plan, taking action

Helping people to stay at/return to work requires a simultaneous combination of work-focussed healthcare and an accommodating workplace. Both need to collaborate, communicate and combine information. The imperative is to prevent development of negative psychosocial influences since these reduce workers' ability and willingness to participate in productive activity (Gifford 2006, Shaw et al 2009).

Chronic pain

Patients with established chronic pain may need help in accepting and managing their pain as chronic.

Addressing negative findings

X-rays, scans and blood tests may show normal results related to past resolved pathology and age-related changes. Focussing (without good reason) on speculative hunts for peripheral tissue-based diagnoses or positive tests, rather than acceptance of chronic pain (a CNS function problem) and self-management is detrimental to patients (Haffner 2002). A cure-based focus encourages fear avoidance, poor self management, and development of chronic disability. It is natural to question a new direction when present skills feel inadequate for dealing with it; to feel angry, distressed and to grieve when a past pain-free life is lost. Further despair will come with every negative test or failed treatment.

Rather than seeking more tests, rely on experience of the wide range of 'normal' and of chronic pain, if uncertain, ask a more experienced colleague. A thorough assessment, clinical reasoning and following guidelines is the recommendation, however if you feel concerned, ask for guidance.

Chronic pain management: a biopsychosocial approach

If pain is determined to be chronic, the focus moves from cure to:

- Acceptance of chronic pain.
- Tissue health, rather than cure.
- Building fitness and the self management of chronic pain.

Patients favouring a medical 'fix it' approach can be a challenge for the physio-therapist promoting a self management approach. Employing psychological models and principles of change helps to facilitate rehabilitation, making sense of the patient's predicament and providing possibilities for change and improved function (Harding and Williams 1995).

Disability level in pain patients is more strongly linked to pain beliefs, expectations, coping styles and perceived control, than to pain intensity, chronicity or pathology. This does not mean patients have mental health problems: feeling depressed, anxious, frustrated or angry is to be expected with chronic pain.

Cognitive-behavioural pain management (C-BPM)

C-BPM is a broad group of interventions involving the application of principles derived from the study of behaviour change or learning, and experimental methods to change the ways in which pain sufferers perceive and react to their pain (Bradley 1996, Turk 2002). It requires patients to be active participants in the process rather than passive recipients, helpful in achieving an increased sense of control. It recognises that there are complex interactions among cognitive, affective (emotional) and behavioural change. Positive change in one of these areas may promote positive change in the others.

The methods involve active problem-solving, applying coping skills, and address-ing unhelpful beliefs and responses. Learning to do this through modelling, role playing, or practice with coaching and feedback is almost certain to help patients think of themselves as more able to deal with problems. The key book for health professionals on C-BPM is Main and colleagues (2008); for patients: Nicholas and colleagues (2011).

Chronic pain model

A chronic pain model useful for patients is that of Nicholas. It helps them see the many consequences of having chronic pain, and patients can be helped to expand on this model themselves: looking at their losses (ranging across work, social life, family life, hobbies and sport), unhelpful consequences and the interactions between them. Although chronic pain itself may not be curable, these factors contribute a large proportion of the suffering associated with chronic pain, and are amenable to pain management (Appendix 13.1).

Chronic pain and depression

Considering the on-going nature of chronic pain, it is not surprising that one con-sequence is a high incidence of suicidal thoughts. Suggest that with ongoing pain it is normal to feel depressed, if the response is affirmative, then enquire whether they have thought of harming themselves.

Your unit's suicide prevention policy will give guidance on assessing risk and what to do if patients are feeling suicidal. First, sensitively find out any meaningful reasons they have for not carrying out such thoughts (e.g. my children need me). If a patient can give you no reasons for continuing and has plans for how to end their life, e.g. a medication stockpile, you need to ensure they:

- Are feeling safe to return home.
- Will seek long-term help and know where to obtain this.
- Have a source of emergency help such as a trusted family member or friend; know how to contact the Samaritans if things escalate.

If patients are revealed to be actively suicidal then obtain professional help immediately. You may need to escort them to A&E or a source of psychiatric liaison. Whenever it emerges that patients are significantly depressed, but not currently receiving help from their local mental health team, inform their GP of your findings, incluing the means of suicide if these are revealed to you. You will need to ensure that you receive a debrief after such an event, as it can have an impact on health professionals too.

There is strong evidence that C-BPM has a powerful positive effect on depression due to pain.

Physiotherapists' 'manner' and interaction with patients: facilitating patient change and empowerment

'Helping' patients by providing physical support, being the sole source of information, and always finding solutions for problems results in patients being disempowered and unlikely to maintain improvement beyond treatment. Instead:

- Use active listening skills, asking about their experiences; check you have understood them. Check how your information fits with their understanding and experience.
- Use a collaborative approach, rather than that of an expert.
- Use operant principles when helping patients practise motor skills or make decisions. Make achievements the focus and the route to improvement rather than 'correcting' patients or pointing out what you don't want.
- Empower patients; let them take the credit.
- Place more emphasis on learning through experiment and reassessing past experience.
- Use clinical reasoning as an evolving process; patients have hypotheses too that will alter as assessment and pain management proceeds. Involve them in this process (Jones 1995, Butler 1998).
- Use Socratic Questioning to help patients discover links and answers they need; see they have this within them. If patients say something you disagree with, don't initially say so. 'That's interesting' then later 'I wonder what would happen if….?' Help patients review their initial assumptions.

Pain behaviour and the physiotherapist

Patients may feel that they have not been believed, this presenting as either seeming indifference or in higher levels of pain behaviour and pain talk. Ask the patient: 'A number of patients report they haven't always been believed about their pain. What is your experience?' Many times patients are not aware of the effect of their pain communication: 'Oh, I was just trying to deal with the pain; it's really bad today'. Acknowledging this and emphasising that you believe them and are aware of particularly bad days is immensely helpful.

Patients may assume that physiotherapists will resort to coercion or bullying when they believe a physiotherapist's expectations are more than they can cope with. The undoubted effectiveness of physiotherapy is testimony to physiotherapists' abilities to teach and improve patients' confidence. However, some patients require special handling, e.g. the very anxious, or those frequently reporting that movement or exercise makes the pain worse or unbearable.

Operant learning

On Monday you go into a shop, wait politely, but don't get served.

On Tuesday you go into a shop, bang on the counter and get served straight away. Which behaviour will you tend to use when you go to the shop on Wednesday?

If patients finish a physiotherapy session with a sense of achievement and that the physiotherapist is pleased, they are likely to do their home programme, look forward to the next session and attend well.

If, however, they finish a physiotherapy session in severe pain and the physiotherapist appears indifferent to how hard they have tried, they are likely to leave with a sense of hopelessness and unlikely to return.

This involves using reinforcement following specific behaviours. A reinforcer is defined by its effect on the behaviour it follows and is usually something 'pleasant', appreciated by the individual (praise, attention and interest, a prise). A child's naughtiness can actually be reinforced by smacking if this produces the attention the child craves. Activities that patients learn to do should eventually be reinforcing in themselves, giving a sense of enjoyment, satisfaction or achievement. Until this occurs, patients need reinforcement from other sources to bridge the gap. This may be provided by their physiotherapist, friends or family, or self-provided: rest, chocolate or time alone to play favourite music.

Cairns and Pasino (1977) studied the effects of reinforcement on LBP patients receiving daily measurement of walking and exercise bike distance. Significantly more performance increases were obtained when patients were reinforced (praise and engaging in desirable conversation only if walking or bike riding distance increased over its previous level).

When starting new exercises with patients, physiotherapists will achieve quicker improvement by reinforcing immediately and frequently. Once this has been established, less frequent praise keeps improvement continuing.

Stopping behaviours (e.g. repeatedly talking about pain) is tackled by removing the reinforcers previously sustaining them. Pain is acknowledged not ignored, but the focus is on change despite it. Faster improvement and less anxiety are also seen when patients observe reinforcement being used with other patients.

Avoid criticising the quality of patients' attempts, e.g.:

'Higher with that leg, keep your weight on that buttock, don't let it lift up, that makes you use the wrong muscles and your back twist'

Use reinforcement to achieve more rapid and enduring improvement, e.g.:

'Great, that leg's higher now, you're putting more weight through your right buttock which makes your back straighter. You're coming on really well with that. I think you're ready for the next stage.'

If no improvement can be discerned, reinforcement can still be given to help confidence and aid progression, e.g.:

'That's a difficult exercise for you, you're doing very well to keep trying and I noticed you're still remembering to keep your left arm relaxed as you do it, great'.

Physiotherapists can use varied non-verbal ways of reinforcement, e.g. hand gestures and facial expression, interest or concern. Reinforcement is also a means for learning, e.g. include what you want in your praise: 'your shoulder muscles look so much more relaxed, looser now; that's really good improvement'. This results in more frequent relaxation than 'your shoulders are very tense, try to relax them'. Information is provided about what is appropriate. Curiosity is a powerful drive, so providing information is also itself a reinforcer. This is a subtle process and more details on how to use operant learning are given in Harding (1998).

Many activities eventually become reinforcing in themselves. More naturally reinforcing social goals such as going dancing, joining a yoga group, or using Nintendo Wii Fit as part of a family 'challenge' may strongly help patients prioritise and maintain activity.

Empowerment, problem-solving and self management

Empowering patients and providing them with opportunities to problem-solve and discover solutions is vital if patients are to take an active role. It helps confidence and increases the likelihood that patients will continue after discharge. It is important to encourage patients to use and develop their knowledge and experience, operantly reinforcing this. See Appendix 13.2.

Social or observational learning: modelling

Modelling is an additional technique to help patients regain past motor patterns or learn new ones, e.g. as you walk with them, emphasise the components of a rhythmical relaxed walking pace such as loose back, knee and ankle movement and free arm swing. Use humans' innate ability to imitate behaviour; your movements helping them see what you mean and initiate new behaviours.

Sometimes patients are unaware of their behaviours. When other methods have been unsuccessful, it is sometimes necessary to 'hold up the mirror'. Video-recording of patients' walking can be reviewed with them to see their achievements and identify areas for progression.

Socratic questioning

Socrates used provocative questions to challenge clients' underlying beliefs about themselves. Using Socratic questioning rather than a didactic approach:

- Helps patients feel respected and capable of understanding and working towards a solution for their difficulties.
- Helps patients counteract and challenge negative thoughts/beliefs.
- Trains patients to think differently, enabling them to feel better and more positive about themselves.
- Encourages ownership of the solutions to their problems.

The goal is to teach patients a process of evaluating their goals, thoughts, behaviours, moods, life circumstances and physiological reactions so that they can learn methods for improving the management of their pain problems.

Socratic questioning involves asking patients' questions which:

1. Patients have the knowledge to answer: What are facts; what are simply perceptions? What evidence supports or contradicts those perceptions?

2. Draws patient's attention to information which is relevant to the issue being discussed but which may be outside their current focus: How else can the situation be perceived? How might an acquaintance or family member see it?

3. Generally move from the concrete to the more abstract so that

4. Patients can eventually apply the new information to either re-evaluate a previous conclusion or construct a new idea.

The questions are less about challenging or changing beliefs as guided discovery. Socratic questioning often goes hand in hand with behavioural experiment; further details can be found at http://www.padesky.com/clinicalcorner/pdf/socquest.pdf.

Coping strategies

Physiotherapists can encourage patients to regain purpose by reviewing their desired goals. Refining and using their more helpful coping strategies, challenging less desirable ones, and practicing new ones will ensure they broaden their expectations and achieve wider goals.

Values, goal setting and pacing

Common changes that some people with chronic pain report include:

- Not working.
- Reduced level of housework or DIY.
- No longer easy to do things.
- Decreased pleasurable and social activity.
- Not trying new activities.
- Rest or reclining frequently during the day.
- Sleep problems.

Finding a focus for moving forwards in pain self management is an essential starting point.

Values

Our behaviour is influenced by what values we prioritise; having a chronic condition may lead to loss of core values. Some patients report putting so much time and energy into hunting for pain 'cures' that they lose sight of the important things in their life.

When setting goals identify the values and areas of life that are important to the individual, so that goals can be based on these, e.g.:

- George exercises because he has been told to by a physiotherapist.
- Geoff exercises because he wants to be able to take his son to the park to play football with him.

Who will continue exercising when the going gets tough?

Helping chronic pain patients to examine their values identifies what they care most about and want their life to stand for. Values provide motivation for behaviour change which is more likely to be sustained. Higher success at living in accordance with values correlates with less physical and psychosocial disability, less depression and interference with functioning, and less pain-related anxiety (McCracken and Yang 2006).

Value domains include:

- Social relationships.
- Family relationships.
- Intimate relationships.
- Education/learning.
- Work/career.
- Growth/self-development.
- Recreation/leisure.
- Spirituality.
- Citisenship/community.
- Health/physical well-being.

Values are the overall direction and goals are the end point, e.g. if a patient's value is being a loving attentive parent, a goal might be to go swimming weekly with their daughter.

Goal setting

Having considered values, then turn to the practical goals they would like to achieve in the future. Goals should be determined in terms of what is observable or measurable (e.g. return to specific duties at work, playing football with my son for 30 minutes). Initially longer-term goals for the next 6 months or more will be chosen and preferably from a range of domains: work, hobbies, social, family/relationships. It is essential that pleasurable goals are chosen as well as more work-focussed goals to ensure life-balance is maintained.

The acronym SMARTER (some use SMART) helps the process of goal setting (Appendix 13.3).

It is often necessary to set short-term goals that are achievable to begin with, e.g. returning to work as a self-employed builder may have short-term goals of decorating the living room within a month or fixing my mother-in-law's leaking taps one by one.

Patients must also consider what is preventing them achieve them, e.g. the fear of jarring involved in travelling on a bus, or lifting.

They then try to work out the steps to achieve their goals, breaking them down into their constituent parts. Outcome goals should be set in combination with performance goals (e.g. exercise and building blocks) providing the mechanism by which to achieve final goals.

Principles of pacing activities

Pacing is the steady build-up of an activity whether increasing the numbers of exercises, distance, or the time spent doing an activity or maintaining a static posture.

Using the goal-setting approach links behaviour change and treatment goals to patients' longer-term goals by means of pacing: a systematic and graded approach to building up an activity. This provides time for changes in strength, flexibility and stamina needed to break habits of overactivity/underactivity. Patients push on with activities on better days (the 'danger' days!) then rest/avoid activity when the overactivity has resulted in pain flare-ups, e.g. the back pain patient who goes shopping on a better day, only to find that the less frequently performed activities such as bending and lifting cause a flare-up in the pain prompting 2 or 3 days being very careful or resting to settle it down.

Pain is not a helpful guide as to when to stop, often telling patients to stop too late, or hurting before they have barely started. By setting baselines, then pacing activity, patients learn what is manageable. It is physiologically more astute to work to physical capabilities than rely on sensation that is fickle and influenced by so many different factors. When helping patients return to or improve activities the following basic principles are useful:

- Patients make all decisions and learn principles for future activity, which encourages ownership.
- Make a plan. Prioritise what has to be done on a daily basis.
- Start activities with realistically low 'manageable' baselines, then build up tolerance to the activities gradually and systematically.
- Take regular rests between activities.
- Change position regularly while performing activities.
- Do small amounts often, rather than doing everything at once.
- Avoid long unbroken periods of either activity or rest.

Pacing from modest baselines is incompatible with overactivity/underactivity cycles so helps change this habit.

It is suggested patients: Make two or three measurements of the activity, ideally at different times of the day.

- Set their first baseline as a 'toe in the water' and all with the intention that they are easily manageable, both at the time and for the consequences.

- Find the average of the baseline measurements and start at 80% of this, reducing the risk of starting too high for confidence or the level of provoked pain. It helps to explain to patients that a baseline cannot be set too low since the amount will build up with pacing, but that if they start too high, they will not be able to maintain activity on bad days and will not have learnt to break overdoing or pushing habits. If patients have had a problem for many years there is no need to rush towards achieving high levels of activity or fitness. It is more important patients learn how to do it, since they can then continue the process themselves over a more realistic timespan with confidence.

An adverse response (severe or unmanageable pain or loss of confidence) to a rapid build-up does not favour long-term progress. Be explicit, e.g. 'You have planned to increase to doing three times as much in a week. If you really think that rate is manageable then try it. Remember though that you have a habit of pushing on and aiming high, which has tripped you up in the past. How about trying this new way? It may be more of a challenge for you to do less than to do more. What do you think might happen if you went more slowly?'

If the patient decides to race ahead, then finds it hard to keep going then this is still an opportunity: 'What have you learnt from this? How about going slower and seeing what happens?'

Paced improvement is not always faster or more. Walking very slowly is much more difficult; starting at a more relaxed, natural speed may actually be easier. When walking is difficult and painful, this does not necessarily mean running is even harder; it is occasionally easier to start with running. In C-BPM it is recognised that confidence or, conversely, fear are the main drivers for progress and sense of achievement. The section on graded exposure will demonstrate how a gradual build-up in activity on a fear scale rather than a physical difficulty scale is more effective in returning patients to function and achieving goals.

Set-back plans

Sooner or later patients need to cope with a set-back. Usually pain flare-ups can be managed with a flare-up plan, reminding patients to utilise helpful coping strategies for a difficult day. Sometimes, however, patients feel they cannot manage this; the flare-up is lasting more than a day or two, or they also have an illness, minor injury or family crisis to cope with. Having a plan for set-backs keeps them in control without feeling that their pain has taken over again.

- Help patients put together a set-back for activity and exercise – cutting back, for example, by 50% and building back up in 5 days, or whatever seems appropriate for the problem they are dealing with.

- Encourage prioritisation, but ensure pleasurable activities remain to help them get through.

- Suggest a flare-up box, e.g. enjoyable DVD/CD, inspiring letter, or engrossing book as a reward for keeping going with their plan. Include reminders: what are the usual risks, how to combat these; ring a supportive friend.

Goal setting has a central role within rehabilitation and C-BPM. This chapter can only touch the surface. More, very readable and practical, insight into goal setting and its process has been written by Gladwell (2006).

Relaxation

Relaxation training involves helping patients learn ways of calming themselves and reducing muscle tension, either by listening to a prerecorded CD or following spoken or written instructions. Patients follow the instruction from memory for everyday situations.

Advice for patients includes:

- Reserve specific, undisturbed times of the day, e.g. negotiate with/tell the family, switch off the phone.
- Begin to learn relaxation techniques using comfortable postures initially, whether sitting or various lying positions.
- Wear comfortable loose clothes.
- Be realistic; don't expect to grasp the skill quickly or completely. Regular practice will make a difference.
- Try out a range of skills. While one or two techniques may come more naturally, persist in practicing a range: backups for challenging circumstances.
- Practise techniques for a range of needs: mental relaxation (e.g. mindfulness), breathing techniques; physical tension release (e.g. progressive muscle relaxation); distraction (e.g. imagined scene).
- Practise when comfortable and quiet, progress to less comfortable, noisier places; learning to both switch these out or relax despite them.
- Some techniques lend themselves to frequent 'take 5' moments in the day to assist pacing and stop a build-up in mental or physical tension.
- Mini-relaxers: briefly scan the body for tension, relax it, return to the previous activity. Patients may notice problem areas (e.g. the shoulders, stomach or jaw), which tense during activities (e.g. driving).

Some useful methods and ideas for patients can be found in Nicholas et al (2011).

Attentional techniques

Another form of relaxation:

- Begin with techniques that distract from the pain through attention to imagined pleasant scenes or future plans, or attention to external stimuli such as music, scenes or smells.
- Patients may then try imagining scenes which, while including the pain, focus on their pleasant or exciting aspects, or change the pain into something more pleasant, e.g. the feeling of a red hot poker becoming a warm evening sun.
- Finally patients use techniques that focus their attention on the pain. It is a way of gradually approaching the pain, even examining it in detail. Patients can explore their response to the pain too.

These techniques tackle avoidance, so may need gradual or graded exposure, but allow patients to explore fears of what would happen if avoidance was gradually discarded: a process of challenging beliefs, desensitisation and habituation.

The cognitive model

This links the thoughts that patients have about their situation with their feelings. Cognitions include pre-existing beliefs, assumptions, expectations and perspectives: patients' 'way of seeing things'. They are self-statements patients think to themselves, often quite fleetingly, and are reflected in what patients say to others.

Some cognitive styles or habits are more unhelpful to pain patients by preventing progress in rehabilitation, adjustment and acceptance. Some common ones can be found in Appendix 13.4.

Cognitive approaches to pain management aim to help patients monitor and capture these thoughts, and link them to their feelings. Patients are then taught how to replace unhelpful thought patterns associated with feelings such as distress, frustration, anger, depression or confusion with more helpful ones. Some examples are found in Appendices 13.5–13.7.

Fear-avoidance

Both fear of pain and fear of harm can be operating in people who have fear of movement. It is the experience of anxious feelings that drives the person to dread and hence avoid a feared activity or situation. This might include lifting/carrying, being jostled in a crowd or bending.

There are two main ways of working with patients on fear of activity: behavioural experiment and graded exposure.

Behavioural experiment

How we interpret situations often guides our behaviour, e.g. chronic pain patients who have quite strong beliefs about their pain: 'Unless I stop moving when I experience pain, I will make it worse and cause more damage', are more likely to restrict activities and come to fear movement.

Therefore it is important we are aware of patients' beliefs and what meaning they attach to activities, e.g. a patient thinks the pain in her hands comes from overusing her computer: 'I have caused the pain and therefore what I do can make it worse.' This can lead to feelings of guilt, fear of damage and avoidance of hand movement. Her negative automatic thoughts could be: 'this is it, my day is ruined', while her assumptions/predictions could be: 'if I don't stop immediately when I feel uncomfortable, my pain will increase'. Behavioural experiments help people challenge these thoughts by trying new behaviours, then looking at evidence from the experience.

Behavioural experiments directly challenge false beliefs, and reinforce how predicting the future is unhelpful and cannot be relied upon. It is usual for elements of doubt to remain, but these can be a focus for further experiment.

Behavioural experiments are performed where the key feature is fear; they would not be done where physical impairment meant that the patient was at risk of failing.

Observing patients while they enter and move around the building, use their aids, and undress for assessment will give you clues for what is feared. It is important not to remark on what they can do: 'Oh, I saw you could stand on your right leg when you step out of your trousers'. Patients might take this to mean you don't believe them, don't understand how painful it is, or are trying to catch them out. Acknowledging the difficulties 'I can see how difficult it is to stand on your right leg: do you have any concerns about walking?' will gradually elicit the fears and move towards material for doing behavioural experiments.

It is crucial to set experiments up as 'no lose'. Whatever the outcome, something important can be learned from it. Even if it does not go to plan, it is still valuable, because we can then look at what happened and adjust future plans accordingly.

Case study 13.2 on behavioural experiment illustrates its practical application. For further reading, Bennett-Levy and colleagues have produced a book on behavioural experiments for those helping patients to manage their emotions (Bennett-Levy et al, 2004).

Graded exposure

Fear of pain can be more disabling than pain itself and frequently needs to be the main focus. To overcome avoidance of anxious situations and activities, they are tackled one step at a time in achievable stages. The method of returning to a safe place should be clear. If patients report frank panic attacks or actual phobias, then graded exposure should begin with a psychologist present.

Teach the rationale and process of graded exposure, so that patients can apply these to other settings:

- The importance of facing feared situations.

- Understanding that avoidance is the main contributing factor. If avoidance continues fear tends to generalise to more settings.

- 'Exhaust' the anxiety by staying with it rather than using avoidance.
- The role of behavioural experiment: rating expectations of pain and anxiety feelings.
- What the 'graded' of graded exposure means, practically.
- Prepare patients for the tendency for fear/anxiety feelings to return, and the need to practise exposure on a regular and frequent basis, even after it appears to have been overcome.

Patients are encouraged to firstly set up a hierarchy of related feared activities from mildly disconcerting to extremely anxiety provoking, rating them 0–100 on provoking anxiety. The example in Figure 13.2 shows the contrast between an activity hierarchy and a fear hierarchy.

It is important that patients are in control. The first steps should be sufficiently challenging, but not so anxiety provoking that patients find them hard to manage. Tasks that do not provoke anxiety at all are not helpful; aim to start around 20–30/100 of anxiety. Try to space the steps evenly in terms of the anxiety they provoke.

Patients need to stay in the chosen anxiety-provoking situation to experience the plateau of this feeling, then stay longer until they discover that it reduces – no more than 10–15/100. With the first time it may take a long time for the anxiety to reduce. The next time, however, the anxiety may not be quite as bad, fading in a shorter time. 'Safety behaviours' will tend to be adopted, e.g. taking the mind away from the feeling of anxiety, using the physiotherapist as a source of reassurance, compensatory movements to avoid weight bearing, bending. These need to be watched for by the physiotherapist and patient so they can be stopped or avoided.

---

100 Running down whole flight of stairs alone
100 Running up whole flight of stairs alone
100 Walk down whole flight of stairs, alone no handrail
 95 Walk up whole flight of stairs alone no handrail
 90 Walk up/down whole flight of stairs hand lightly on the rail
 85 Walk up/down whole flight of stairs, no-one there in earshot
 70 Walk up/down whole flight of stairs, friend in next room
 70 Walk up/down small flight of stairs, no-one in earshot
 50 Walk up/down small flight of stairs, friend in next room
 50 Walk up whole flight of stairs, friend wait at the bottom
 30 Walk up/down whole flight of stairs, friend behind me
 30 Walk up/down small flight of stairs, friend wait at the bottom
 20 Walk up/down small flight of stairs, friend behind me
 10 Step up and down 2 steps, friend behind me in case

Graded Fear Hierarchy

Run up 2 at a time and run down 1, 2 then 3 times
Run up/down 1 flight of stairs 1, 2 then 3 times
Walk up and down 2 steps at a time going up 1, 2 then 3 times
Walk up and down 1 whole flight of stairs 1, 2 then 3 times
Walk up/down small flight of stairs 1, 2 then 3 times
Step up and down bottom step 1, 2, 3, 4 5 then 6 times

Figure 13.2 Graded activity versus graded exposure.

It is essential patients finish each session with a sense of achievement. Explain that the fear feeling tends to return; it will be there again next time, but will go a bit faster. Gradually, patients tackle increasing amounts of the feared activity, and deliberately integrate it back into everyday life: gaining a sense of achievement. The fear hierarchy will also change, the higher scores beginning to reduce.

It can be seen that time needs to be set aside to do graded exposure since it is imperative that patients stay with their anxious feeling until it subsides, and finish a session with very low levels of anxiety.

Occasionally a task is started that despite a prescore of 30/100, proves to be much more when attempted. The task should immediately be stopped then rescored and restarted based on this experience.

If patients deny fear but still wish to avoid 'unnecessary' pain, introduce them to desensitisation: working towards normalising the sensory cortex input and gradually altering its output. Hearing of other patients' achievements in similar situations will help them believe this is possible, and worth working at to avoid increased pain and hypersensitivity in the long term. Frequently, when desensitisation begins, then fears emerge. This can be acknowledged and tackled with graded exposure.

Treatment specific to pain type/syndrome

As well as C-BPM there are specific treatments or advice for various pain syndromes.

Neurogenic pain: slowly developing regional musculoskeletal or 'neuralgia-like' pains

Gross signs of nerve conduction problems will be absent, but subtle changes can occur such as the reduced vibration sense found in work-related upper limb disorder, carpal tunnel, capsulitis, epicondylitis and osteoarthritis (Laursen et al 2006). The mechanism here is not fully known, only that it is considered central since these changes are bilateral in unilateral conditions. Axoplasmic transport stops when a nerve receives insufficient oxygen/blood supply: a consequence of sustained posture and unvaried overuse, influencing the chemicals received in target tissues. Patients may appreciate this information about their otherwise mysterious condition. Now it is chronic however, reviving axoplasmic transport would not bring *complete* resolution; the die is cast in the CNS so pain management needs to be the focus.

Neurogenic pain: fibromyalgias

There is no intervention that eradicates fibromyalgia syndrome (FMS) symptoms. Nevertheless, some treatments may be helpful even if they do not offer a cure: regular physical activity supports a favourable long-term outcome. Belief that pain is due to damage however, prevents patients from discovering this. Stress management, education, self-management and C-BMP strategies help achieve good results in FMS management (see Moores 2002).

While joint hypermobility confers benefits – for sports such as swimming, dance and gymnastics, and for knee arthritis and bone mineral density in older age (Dolan et al 2003) – a few people with joint hypermobility seem to be prone to spasm flitting to many muscles, and symptoms of fibromyalgia. It has been observed that they tend to need to build up (pace) new physical activities more gradually, and generally tend to have higher levels of training pain with new activity (Harding 2003). These patients frequently report stretch is beneficial for symptoms (Harding 2003).

Neuropathic pain: complex regional pain syndrome (CRPS)

There has recently been an explosion of research into effective methods of treating this terrible condition. This is a specialist area which you may take future interest in. Moseley's study (2005) demonstrated that sequential activation of cortical motor networks using hand laterality recognition, imagined movements and mirror movements, is the most effective management progression. It gives insight into why and how CRPS can be helped. The NOI website (http://www.noigroup.com/) gives a wealth of clinical guidance and support in this area. CRPS however can be severely impacted on by inappropriate management. 'Dabbling' is not recommended; a thorough immersion in the literature and clinical training in application of these evidence-based techniques is.

Treatment formats

Individual versus group

Individual patients appreciate learning from their physiotherapist about the experience of other patients. However, while physiotherapists can do really helpful work with individual patients with chronic pain disability, the advantages of group work make it worth finding an appropriate group for these patients. Patients learn from each other: group work is powerful for change, helping patients shift their beliefs through social learning via others' and their own experiences. There are many groups around the country that can be utilised.

Expert patient groups

These were set up nationally, with training for patients with chronic conditions to teach others in self-management. Pain is the most common condition within a range of others seen by these groups. There is much we as professionals can learn from them. A local group may allow you to observe their sessions, giving you insight into which of your patients could benefit. Useful details and patient literature can be found on http://www.expertpatients.co.uk and http://www.paintoolkit.org.

Back to work and functional restoration programmes

These are outpatient groups run usually by physiotherapists, though some have psychologists who do teaching sessions to specifically work with patients on their cognitions and mood.

Outpatient pain management groups

These are interdisciplinary: professionals from a variety of disciplines working together in an integrated way with the same model and approach (usually C-BPM), joint goals and ongoing communication. These can range from daily to weekly and it is usual for a programme at a centre to have a standardised format and length. Patients need to be able to travel to and from the unit each day of the programme.

Intensive pain management programmes

Similar to outpatient programmes, these are generally more concentrated, lengthy and expensive. Patients may attend as a resident or out-patient. They are designed for patients who on the whole are more disabled and distressed by their pain. Patients are expected to attend each session every day during the week. For some patients it is an opportunity for them to be in an environment away from the influence of family members so they can focus on learning pain management skills.

Support for physiotherapists working in pain

Physiotherapists with an interest in pain may join the Physiotherapy Pain Association (PPA). Full membership is available to CSP members though other practitioners may join as associate members.

The references for this chapter can be found on www.expertconsult.com.

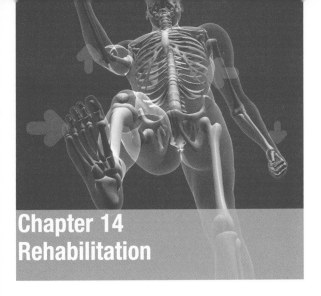

Chapter 14
Rehabilitation

Introduction

- Rehabilitation has many definitions, most of which include the terms optimising function, multidisciplinary, quality of life and patient-centred (Sinclair and Dickinson 1989).

- It might be helpful to consider the word as an umbrella term covering many aspects of patient care.

- Traditionally rehabilitation has focused on the restoration of function as seen in many areas of sports medicine where full recovery is anticipated.

- Many of the patients that physiotherapists work with have progressive long-term conditions where the nature of the injury or illness results in a permanent changes in the structure and function of the body (impairments) (DOH 2005, WHO 2001).

- All therapists will encounter patients where age-related changes have occurred, some of which may be irreversible.

- In these presentations the restorative approach cannot fully meet the needs of the individual.

- Contemporary rehabilitation needs to be able to cover a range of care aims that together make up holistic patient-centred rehabilitation (Table 14.1).

Rehabilitation of patients with neurological presentations

- The rehabilitation of patients with neurological issues will require the physiotherapist to follow a problem-solving, multidisciplinary approach in order to ensure that the patient receives effective management.

Table 14.1 Holistic patient-centred rehabilitation

Rehabilitation focus point	Intervention and treatment possibilities
Assessment and review	Use ICF to identify the impairments and activity limitations and participation restrictions to ascertain the nature and severity of the presentation
Empowering	Education and support to individuals and their carers about the situation to allow them to take an active role in their care
Supportive	Provision of appropriate support strategies to help the patient and family cope with their condition/presentation
Restorative	To promote/encourage/facilitate improvement in function for patients with new deficits resulting from a disease process, trauma or surgery
Maintenance	Provision of treatments, equipment, care and guidance to maintain gains made by the individual
Preventative	Anticipation of potential complications and difficulties
Palliative	To improve comfort and reduce discomfort, e.g. pain
Enablement	To maximise the use of existing functions
Conditioning	To improve endurance and strength in activities for patients who have become de-conditioned by poor nutrition or prolonged acute/chronic illness

- The principles of assessment, team working, patient-centred care and goal setting will assist the physiotherapist to develop a timely, appropriate, patient-centred treatment plan for the rehabilitation of each patient.
- It is important to remember that treatment and intervention can be required at any stage in a person's life. Rehabilitation may be needed following an injury and initial diagnosis or for many reasons including end-stage palliative care.
- Treatment can be provided in a variety of settings including outpatient clinics, acute hospital wards, intensive care units, community day hospitals, schools, at work and in the home and private services.
- Many of the patients and their families or carers will have encountered many different health care professionals and will have become experts in their condition. They may be seeking advice and guidance on how best to manage their condition at any one time. Long-term conditions require long-term management.

- Working in partnership and listening to what the patient says are essential to the effective management of their problems. As the expert in physical therapy the physiotherapist will be able to identify appropriate treatment or care plans with the patient, based on the findings of the assessment.

- The individual may require the services of several different members of the health and social care team at any one time, therefore the skill of the individual member of the team is to identify the most appropriately skilled health or social care professional for each patient. This requires ongoing communication over time, across service settings, with the need to access reviews both in the community and in the hospital being integral to the patient's programme of rehabilitation.

- It requires health care professionals to have a knowledge and understanding of what their colleagues can offer and how to access their services and how to make onward referrals.

- In summary it's about accessing the right services at the right time. Physiotherapy is often only part of the solution.

- Using a case history and referring to the International Classification of Function (ICF) the physiotherapy management of a patient presenting with neurological problems will be outlined in the following section (WHO 2001).

- To ensure that each patient has an appropriate treatment plan all of the components of the ICF must be included in the assessment.

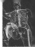
ICF-based patient case study

- A 28-year-old male suffered a traumatic brain injury following a road traffic accident.

- He underwent neurosurgery to remove an intradural haematoma and suffered further anoxic brain damage during a postoperative cardiac arrest.

- Initially he was intubated and ventilated for 2 weeks and then had a tracheostomy.

- He had abnormal levels of consciousness for several weeks with a fluctuating Glasgow Coma Scale score ranging from 3/15 to 9/15 (Teasdale and Jennett 1974).

- He was weaned off the ventilator after 1 month, spontaneously breathing and opening his eyes.

- He had poor swallowing ability and dysarthric speech.

- A percutaneous endoscopic gastrostomy (PEG) was inserted to maintain his nutritional status (Kirby et al 1991).

- He was managed on a general neurological ward for 8 weeks and referred for rehabilitation.

- Following this he was transferred from the acute hospital setting to a specialist neurological rehabilitation inpatient setting with the PEG in situ.

- At the point of discharge from the acute setting the tracheostomy was removed and some verbal output was noticed with single words being uttered.

- Abnormal tone was present in all four limbs and he was unable to move independently in bed, e.g. rolling, lying to sitting.

- He demonstrated no ability to balance in sitting and had poor head control requiring specialist seating and support.

- Then followed 18 months of inpatient rehabilitation, involving specialist seating, splinting, swallow assessments, the use of communication cards, prevention of contractures, maintenance of range of movement, control of movement and strengthening.
- He was then moved into a long-term residential placement for fully supported living and was dependent for all personal activities of daily living.
- At this point he continued to need the PEG to maintain adequate nutrition, but was starting to take oral food and fluid as his swallow had improved.
- Behaviourally he often spat out drinks and would not take adequate volumes to maintain hydration.
- After 6 months in his long-term residential placement his family requested that he return home with support from health and social services.
- At this point 27 months after the initial injury the social worker who was supporting the re-settlement into the community requested involvement of the community rehabilitation team and made a referral to physiotherapy.

Assessment of the patient (using the ICF classification model)
See Tables 14.2 and 14.3.

Interventions and treatment plan
Prioritising the interventions

- Using the structure of the ICF gives an overall picture of the patient's issues and highlights the specific problems.
- The important issue for the rehabilitation team is to determine what they can influence most effectively and which area will have the biggest positive impact on the individual.
- Identification of which problem to tackle first may require careful discussion with the team and with the individual and the family.
- It is possible to work on several areas at once. Experienced clinicians will consider the risks involved in not addressing an issue and the consequence and likelihood of there being unacceptable risk if an area is not addressed.
- In this case the risks of social isolation, increasing frustration and disruptive behaviour as a result of being unable to access more than one room were deemed to be the priority issue.
- There was a high likelihood of isolation occurring and the consequences to the individual would impinge on his ability to improve during rehabilitation.
- The importance of giving him some control was also considered to be of high importance to facilitate improvements in his behaviour.
- Removal of the PEG was viewed as being low priority and low risk, but it was something that could have been addressed relatively easily.
- In summary, this case illustrates the type of patient that may be encountered and the multiple issues that they may be associated with. Logical organised assessment and effective communication with other team MDT members will ensure that patients receive an appropriate treatment plan and effective interventions.

Patient-centred care and team working

- Considering activity and participation issues in the case can be used to illustrate patient-centred care and team work.
- This young man is fully dependent on others and at the time of assessment had difficulty communicating his needs to others.

Table 14.2 Body structure and function, activity and participation

Impairments (body structure and function)	Activity limitations	Participation restrictions
Limited concentration Behavioural issues, shouting out	Difficulty following commands and listening	Limited options for social interactions. Unable to get outside bedroom easily
Poor memory Dysarthric speech Poor planning	Difficulty communicating his needs	
Slow oral phase of swallow	Difficulty learning new tasks Unable to maintain fluids without use of PEG	Difficulty getting carers that will look after the PEG site
Abnormal voluntary control of his trunk	Unable to sit independently without full support	Fully dependent for all activities of daily living
Abnormal voluntary control of his hands	Unable to manipulate objects effectively	
Abnormal voluntary control of the left leg, extensor spasms	Unable to keep feet on foot plate	Has limited control over his environment
Contracture of the left foot into plantar flexion and inversion	Unable to be placed in a standing position	
Contracture of the right knee (30° flexion)	Unable to straighten the right knee to assist with washing and dressing	Unable to shower dependent on bed wash only
Incontinent of urine and faeces	Unable to toilet himself or indicate when he requires toileting	
Fear of new movement	Takes time to get to know new care staff	

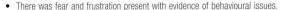

- There was fear and frustration present with evidence of behavioural issues.
- A patient-centred approach should explore the appropriateness of the environment, control over the environment and the communication difficulties and access issues.

Table 14.3 Contextual factors: environmental and personal

Environmental	Personal
Living in council accommodation in one room with hospital bed, hoisting equipment and specialist seating	Much loved by family and friends, young, full of energy, high spirits and lots of laughter
Supportive family with friends and relatives	
Lots of people coming and going visiting him	Young man with a history of traumatic brain damage
Awaiting rehousing	

Actions for the health team

- Submit reports to housing and social services to ensure client becomes a priority for re-housing. Information sharing between health and social services is important to ensure that the impact of the housing issue is understood in terms of its impact on the individual's potential for recovery and improved health status.

- These reports are best compiled as an MDT report.

- The physiotherapist information should focus on the mobility issues, e.g. wheelchair dependence and need for a hoist for transfers from bed to chair and chair to commode.

- The occupational therapist will report on other equipment issues, e.g. the need for a wet room that is wheelchair accessible, and that will allow a carer to shower the patient using a specialist shower cradle.

- The report will identify that the patient requires specific access in and out of the property to facilitate the care plan, which includes 3-weekly trips to a day centre for therapy intervention.

- Education and advisory role for the family, to explain why the patient needs accommodation that does not impose restrictions on the way in which he is managed at home.

- To review the need for a PEG feeding system.

- The PEG feed was inserted over 2 years previously during his acute care in the hospital setting to maintain adequate nutrition, when swallowing and speech was negligible.

- During the physiotherapy assessment of impairments, activities and participation it was identified that the individual was now taking in a reasonable volume of food and fluid.

- The family reported that the PEG had not been reviewed for some time and at last review a decision was made to retain it in order to ensure adequate hydration due to his occasional refusal to drink.

- For several months now he was taking oral fluids well with no issues.

- The PEG had become an ongoing source of difficulties for the patient as it frequently became infected and sore.

- A referral was made to the community dieticians for a review.

- The Community team requested a review from the acute services who had put the initial PEG in situ to request if it could be removed.

- This involved an assessment period where the PEG was not used to see if the patient would co-operate and tolerate taking sufficient oral fluids on a daily basis.

- Speech and language therapists reassessed swallowing.
- Once it was established that the patient could eat and drink adequately the PEG was removed.
- Control over the environment and communication of needs (Barnes 1994, Young 2003).
  - A detailed assessment of his cognitive ability, upper limb movement, trunk control, sitting postures and positioning was completed by the occupational therapist and physiotherapist.
  - It was identified that a switch system might provide some control over the environment and assist with communication of needs.
  - The team contacted the regional environmental control assessment team for them to undertake a specialist assessment.
  - A period of training and evaluation was discussed with the family and a system was installed.
  - The patient's wheelchair was reviewed by the occupational therapy team and a suitable lap tray was identified on which the switch could be place. The system had facilities such as a buzzer system to call for help and assistance and the ability to control his music system enabling the patient to regain some control over his environment and care needs.
- During this time the patient was re-housed and further assessments for equipment needs to assist the issues the patient had with limited balance and mobility.
- A problem identified in the new accommodation was a difficulty with showering, the patient required 2-3 people to be able to shower due to the risk of slipping out of the shower chair.
  - The patient's sitting balance was re-assessed and identified as being a high risk.
  - Examination of a shower cradle, previously used in the residential setting, identified the need for this equipment to be installed in the patient's home.
  - The team ordered the equipment and then it was possible for the patient to safely shower with members of the family or 2 carers only.

SMART goals for the patient and his family

- To drink sufficient fluid over a 24-hour period to maintain adequate hydration on an ongoing basis.
- To be able to operate a lap switch when sitting in the wheelchair and be able to turn the television on and off consistently in 2 months time.
- To shower in safety with assistance of two people in 2 months time.
- The goal attainment scale was used to evaluate the input, with goals set and achieved (Turner-Stokes 2009).
- All the goals required input from the patient, family and team.
- The team worked together to share skills and knowledge for the benefit of the patient.
- The case is ongoing with long-term monitoring and support available for the patient.
- Chronic conditions require ongoing assessment, patient-centred goal setting and involvement of the multidisciplinary team.
- The goals need to be reviewed and progressed as needed following reassessment.

Treatment of complex trauma

- Rehabilitating complex trauma patients can be a daunting undertaking when the patient presents with multiple injuries, both physical and psychological.
- This section provides an indication of the framework with which to progress the patient through the stages of recovery.
- Guidance is provided to assist the reader to recognise when it is appropriate to take the next steps in rehabilitation and when the progression has been too rapid.

Getting started

- The trick to getting this right is in the assessment, planning, and being logical in the way treatment is applied.
- Tips:
- Be methodical and through and allow sufficient time
- Write plans down (there is often too much to remember)
- Goal setting initially with the patient is key, make sure this is managed in small chunks, ensure the patient knows what is happening
- Set short-, medium- and long-term goals
- Frequently reassess progress, record it and modify the programme according to the results
- Think of the whole patient and do not get caught up focussing on one area
- Do not let treatment preferences dictate how a patient should be treated
- Uncertainty about how to tackle a problem should be managed by reading around a topic or asking for help
- Do not try to ignore problems and hope that they will go away!
- Accept limitations of knowledge and experience and accept help from others, who may be able to provide ideas that will provide inspiration.

Things to consider when planning a rehabilitation programme

Severity, irritability and nature of the problems

- Treatment should not:
- Make the patient's symptoms worse
- Make the patient more tired than is necessary
- Make the patient feel that the mountain is too high to climb!

The ability of the patient to learn and retain information

- Have they had a traumatic brain injury?
- Are they able to process the information they have been given to aid their recovery?
- Are they able to remember the information, exercises and treatment in their planned programme?
- Is the medication they are taking having an influence on their mental state/ memory/processing ability?
- There is no point in giving the patient verbal information if they have poor short-term memory, and are likely to forget.

- Think of the alternatives, e.g. write plans down, write instructions for exercises or provide the patient with pictures of the exercises they need to do.
- A good idea is taking pictures of the patient doing their own exercises using their camera or mobile phone, it can be a fun activity and helps to remind them what to do.
- They will need to provide consent for copies of the photographs of their exercises to be included in their patient records.
- Use visual cues to remind them to actually do their exercises or treatment, e.g. sticking post-its or coloured stickers around the room in key places, can help to jog the patient's memory.

Ensure the patient is ready to undertake treatment
- Agree the plan, stick to the plan initially and modify the plan if results are not forthcoming.

Key Points
Make sure that the patient is:
- not overtired
- not in too much pain
- in the right state of mind to progress

Goal setting
- The setting of long- and short-term goals and making them specific to the patient is key to achieving a successful outcome in rehabilitation.
- A problem-orientated approach to goal setting is most commonly used, with rehabilitation teams defining specific, measurable goals that have been developed in conjunction with the patient.
- Patients often pick a goal which is difficult to achieve in the short term, e.g. climbing stairs in their house, so they can go home from the hospital.
- Break down the task for them into smaller goals, which they can realistically achieve.

Goal-setting example
- To get up stairs a patient needs to be able to flex their knee and hip to 90°, currently they are able to flex to 20° in each joint.
- Grade 4 quadriceps, gluteal muscles and good balance are required to achieve this.
- Setting them a goal of increasing their ROM by 10° increments per week, their power and balance in similar increments, is achievable.
- If they are given a time line (Table 14.4), they will have an idea about how long it will take to reach their target.
- Warning! Before setting goals and targets are set ensure all pathology and healing times and possible setbacks are taken into consideration.
- If more than one pathology is in existence at any one time, things will often not go according to plan.
- It is essential to constantly reassess and redefine goals as necessary.

Table 14.4 Example of timeline for increasing functional activity in the lower limb

Today	2 weeks	4 weeks
20° at knee	40° at knee	60° at knee
Unable to use own strength to straighten knee	Can lift leg to 40° against gravity	Can lift leg to 60° against gravity
Unable to stand on 1 leg	Can stand on 1 leg holding on to support firmly	Can stand on 1 leg support through finger tips

5 weeks	6 weeks	Get to go home
Can do 5 step ups	Able to climb whole flight of stairs	

Stages of rehabilitation in complex trauma

Early stage

- Immediately following admission and in the early stages the patient may be unable to undertake an active part in the rehabilitation process, therefore treatment is concentrated around the following:

The vitals

- For example respiratory function.

Circulation

- Management of swelling, skin condition, prevention of breakdown and pressure sores.
- This should be aggressively managed.
- Consider pressure control measures and a positioning chart to aid nurses and to remind the patient to change positions.

Bed mobility

- Enabling the patient to do as much as they physically can, and teaching them tips and tricks to make moving around easier and more comfortable.

Maintaining joint range of motion (ROM)

- Using passive stretches and positioning techniques.

Offering psychological support

- Advice and reassurance should be offered early on.

Middle stage

- This period can go on for a very long time depending on the extent of the injuries, the complications and the patient's willingness to engage in treatment and work hard at it.
- This may be as an inpatient or outpatient and this stage requires regular revision of the patient's goals.

- Be prepared for setbacks that occur, e.g. poor healing in bones, skin or scars or even the need for further surgery.

End stage

- This is the most rewarding phase and yet the most difficult.
- It can require diplomatic discussions around the following:
- Relationship issues
- Plans for work or the future
- Vocational plans/retraining
- Plans for sports/running/adventure/travel and the opportunities available
- The practicalities of living with disability
- Driving.
- Team working is crucial at this stage, bringing in others, e.g. occupational therapists, who have training in psychological support and vocational planning.

Key Points

- During the early stage of rehab be open and honest about what is realistic in the future.
- This is crucial, as not everyone will be able to be a paralympic athlete, and not everyone will go back to the job they used to do.
- Guidance in these subjects is key to being able to set realistically achievable goals that will not set the patient up for a huge disappointment in the future.
- Learning to balance between reality and overoptimism is a key skill for a therapist to acquire.

Importance of diet

- Provide the body with adequate energy during rehabilitation!
- Healing requires more energy than might be expected.
- It is appropriate to increase caloric intake to promote healing.
- Patients that have received traumatic injuries, e.g. fractures of the long bones, have an immediate increase in metabolic demands, that can translate into a caloric demand three times that of normal.
- Many patients will be undernourished when they get to see a physiotherapist, so they need education about their protein needs and calorie intake, and advice about how much and how often to eat in order to help the healing process.
- Boosting mineral intake can help with the healing process of the bones, muscles and skin.
- However care must be taken to ensure that the dosages are appropriate, especially in the presence of a head injury, when high doses may be toxic to the patient.

Promotion of the healing process

Smoking education

- A recommendation is that those who have traumatic injuries cease smoking for the full rehabilitation period; this is particularly pertinent for those with inhalation injuries.

- Current and previous smokers were less likely to achieve bony union than non-smokers and twice as likely to develop an infection.

- Previous smokers are 2.8 times more likely to develop osteomyelitis (bone infection) and soft tissue healing is adversely affected (Bartsch et al 2007).

- It is important to remember that alcohol intake has also been linked to similar problems in the healing of soft tissue following traumatic injury (Radek et al 2005).

Pain management

- It may be necessary to produce discomfort, as tight structures are mobilised and muscles are worked; however, it is important to know the difference between acceptable levels of treatment soreness and provoking the patient's symptoms.

- 'No pain, no gain' is not appropriate as a mantra to follow, just as it is impossible to effectively treat patients without inducing some soreness.

- Be conscious of the patient's symptoms and make sure they are working with the medical staff to take their medication correctly and they are being prescribed adequate levels to enable them to achieve the treatment goals.

- Always allow enough time for pain medication to work.

- Have a working knowledge of what they are taking to control the pain, when they took it and how long it will last.

- Do not start a treatment session if the pain relief is about to stop working or has not started to take effect.

- Plan ahead and make sure you work with the patient to get the most out of the time you spend with them, maximising your effectiveness.

- Ask the patient when they feel they are most awake, in the least amount of pain and most receptive and then plan the treatment time around this.

Key Points

- Make sure you understand what medication the patient is on, how it works and how long it takes to have an effect.

- Read around the subject and refer to the British National Formulary (BNF) to develop appropriate pharmaceutical knowledge.

Management of traumatised muscle

- Assessment of the strength of all muscle groups is essential for treatment planning.

- It is essential to ensure the muscle is fully innervated and the muscle is free from scarring in the fascia and skin that can affect joint motion.

- Some patients will have a huge loss of muscle bulk as a result of tissue loss and atrophy (Figure 14.1).

Tendon damage

- Repair and treatment should include stabilising the tendon allowing it to heal, providing an environment to promote healing and reducing swelling in the area.

- Patients should be provided with a protocol and guidance for the rehabilitation of each tendon repair.

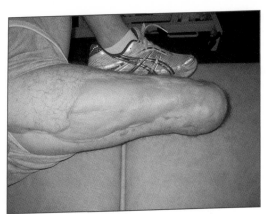

Figure 14.1 Soft tissue involvement in a traumatic injury.

Muscle strength

- Muscle strength may be increased with progressive resistive exercise.
- The progression of strengthening exercises, from those provided for a flickering muscle (grade 1, Oxford Scale), through to the heavy loading that may be achieved at end stage rehabilitation will be determined by continuous assessment of the muscles and determining their ability to be able to benefit from working against a greater resistance or for a longer duration.

General conditioning

- Combine various exercises to treat the effects of debilitation, prolonged bed rest, or immobilisation.
- The goals here are aimed at re-establishing haemodynamic balance, increasing cardiorespiratory capacity and endurance, and maintaining range of motion and muscle strength.

Exercise considerations when planning the rehabilitation programme

Active and passive exercises

- Can overcome loss of articular and muscular movement.

Exercises performed independently by the patient

- Can improve circulation and metabolic improvement.

Exercises performed against resistance by a physiotherapist

- Counteract muscular atrophy and restore the neuromuscular memory.

For patients with a neurological injury

- Provide exercises that produce precise movements, using the whole kinetic chain.

Exercises for postural sequences

- Can help recover normal movement/motor memory, e.g. moving from sitting to standing.

Static-dynamic exercises

- Can be used to counteract hypertrophy and scar contractures, by using forces that release scar tension in a constant, continuous, and adjustable manner.

Proprioceptive neuromuscular facilitation (PNF)

- Can help to re-establish functional patterns of movement.
- Table 14.5 indicates the types of exercises that can be used for a patient who has sustained a mild head and soft tissue injuries.
- Each exercise should be specific to the patient and have purpose, direction and be graded at the correct level, so that the patient may achieve their goals within the projected timeframe.

Key Points

- The use of gravity-assisted, eliminated, gravity-resisted, moving on to weight resisted exercise is vital to the patient's progression.
- The same progression should be applied with balance, hydrotherapy and cardiovascular exercises.

Table 14.5 Example of exercises for patient with mild head injury and soft tissue trauma

Assessment findings	Type of exercise to consider
Quadriceps power, Oxford Scale Grade 3	Resisted knee extension Thera-band Ankle weights PNF half leg patterns Hydrotherapy buoyancy resisted knee extension Kinetic control and muscle balance exercises
Poor balance and proprioception in standing	Balance exercises in different positions with eyes open and closed Wobble board exercises and games PNF Nintendo Wii Fit
Unable to sit to stand with normal movement	Normal movement/Bobath techniques
Low endurance for walking and results for multistage walking/'timed up and go' test poor	Paced walking programme Gentle cardiovascular programme, including swimming, cycling and aqua jogging, with heart rate at 60% of maximum

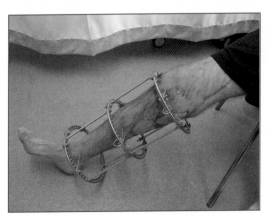

Figure 14.2 Extensive lower limb damage and scarring.

Management of the skin

- Skin is nearly always affected in trauma and excessive swelling and oedema, and open wounds can all cause scarring (Figure 14.2).

Oedema

- Control oedema using the RICE principles, 'Cryo-Cuff' or 'Game Ready' if available (www.cryocuff.com, www.gameready.com).
- Reducing oedema can result in reduced scarring, improve joint function and ease pain.
- Consider using graduated bandaging, tubigrip and pneumatic pressure therapy.

Scars (Figure 14.3)

- Patients will often present with multiple scars, which will respond to different treatment modalities, that may include manual therapy, electrotherapy, the application of gels, lotions, splints and bandaging.
- Refer to Chapter 4 in this volume and in Volume 1.

Management of nerve injuries

- Nerve injury is divided into peripheral and spinal, with some patients presenting with a combination of both.

Assessment of the ongoing recovery of peripheral nerves

- Testing the muscles which are innervated by recovering nerves informs the treatment plan, especially the progression of exercises for the involved muscle groups.
- Examples of treatment modalities for recovering nerves are outlined in Table 14.6.
- Patients that sustain a spinal cord injury are treated in specialist units.
- The reader is referred to the assessment volume chapter on spinal injuries and to the treatment chapter in this volume.

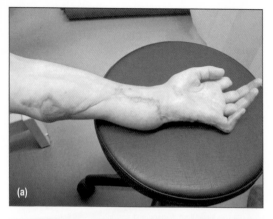

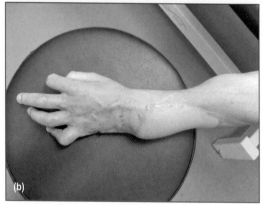

Figure 14.3 (a and b) Extensive skin damage and scarring.

Hypersensitivity and allodynia

- Can be treated by using:
- Neural suppressing drugs (medical team involvement required)
- Desensitisation techniques – using different textures, temperatures and constant stimulation of the skin
- Contrast baths
- Acupuncture
- Neural mobilisations
- Pain management education.
- If a nerve reconstruction has been performed, guidance should be sought from the consultant as to when to remove the splint and when to start stretching and mobilising.

Table 14.6 Treatment interventions at each stage of nerve recovery

Activity of muscle	What to try	Results
No muscle activity	Splint and protect the area Refer to a peripheral neurologist for further assessment, e.g. nerve conduction studies Educate the patient about the healing process	Soft tissue remains in good position and does not contract during the period that the nerve is recovering
Flicker of activity in the muscle	Continue to splint and protect Active assisted exercise Gravity/buoyancy assisted exercise Functional electrical stimulation (FES) Adverse neural dynamic exercises (AND) Soft tissue work around the area of the suspected interface of nerve and restricted tissue	Maintains soft tissue in a good position and prevents contractures Exercise helps normal movement to occur FES encourages nerve activity in the recovering nerve Encourages neural mobility Allows soft tissue to move freely
Grade 3 and higher muscle activity through Range	Normal movement exercises Resisted/buoyancy resisted exercises Progress to functional exercise Increase the range of AND exercise	Normal return to function

Psychological management

The use of imagery

- Imagery involves the use of several techniques and may be referred to as guided imagery, mental rehearsal or self-hypnosis.
- This involves the patient creating mental images, feelings and sensations related to a desired outcome, as though it is actually happening or has happened.
- An analysis of the use of imagery by injured athletes concluded that 'The implementation of imagery alongside physical rehabilitation should enhance the rehabilitation experience and, therefore, facilitate the recovery rates of injured athletes' (Driediger et al 2006).

Characteristics of patients who recover faster (Michaels et al 2000)

- There are identifiable differences between people who recover quickly and those who don't.

- They:
- Take personal responsibility for their recovery process
- Have high motivation, desire and determination
- Have excellent social support
- Maintain a positive attitude
- Frequently use imagery and other visualisation techniques
- Expect a full and successful return to functional activities.

Positive effects of using imagery (Driediger et al 2006)

- Injured athletes, cancer patients, and those undergoing physical rehabilitation indicate that the use of imagery:
- Increased feelings of control
- Increased rate of healing
- Increased ability to cope with therapy
- Increased motivation to participate in self-care
- Improved mood
- Improved quality of life
- Decreased post-operative pain
- Decreased post-operative anxiety
- Decreased amount of pain medication taken
- Reduced length of time in the hospital.

Application of imagery

- If a patient wants to climb the stairs, get them to imagine that they are at the bottom of the stairs looking up.
- Ask them to close their eyes and picture in their mind's eye, either themselves doing the task, or watching themselves doing the task, as if seeing it happen on a television screen.
- Talk them through the process of what they would feel under foot, how they should feel their leg move up onto the step, what they would see, what they would hear and even what they would smell.
- Get them to rehearse this in their head before they start the task, as it will help the process to happen more naturally.
- Telling them that top professional golfers use the techniques to control the 'yips' (a state experienced by golfers that causes them to miss important shots), this may get them to buy into the concept of imagery.
- You can use it for any movement that they need to practise.

Other psychological techniques

- Other techniques which can be used to good effect in the rehabilitation of the trauma patient include cognitive behavioural therapy (CBT) and eye movement desensitisation and reprocessing (EMDR).
- These skills are specialist in nature and require additional training.

Post-traumatic stress disorder (PTSD) and other associated issues

- Being aware of the psychological effects of trauma, including adjustment stress, anxiety and the effects of minor traumatic brain injury is crucial.

- If you become aware of problems, refer on to a specialist, such as a community psychiatric nurse (CPN) or a psychiatrist.
- There are many organisations such as 'Changing faces' and 'Combat Stress' who can help patients with adjustment to disfiguring injury and PTSD.
- Patients present in lots of different ways if they have PTSD, often they are angry and aggressive, pick arguments with their friends and family and use alcohol or drugs to help them sleep or just 'forget'.
- They can have poor concentration, are withdrawn, have low mood and often report that they get flashbacks or nightmares.
- They are often hypervigilant and sleep very poorly.
- If the symptoms are going on for longer than 6 weeks and are not improving further help should be sought from a professional in this field.
- Often the only person they will tell is their physiotherapist and you should act before the situation deteriorates.

> **Key Points**
>
> - Refer the patient to a specialist if psychological problems are suspected
> - Consider CBT to enhance the rehabilitation
> - Remember this chapter provides preliminary guidance, further reading will enhance your knowledge base and your ability to manage your patients more effectively

Treatment of the musculoskeletal sports patient

Introduction

- Rehabilitation of a patient with a musculoskeletal sports injury encompasses a wide range of presentations from a grade I calf strain to a dislocated shoulder.
- The process of taking an athlete from point of injury to full fitness has many points to consider:
- The journey usually starts with 100% treatment and 0% rehabilitation and then gradually over time this ratio changes to become predominantly rehabilitation.
- There is always a need for active treatment, e.g. to maintain range, reduce morning stiffness and to assess progress. Even when the athlete has been back in full activity for some time, daily assessment and treatment may still be needed.
- The process of progressing a patient through a rehab programme can be monitored using a traffic light system for daily assessment (the reader is referred to the assessment volume for details of this process).
- Historically patients have been treated with a period of rest, followed by activity where rehabilitation is introduced. However, for an athlete rehabilitation can, and should be started as soon as possible.
- This can start with simple bed exercises, e.g. isometric toes, ankle and quadriceps contractions to aid blood flow or the use of an arm ergometer, sitting down boxing, static bike work. This early work is important both physically and mentally for the athlete.
- Following the ethos that every injury is an opportunity to return stronger, faster, fitter, more agile, more stable and less likely to get another injury puts a

positive spin on an injury, it shows the athlete from an early stage that they will be considered holistically as an athlete and not just a hamstring tear for example.

- An injury can often give an opportunity to correct other issues, such as poor core stability or muscle tightness in other areas.
- Early, mid and late stages of rehabilitation will be considered under the following headings:
- Joint homeostasis
- Range; joint movement and muscle length
- Strength
- Restoring balance
- Restoring function.
- It is not to provide the rehabilitation pathway for all injuries but the reader is provided with a framework which can be used to help plan and develop a rehabilitation programme for an athlete with any injury.

Early treatment phase

- The priorities in this phase are homeostasis and range of joint movement and muscle length.
- The early phase has no timeframe, it starts as soon as the injury occurs and never really finishes, because even at end stage rehabilitation modalities used in the early stage may also continue to be required.

Injured area homeostasis

- Following an operation or after any injury, the initial phase concentrates on creating an environment which is optimal for healing and stopping further cell damage, this is often referred to as homeostasis.
- This involves the use of PRICE (protection, rest, ice, compression and elevation) to avoid further injury (ACPSM CSP 1998).
- The protection element puts the injured area in a position which avoids undue stress that could disrupt the healing process and it also helps with pain control.
- This may involve the use of a sling, splints or crutches or simply advice on what movements to avoid.
- Rest is very much associated with protection, and avoids placing undue stress on injured tissues which may disrupt the early elements of tissue repair.
- Rest can also reduce the metabolic demands of the injured area and thus aid healing.
- Advice on why this is important must be given as the athlete may want to get back to training.
- Ice is used initially to provide some pain relief and to set up a hypometabolic state which has been shown to reduce secondary cell damage (Fevre 1998).
- There is debate about how best to apply cryotherapy.
- Currently, 10 minutes of ice massage followed by 10 minutes rest and then another 10 minutes of ice massage seems to be the popular method.
- Compression can be in many forms, e.g. strapping or elastic bandages.
- It is used to limit the amount of oedema caused by exudation of fluid from the damaged tissue.

- Elevation of the injured body part lowers the pressure in local blood vessels and helps to limit bleeding, it also aids the drainage of inflammatory exudates through the lymph vessels.

- This element is often more important for lower limb injuries, the injured area should be placed so that it is above the level of the heart.

- Visiting the athlete at home can be important at this stage to ensure that they are resting appropriately.

- Accurate diagnosis can be difficult due to swelling and pain, therefore the position of rest may have to be maintained for the initial 72 hours until an accurate diagnosis and treatment plan can be made.

Range: joint movement and muscle length

- The final goal is for the athlete to resume full activity in their sport.

- In the early rehabilitation phase full range of the affected joints or full mobility of the affected muscles and neural tissues must be achieved.

- To start this process some Cyriax grade 'A' mobilisations (Kesson and Atkins, 1998) or Mulligan mobilisations with movement (Mulligan 2010) can be used, these active assisted movements are pain free.

- To progress the treatment passive mobilisations can be introduced to improve both accessory and physiological movements.

- Where appropriate some stretching techniques may be included at this stage.

Strength

- One of the main issues post injury is the loss of muscle strength.

- This occurs quickly due to pain inhibition and joint oedema, therefore as soon as possible isometric contractions should be undertaken and exercises for unaffected areas should be carried out to prevent muscle atrophy and to help maintain a positive psychology in the patient.

- Isometric can be progressed to concentric contractions and manual resistance can be a good way to start muscle activity, as the therapist can feel the quality of the muscle contraction and can carefully increase the work load.

- If the injury is a lower limb injury exercises can be carried out on the non-injured leg as this will facilitate strength development.

- If the injury is an upper limb injury then the non-injured side can be worked and of course the lower limbs.

Balance and function

- This area of treatment may be more difficult to begin as early as improving range or strength, but balance can begin with the facilitation of joint position sense.

- Depending on the injury and the functional status it is good to get the athlete moving about as soon as possible in a professional setting.

- A home visit can be useful early on and it can also be good to get the athlete to their usual place of work and environment to aid recovery enabling them to feel part of a group.

- In this period the athlete can watch videos with a coach which can be useful for skill development and psychologically to make the individual continue to feel part of a team.

Mid treatment and rehabilitation phase

- This phase is where joint homeostasis and range, i.e. joint movement and muscle length become less of a priority because the goals will have been successfully achieved earlier in the rehabilitation process.
- The range and muscle length will need to be checked on a regular basis and maintained.
- Joint homeostasis will need to be monitored after an increase in work load or a change in work, as it is these changes which can upset the homeostasis.

Strength

- The approach to treatment or rehabilitation is very individual and strength training in particular can be carried out in many ways.
- A progressive system of stages can be very good, this means that every exercise that is chosen is progressed only after assessment and when the athlete can complete the exercise in a satisfactory manner (Table 14.7).
- An exercise is chosen and to begin with there will be no weight and nothing else to concentrate on.
- This simple exercise requires the patient to demonstrate good control and movement patterns (level 1).
- When this is achieved some loading can be added (level 2)
- When this is achieved this load may be increased (level 3).
- When the exercise can be carried out with some load or resistance then a proprioceptive challenge can be added and at the same time the load is removed (level 4).
- When the balance challenge can be achieved with ease the load is reintroduced (level 5).
- The balance challenge and load can be gradually increased (level 6).
- The final stage involves the patient undertaking the exercise with a balance challenge, load and with an extra demand being introduced (level 7).
- Levels 1 to 3 are considered to be mid phase, as they are concerned with quality of movement, range of movement and control.
- Levels 2+3 are concerned with keeping this quality of movement as load is introduced and gradually increased.
- Level 4 is the transition zone where the load is removed and the quality of movement is subjected to a balance challenge.
- The introduction of a balance challenge to these exercises is where there may be some overlap of the areas of rehabilitation.
- The balance challenge can be the introduction of a gym ball into a Bulgarian squat avoiding the patient lying on a hard surface or it can be performing a gluteal bridge, moving from 2 legs on the ground to 1 as the gluteal bridge progressions show (Table 14.8).
- Levels 5 to 7 make up the late phase.

Restoring balance and restoring function

- This is the area of rehabilitation where all the other factors required for success are needed, e.g. the use of pool sessions, balance training, jump work, movement work, and resistance band work.
- As for rehabilitation of strength the use a progressive system of stages is used.

Table 14.7 Table to demonstrate the progressive system for developing exercises

	Mid Rehabilitation Phase			Transition zone		Late Rehabilitation Phase		
Level 1	Level 2	Level 3	Level 4	Level 5	Level 6	Level 7		
Exercise	Exercise	Exercise	Exercise	Exercise	Exercise	Exercise		
	With load	Increase the load	No load	With load	Increase the load	With load		
			Balance challenge	Balance challenge	Balance challenge	Balance challenge		
						An extra demand		

Table 14.8 Examples of how the progressive system can be incorporated into exercise provision

Bulgarian squat	Add weight	Increase weight	Back foot on gym ball, no load	Back foot on gym ball, with load	As level 5 and Increase the load	Add in front foot on bosu
Double leg gluteal bridge	Add weight	Progress to single leg, free leg held still	Single leg, free leg counter movement	Add load	Foot on floor, now on a ball	After a set have to jump up and run
Bench press	Add weight	Increase weights and reps	Gym ball under back	Single foot on floor	Foot on floor, now on a balance disc	After 1 set get up and do another exercise

- An example of balance training is outlined in Table 14.9.
- The example in Table 14.9 demonstrates the progressive system for balance training, where instead of introducing different exercises or different loads as happens in the development of strength, the balance work uses the same exercises, with the use of equipment being progressed.
- Level 1 may start in double leg stance with the patient catching a ball on firm ground, which may be progressed to being performed on a trampoline.
- Level 2 progresses the work on a trampoline to single leg movements such as toe touch and the use of a balance pad is introduced with double leg ball catching.
- This is gradually developed with the athlete demonstrating that they can comfortably perform the exercises using the equipment.
- Eventually the patient progresses to level 8 where they undertake a dynamic circuit, e.g. using a series of bosus medicine balls placed in a row, bouncing on to a balance beam and then hopping over hurdles.
- Another area involved in restoring function is movement and fitness.
- This area probably more than any other is sport-specific and where the physiotherapist knowledge of the sport is essential.
- This area changes greatly depending on injury type and sport involved, however, once again the physiotherapist is encouraged to follow a progressive process, similar to that outlined in Table 14.7.
- A progressive process for movement could begin with some jogging or simple warm up procedures, then it could be developed by introducing some straight line running, followed by some multidirectional work.
- After this some reaction work may be appropriate for a sprinter for example.
- This can be further progressed by adding in some work with an unpredictability element, for sports such as squash or rugby, so the athlete can learn how to react to specific stimuli.

Late rehabilitation phase

Joint homeostasis and range; joint movement, muscle length

- At this stage these need only be assessed and maintained and action will only be required if a problem occurs.

Strength

- This is often the main priority at this stage, but there is much more to the rehabilitation of an athlete than improving their strength.
- As outlined in Table 14.7 levels 5 to 7 constitute the late phase.
- Level 5 involves the patient exercising with a load and a balance challenge.
- Level 6 is run at the same demand level as level 5 with gradually increasing load. Level 7 includes the use of load, balance challenge and an extra demand.
- The extra demand in level 7 is where the element of fun can be included in the process.
- The physiotherapist needs to use their imagination and knowledge of the patient's sport.
- The extra demand could be the introduction of a movement in addition to an exercise, e.g. the patient carries out a set of exercises and then is required to turn and catch a ball, or to run a set distance.

Table 14.9 The progressive system of stages for balance training

| | Mid Rehabilitation Phase | | | Transition Zone | | Late Rehabilitation Phase | | |
	Level 1	Level 2	Level 3	Level 4	Level 5	Level 6	Level 7	Level 8
Hard surface	Introduce work							
Trampoline	Introduce work	Increase work						
Balance pad		Introduce work	Increase work					
Balance disc			Introduce work	Increase Work				
Bosu hard side up				Introduce work	Increase Work			
Bosu soft side up					Introduce work	Increase Work		
Bosu in a row					Introduce work	Increase work		
Complex beam work						Introduce work	Increase work	Increase work
Complex dynamic							Introduce work	Introduce work

345

- Up to this point the exercises may have been sets and repetitions (reps) based, this can be built towards using circuits.
- These are more stimulating and fun for the patient as they tend to be more dynamic, including running, skipping or hoping between stations.
- By manipulating the work to rest ratio the exercises can be made more sports specific.
- Another very useful progressive series of work can be lower limb band work.
- This involves the patient undertaking a programme of work that uses a resistance band to make movements such as stepping up more difficult or uses a band around the knees while walking to increase gluteal strength.

Restoring balance and restoring function

- The balance sequence covered in Table 14.9 progresses the patient from static exercises on different surfaces to more dynamic activities.
- Initially the patient balances on a bosu, with the soft side up.
- The progression involves a line of bosus and a balance beam to increase the demand of the exercise.
- The final progression may involve a combination of all these pieces of equipment and ultimately even more dynamic equipment can be used.

Final rehabilitation considerations

Sport-specific activities

- There are other areas which may need to be worked on to improve the sporting function.
- These depend very much on the patient's specific sport.
- One area that may be used in many sports is jumping, which can be progressed through a carefully devised programme.
- Jumping is a part of the overall rehabilitation that may be neglected.
- By concentrating on ensuring the patient uses correct technique during their rehabilitation future injuries can be decreased.
- Jumping can be commenced with the patient carrying out a double leg jump from the ground to land on a small box.
- By using an upward jump with a small landing height there is decreased pressure taken through the lower limb joints on landing.
- This can be progressed as follows:
- Using a higher box
- One-footed take off and a 2-foot landing can be used to develop power
- Higher boxes can be used and 1 foot landings undertaken
- If there is no effect on joint homeostasis the athlete can begin to jump down
- Eventually plyometric activity can be included.

Fitness and movement

- Fitness and movement work is very sport specific, and it is in this late stage that movements, distances and rest periods can be fine tuned to be sport specific and even position specific.

e.g. a football player who plays as a forward completes approximately 300 metres of sprinting during a game, whereas a central defender only sprints for around 170 metres and yet the total distance covered by a central midfield player is far greater than that covered by players from any other position.

Joint tolerance

- At some stage it may be necessary to work on the tolerance of a joint.
- If a sport lasts for 80 minutes or longer it is important to know that the previously injured area can cope with being loaded for a prolonged period of stress.
- Joint tolerance is often tested during the very late rehabilitation process.
- Games such as badminton or squash can be used to improve strength, co-ordination and endurance and because they are different to many other sports they help to prevent pattern overload.
- The use of circuits is another way of avoiding pattern overload and they can be fun, used to reintroduce the athlete to competition and to incorporate the athlete back into team activities.

Summary

- The rehabilitation of athletes should incorporate a progressive system.
- There are many advantages to using a progressive system which has been covered in this section (Box 14.1).

Box 14.1 Benefits of using a progressive system for the rehabilitation of athletes

- It allows the athlete to see gradual improvements as the system develops
- This system can be used for all athletic development
- If the injured site homeostasis is disturbed the therapist knows exactly what load was put through the area during the last session
- Each session must be notated accurately because in a world of increasing litigation this progressive system of only moving the athlete on when they can easily cope with the previous stage can help protect the clinician if it ever becomes necessary

---

The references for this chapter can be found on www.expertconsult.com.

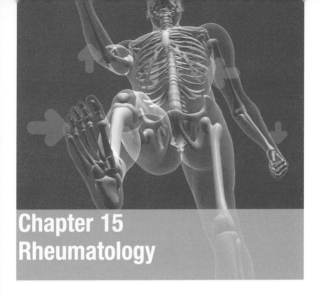

Chapter 15
Rheumatology

Introduction

- Inflammatory arthritis includes rheumatoid arthritis, systemic lupus erythematosus, scleroderma, polymyositis, vasculitis, spondyloarthropathies and gout, with rheumatoid arthritis being the most common form of inflammatory arthritis. Inflammation may be seen in osteoarthritis, but this is due to a degenerative rather than an auto immune process.

- Rheumatoid arthritis is a chronic unpredictable inflammatory disease of multifactorial origin; it is marked by a variable course, involving exacerbations and remissions of disease activity and often leads to joint damage and functional impairments.

- People often experience pain, joint stiffness, joint swelling, reduced muscle power, loss of joint range of motion, fatigue and extra-articular complications, which can lead to a significant loss of function and independence.

- Management should be patient-centred while taking into account each patient's individual needs; therefore a thorough patient assessment must be completed before any treatment is undertaken.

- The multidisciplinary team (MDT) has been shown to be effective in optimising the management of patients with rheumatoid arthritis (SIGN 2000, Luqmani et al 2006) and patients should have access to all members of the team as necessary. There should be good communication and co-operation between all team members, as it may be necessary to refer onto another member of the team if the problems the patient is experiencing fall outside the scope of physiotherapy practice.

Aims of physiotherapy intervention

- Physiotherapy aims to reduce pain and stiffness, stabilise joints, prevent joint deformity, improve exercise tolerance and muscle power, maximise function, independence and quality of life and promote self management, by utilising a number of various treatment modalities available; education and exercise are the important active aspects of physiotherapy intervention (RCP 2009). Contraindications for each modality should always be considered.

Patient education and self management

- As with any long-term chronic condition, it is essential that patients undertake self management; patient education is therefore an important aspect in the management of rheumatoid arthritis, thus empowering patients to manage their own situation.

- Bandura (1977) in the theory relating to self-efficacy stated that: 'the strength of belief in one's own capacity is a good predictor of motivation and behaviour'. Within groups of rheumatoid arthritis patients, studies have shown that stronger self-efficacy correlates with better health status. It has also been found in some studies, that self-efficacy can reduce the number of visits to health care professionals (Cross et al 2006).

- Many rheumatology units will have a formal group patient education programme, these generally run at regular intervals throughout the year and involve various members of the MDT, who each deliver relevant information. Physiotherapists provide information related to exercise, function and self management strategies, e.g. goal setting, which can help to change patients behaviour (Barlow et al 2005). It has been reported this particular mix of education and advice can improve knowledge, self worth and early morning joint stiffness for up to 1 year post intervention (Bell et al 1998, Lineker et al 2001).

- Primary care trusts run the expert patient programmes for people with long-term chronic conditions and are not disease specific. The patients are facilitated to develop their communication skills, manage their emotions, manage daily activities, interact with the healthcare system, find health resources, plan for the future, understand exercising and healthy eating, and manage fatigue, sleep, pain, anger and depression (Department of Health 2006).

- Any patient contact can be used as an opportunity to enhance patient knowledge and understanding of their disease and self management and can be personalised for each patient, so that each individual has their specific needs met.

- Joint inflammation can cause tiredness and a general feeling of being unwell, therefore advice about pacing should always form part of a patient's rehabilitation (Braun and Sieper 2006, Vlak 2004, Liu et al, 2004).

- Patient education has been shown to:
- Increase patient knowledge about their disease
- Help patients to make informed choices
- Encourage self management
- Empower patients
- Improve self confidence (Schrieber and Colley 2004).

- Education should be made available in different languages and styles to suit the local population (Luqmani et al 2009).

Patient support groups

- Voluntary organisations such as National Rheumatoid Arthritis Society (NRAS), Arthritis Care and Arthritis Research UK (formally ARC), all provide excellent written information for patients with rheumatoid arthritis.

- Information on the NRAS and ARC sites are written by health professionals and are regularly reviewed to ensure up to date evidenced based and accurate information is provided specifically for UK residents (Luqmani et al 2009). The organisations provide help lines for patients and NRAS are able to put patients in touch with one another. It is seen to be helpful for patients with the disease to talk to others with the same condition.

- NRAS will also provide support for units to set up patient support groups; these are groups run by the patients for the patients and provide a continuous source of information and education, enabling patients to support one another. The format of the meetings tends to vary according to the population that attend the groups (www.nras.org.uk).

Exercise therapy

- Exercise is the foundation of physiotherapy and should be utilised and encouraged in the treatment of patients with rheumatoid arthritis.

- Exercise therapy can be delivered on land or in water and research supports the use of aerobic activity, improving range of movement, muscle strengthening, stability (balance) and promotion of physical activity.

- When treating patients with a diagnosis of rheumatoid arthritis, it is important to remember that studies have shown that this group of patients tend to be more sedentary and are at greater risk of cardiovascular disease, (Luqmani et al 2006, Sokka and Hakkinen 2008) and osteoporotic fractures than the non-rheumatoid arthritis population (Turesson and Matteson 2007).

- Loss of body cell mass has been described in rheumatoid arthritis (Rall & Roubenoff 2004). The reasons for weight loss in rheumatoid arthritis include factors such as mechanical problems leading to muscle wasting, poor appetite and the metabolic drain of the inflammatory response (Munro and Capell 1997).

- Many factors may lead to reduced activity in this population group including: joint pain and stiffness, loss of body cell mass and disuse of muscles leading to loss of strength and possibly a fear of causing damage through over activity.

- Patients with RA therefore may have reduced:

- Muscle strength

- Aerobic capacity and endurance (Hakkinen et al 1995)

- Limited flexibility and poor standing balance (Eurenius and Stenstrom 2005).

- In addition to its general effects of reduced risk of coronary heart disease, hypertension and diabetes, exercise has shown to improve function in rheumatoid arthritis. (De Jong et al 2004, Van den Ende et al 1998). Dynamic exercise, that is: exercise of sufficient intensity, duration and frequency to establish an improvement in aerobic capacity and/or muscle strength, has been shown to be efficient in increasing muscle strength and aerobic capacity in patients with stable disease (RCP 2009).

- For some time, it was thought that dynamic, active exercise would cause increased pain, prolong active disease and lead to joint destruction (Hurley et al 2002). There is evidence to show the usefulness and safety of dynamic exercise in the rheumatoid arthritis population. Self-management and exercise has been shown to improve physical and psychological wellbeing. Aerobic exercise is known to improve health related fitness, reduce pain and fatigue, and improve function without aggravating or hastening joint destruction. Joint range of motion and specific strengthening exercises are beneficial (RCP 2009). Most of the evidence is obtained from chronic stable rheumatoid arthritis patients. Recorded improvement in muscle strength, aerobic capability, endurance, function, self value and well being have followed participation in dynamic exercise (Hurley et al 2002).

- No adverse effects on the disease activity or pain have yet been observed (SIGN 2000).

- Patients with rheumatoid arthritis have an increased risk of developing both generalised and juxta-articular osteoporosis and associated osteoporotic fractures (Deodhar and Woolf 1996, Lodder et al 2004). Juxta-articular osteoporosis is thought to be due to an increase in local vascularity and direct invasion by the pannus; in addition, the inflammatory mediators are also implicated. Systemic inflammation and reduced mobility due to functional impairment (Deodhar and Woolf 1996) are thought to be factors which can lead to generalised bone loss. Weight-bearing exercise can be beneficial in helping to prevent bone loss and improve balance (De Jong et al 2004). Lemmey et al (2009) were able to demonstrate increased muscle mass, reduced fat mass and restoration of function in their study of supervised progressive resistance training.

- Exercises and exercise advice should be modified for each individual patient and can be adapted to aid functional activities in which the patient may be experiencing a particular difficulty.

- Exercise should be encouraged in patients with rheumatoid arthritis to reduce the risks that the disease can cause as outlined above. Exercise does not exacerbate disease activity or cause joint damage in the short term (Luqmani et al 2006).

- Exercise regimens have been shown to be more successful in patients where personalised contact with a health professional occurs, where the benefits of exercise can be discussed (RCP 2009). Government recommendations for the amount of exercises a healthy adult (16-64 hears old) should undertake is 30 minutes of moderate intensity (cycling or fast walking) on 5 days of the week (www.patient.co.uk).

Exercises to be included in a patient's programme

Range of movement exercises

- Used to maintain or improve range of movement and flexibility of joints and to relieve joint stiffness.

Strengthening exercises

- To improve motor function, by maintaining or improving muscle strength, improve function and aid joint protection.
- This can be achieved by:
- Using free weights: such as a used plastic bottle (filled with varying amounts of tap water) or dumb bells

- The patient's own body weight against gravity
- Thera-Band (resistance band)
- Resistance machines
- Exercise in water. In their progressive resistance training study Lemmey et al (2009) used 80% of one repetition, maximum of 3 sets of 8 repetitions. Starting at 1 set in the first week, and 2 sets in week 2, to reduce the risk of muscle soreness. Exercises were performed on a multi-stack machine.All subjects had established, stable RA.

Aerobic, dynamic exercises

- To improve cardiovascular fitness, maintain optimal weight, maintain or improve function, improve psychological fitness and reduce pain and fatigue. It is also known to have a positive effect on function without exacerbating disease activity or causing joint damage in the short term.
- Aerobic exercise can include activities such as:
- Brisk walking
- Cycling
- Swimming
- Aerobic dance
- Water aerobics
- Stair climbing
- Jogging.
- Aerobic exercise should be carried out at low to medium intensity (SIGN), sufficient to increase the heart-rate to a higher level, allowing the patients to carry on a short conversation whilst exercising. Exercise that fits into the patient's daily routine and something which they enjoy doing will help them to maintain their programme.
- Encourage patients to try something new. Local areas will usually have various exercise programmes for all abilities and interests; look at what is available locally.
- The amount of exercise will vary from patient to patient. Patients should develop and monitor their own progressive exercise programme.
- Patients should understand the importance of exercising so that they do not over- or under-exercise.
- It is important to build up exercise gradually, to prevent the possibility of causing increased joint pain, at the same time; patients should be advised about the increased muscle pain often associated with starting a new exercise. It is important to set appropriate goals with the patient before starting exercise.

Setting a baseline

- Prior to starting any exercise programme, a baseline will need to be determined.
- Establishing a manageable baseline for exercise or activity can be achieved by asking the patient to decide for themselves how much exercise/activity will be suitable for them, e.g. cycling on a static bike for 8 minutes.
- The following day, the patient assesses how they feel following the exercise: Did I overdo it? Was it too easy?

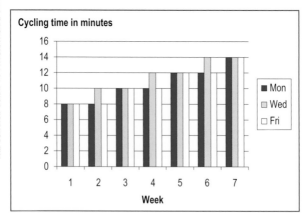

Figure 15.1 Example of exercise baseline.

- They will then adjust the exercise/activity, based on their own judgement; it might be more. For example cycling for 12 minutes on a static bike.
- The average time for the two days is then calculated, minus 20%.
- This will ensure that the exercise is manageable on days when the patient does not feel quite so good.
- For this example:

$$8\ mins + 12\ mins = 20\ mins,\ 20\ mins \div 2\ days = 10\ mins,$$
$$10 - 20\% = 8\ minutes\ as\ a\ baseline.$$

- Exercise can then be increased from this baseline, with the patient avoiding doing too much on a good day with the possible consequence of being unable to do much on the following day.
- The patient can then work towards their goal as per the following example:
- Week 1: the patient could exercise Mon, Wed, Fri for 8 minutes on the bike,
- Week 2: Mon and Fri 8 minutes. Wed 10 minutes.
- Week 3: Mon, Wed, Fri for 10 minutes.
- Week 4: Mon and Fri for 10 minutes on Wed for 12 minutes (Figure 15.1).
- This ensures consistent and gradual increase in exercise.
- An alternative method is to work out using maximal heart rate.
- The recommended aerobic exercise is 60–85% of maximal heart rate for 30–60 minutes, 3 times a week.
- For patients to determine their baseline aerobic exercise capacity, they will need to subtract their age from 220, this will give them their approximate maximum heart rate, e.g. for a patient aged 55 years, 220 − 55 = 165 beats per min.
- If the patient has been fairly sedentary, it may be appropriate to suggest them working at 55% to 65% of that number during their exercise session, e.g. for a patient aged 55 years old, maximum heart rate is 165 (220 − 55), they

would exercise for 20 to 30 minutes with their heart rate between 91 and 107 beats per minute:

$$55 \times (165/100) = 91 - 65 \times (165/100) = 107$$

Aquatic Physiotherapy in the treatment of rheumatoid arthritis

- A working knowledge of Aquatic Physiotherapy, including safety issues, contraindications, precautions, how to utilise the properties of water and local guidelines is required before treating patients in a therapy pool (Bruckner & Khan 2005).
- Aquatic physiotherapy is one of the oldest and most frequently used treatment regimes for rheumatoid arthritis.
- In the long term Aquatic Physiotherapy has been shown to reduce hospital admissions and has few if any negative effects (Hurley et al 2002).
- It is essential that patients are assessed for contraindications to Aquatic Physiotherapy, which may prevent some patients with rheumatoid arthritis from accessing the modality.
- Clinically, patients can move more readily in water and are able to perform activities which they cannot perform on land, e.g. walking or muscle strengthening.
- Loading across joints is reduced by buoyancy which allows functional exercises to be undertaken (Harrison and Bulstrode 1987, Harrison et al 1992).

Therapeutic effects of Aquatic Physiotherapy

- These include:
- Relief of pain
- Maintenance or improvement of movement
- Reduction of muscle spasm
- Strengthening of weak muscles
- Increasing tolerance to exercise
- Re-education of functional activities (Minor et al 1989, Stenstrom et al 1991)
- Enhanced cardiovascular fitness (Chu & Rhodes 2001)
- Progressive weight bearing
- Enhanced wellbeing from enjoyment, social interaction and sense of achievement (Hall et al 1996, RCP 2009).
- Improved balance and proprioception (Hinman et al 2007, SIGN 2000, Luqmani et al 2006, Hurley et al 2002).

Joint protection

Application of core skills

- It is important to remain focussed on the core skills within physiotherapy that can be used to protect joints.
- It may be necessary to refer onto another member of the MDT, e.g. occupational therapy or a specialist hand therapist.

Joint changes

- Normal joints are stable because of the conformity of the bone ends, surrounding capsule and ligaments and the muscles and tendons that move the joint.
- Where there is frequent inflammation of a joint, the surrounding soft tissues become stretched, ligaments are disrupted and invasive pannus erodes cartilage and subchondral bone.
- The results of repeated inflammation are pain, joint stiffness, loss of muscle power, instability as a result of the joint erosion and ultimately deformity.

Process of joint protection

- Patients must be taught how to perform daily activities while placing minimal stress on joints in order to reduce pain, preserve joint structures and conserve physical energy.
- Altering the way, in which people perform certain jobs together with the use of aids and gadgets, can help to maintain independence and protect joints.
- The level of activity can be adjusted according to the level of pain the patient is experiencing. Where possible:
- Advise spreading the load over several joints, e.g. using two hands to carry an object, rather than one.
- Use larger, stronger joints, e.g. the hip or shoulder to shut a door, or forearms to 'hug' objects close to the body.
- Reduce of the effort needed to perform a task by using aids and gadgets e.g. electric tin openers or jar openers.
- Change position at regular intervals avoiding prolonged static postures.
- Avoid positions such as wrist flexion and ulnar deviation at the MCP joints, which may increase the risk of joint deformity (Hammond and Freeman 2001, O'Brien et al 2006, ARC 2007).
- Certain types of grip may present a risk to joints, a tight or prolonged pinch grip or a static grip (as in knitting), places an increased force on the MCP joint and the palm, pulling on the MCP joint, tight or prolonged static grips should be avoided.
- Exercise has an important role in joint protection and should be part of a daily routine, which will help to maintain range of movement, enhance muscle strength and promote general well being.

Fatigue and pacing

Fatigue

- Described as physical and mental weariness and can affect quality of life (Luqmani et al 2009).
- It has been reported that 40–80% of patients with rheumatoid arthritis experience fatigue day after day, irrespective of what they have been doing (Pollard et al 2006, Van Hoogmoed et al 2010).
- Disease activity is thought to be a factor in fatigue allied to other influences such as; pain, psychological and social factors, health beliefs and illness perception, there is also a suggestion that this may be centrally mediated (Pollard et al 2006).

Pacing

- Patients must find a balance between rest and activity by pacing themselves.
- The appropriate amount of rest and relaxation during daily activities can be significantly effective in helping patients to manage the disease.
- Advising patients to recognise their limitations is important, e.g. If an activity 'feels like it's too much', then 'it is too much'.
- Planning which jobs can be eliminated, made simpler, finding the most economical way of performing the activity, using gadgets and aids to assist or enlisting the help of others will all help in conserving energy for the things which are really important to the patient.
- Clinically, it is often difficult for patients to readjust to their disease particularly at the onset, as fatigue is often a problem and will influence the amount of activity undertaken.
- Exercise has been shown to improve physical fatigue as well as psychological wellbeing and self efficacy, encouraging exercise in this patient group allows them to take more responsibility for their own management (Luqmani et al 2009).

Managing a 'flare'

- Rheumatoid arthritis is an unpredictable disease and many patients will experience times when their arthritis worsens, with increased pain and stiffness, this is often referred to as a 'flare' and can last from a few hours to several days. Patients may also experience increased fatigue, appetite loss and low mood during these periods.
- Patients need to be advised about a number of management strategies in order that they can choose what works the best for them.
- During a flare, patients should still move the affected joint(s) within a comfortable range of movement, several times a day, to relieve stiffness and maintain muscle tone.
- Force or resistance should not be applied to the affected part.
- If able, gentle exercise for the rest of the body can be carried out, ensuring that the activity is paced.
- If the wrists are affected, wrist splints may help to rest and support the joint, relieve pain and keep the wrist in a good functional position.
- Relaxation may be of benefit, but it can take practice. Patients can learn how to let go of physical muscle tension and release physical stress.
- Cool packs, for red, hot, swollen joints, or heat for painful joints can be used to relieve joint signs and symptoms.
- Some patients may find transcutaneous electrical nerve stimulation (TENS) useful.
- Establishing a good sleeping pattern may help reduce muscle tension and pain.
- Patient support groups provide excellent advice on coping with flares (Appendix 15.1).

The cervical spine in rheumatoid arthritis

- Cervical spine involvement is often seen in rheumatoid arthritis and other inflammatory diseases such as psoriatic arthritis, ankylosing spondylitis and juvenile idiopathic arthritis.

- Joint, bone and ligament damage can lead to subluxations, which are reported to occur in 43–86% of all patients with rheumatoid arthritis (Roche et al 2002).
- There are indications that subluxations begin soon after the onset of disease.
- A study of patients admitted to hospital for hip or knee surgery showed that 61% had cervical instability and longitudinal follow-up at autopsy indicates that cord compression is the cause of death in approximately 10% of patients with rheumatoid arthritis and cervical spine involvement (Luqmani et al 2009, Roche et al 2002).
- The severity of cervical spine involvement correlates with the duration and severity of the disease, resulting in varying degrees of instability in the cervical spine.
- Approximately 30% of patients with cervical instability will be asymptomatic and it may be difficult to detect signs of neurological deficit in the presence of a painful arthritis, with associated muscle atrophy or weakness (Luqmani et al 2006).
- Anterior atlantoaxial subluxation is the commonest form of subluxation seen in this patient group, followed by subaxial subluxation of the lower cervical vertebrae.
- Basilar invagination (or vertical subluxation) is the most dangerous form of subluxation and posterior and rotatory atlantoaxial subluxations are rare (Roche et al 2002).

Anatomical considerations

- Rotation of the head is performed at the atlantoaxial C1 atlas and C2 axis, vertebral segments.
- The odontoid peg (dens) acts as an axis of rotation and the odontoid peg is held against C1 by the transverse ligament, which runs from one side of C1 to the other.
- The odontoid peg prevents forward slipping of C1 on C2.
- Alar ligaments pass upwards and outwards to attach to the condyles of the occiput from either side of the odontoid peg.
- Synovial joint effusion, proliferation of synovial tissue together with osteoporosis combine to destroy the odontoid peg as well as the transverse and alar ligaments, resulting in atlantoaxial subluxation with concomitant/coexistent narrowing of the spinal canal.
- When the ligaments are damaged, the head will tend to pull the atlas away from the axis during flexion and cause the subluxation.
- Vertical subluxation (basilar invagination), as a result of destruction of the lateral atlantoaxial joints and atlanto-occipital joints leads to upward migration of the odontoid and surrounding pannus into the foramen magnum, compressing the brainstem and spinal cord.
- In these patients sudden death may occur after unexpected vomiting of physical trauma. Basilar-vertebral insufficiency may also occur in these cases, with syncope after flexion.
- Vertical subluxation and atlantoaxial subluxation may occur together.
- Patients may present with symptoms such as new cervical and/or head pain, C2 neuralgia or cervical spine stiffness.
- Hakkinen et al (2005), found that patients with atlantoaxial disorders had reduced muscle strength in flexion, extension and rotation.

- Treatment of rheumatoid cervical spine involvement is usually conservative.
- For patients who present with severe intractable pain or myelopathy, surgery is usually indicated (Choi et al 2006, Kauppi et al 2005).
- Diagnosis of cervical spine involvement is by plain X-ray, with lateral views of the cervical spine taken in full flexion and full extension (Kauppi and Neva 1998) and through the mouth views for C1/C2 specifically (Geusens et al, 2005).
- MRI is commonly used to assess the degree of degeneration in the articular cartilage.

Physiotherapy management and treatment of cervical spine problems in rheumatoid arthritis

- Patients with cervical spine involvement may report symptoms which include headaches and pain extending from the cervical spine to the posterior aspect of the head and into the shoulders. It is thought that these symptoms are as a result of muscle spasm and weakness of the muscles of these areas (Kauppi et al 2005, Luqmani et al 2009).
- The limited evidence to support the physiotherapy management of instability in the cervical spine in rheumatoid arthritis indicates changes in patient behaviour, with clinical and statistical reduction in pain (Kauppi and Neva 1998).
- Kauppi et al (1998, 2005) suggest that treatment is multidisciplinary and should include: patient information, disease activity control, symptomatic treatments and physical exercises, e.g. isometric muscle training, posture advice, provision of practical aids and ergonomic advice.

Muscle re-education

- Specifically treatment should aim to reduce muscular tension in the occipital triangle, and increase strength and endurance of this group of muscles and their antagonists, the deep flexors.
- Isometric or slightly dynamic, flexion, extension and rotation exercises can be taught, against yielding resistance (a finger).
- The introduction of proprioceptive neuromuscular facilitation techniques (PNF) such as contract relax can be used to improve the functional control of these muscle groups.
- Larger muscles of the cervical spine and shoulders should be exercised to ensure control and power is developed throughout their functional range.
- Dynamic flexion and full rotation of the spine were avoided.

Collars

- Cervical collars can be provided to relieve symptoms of neck pain (Kauppi and Anttila 1996).
- It is thought that these warm the cervical muscles and reduce painful tension and have psychological significance for patients.
- Collars made of closed-cell foam polyethylene, strengthened to prevent forward flexion, can be given to provide support for patients with atlantoaxial instability (Kauppi and Anttila 1996, Kauppi et al 1999).
- These patients must be advised to avoid flexion during daily activities, a collar can remind the patient to avoid this movement. They can be weaned off the collar as they get used to avoiding flexion (Luqmani et al 2009).

- Collars should not be used continuously and not when it would increase the risk of falling.
- A collar can provide support when in a car as a passenger, as even a minor injury or accident may have serious consequences for a patient with upper cervical instability. Muscular strength must be maintained and range of movement exercises should be performed, as discussed above (Kauppi and Anttila 1996).
- Specific written instructions should be provided and the patient is also required to inform the DVLA if intending to continue driving.

Other modalities
- Electrotherapy, e.g. TENS, can provide symptomatic relief.
- Heat, hydrotherapy and relaxation may also be useful in the reduction of unwanted muscle tension and the relief of pain (Kauppi et al 1998).

The shoulder in rheumatoid arthritis
- Painful shoulders are often reported in patients with rheumatoid arthritis.
- Problems which occur commonly include: impingement, acromioclavicular arthritis, degeneration/erosion of the glenohumeral joint, rotator cuff tears, deficient rotator cuff, and long head of biceps involvement.
- Exercise has been shown to be effective in the management of rotator cuff disease including longer term functional benefits.
- Maitland's mobilisation and exercise used in conjunction have been found to be beneficial for rotator cuff lesions.
- Ultrasound is often used clinically; however, there is little evidence to indicate that this influences shoulder pain, adhesive capsulitis or rotator cuff involvement.
- There is some suggestion that corticosteroid injections are beneficial in rotator cuff lesions and adhesive capsulitis, therefore the physiotherapist should ensure that they liaise with a rheumatologist if this may be indicated (Buchbinder et al 2003).

The elbow in rheumatoid arthritis
- Elbow involvement may result in loss of extension early in the disease, supination may also be a problem.
- Patients may adduct the elbow across the abdomen in order to rotate the ulnar and obtain supination.
- Epicondylitis and olecranon bursitis may be present.
- Loss of flexion may occur late in the disease and upper limb function may be severely limited. (Isenberg et al 2004).

The hand in rheumatoid arthritis
- The hands are affected in up to 90% of patients with rheumatoid arthritis.
- Patients who undertake hand strengthening and hand mobilising exercises improve their upper limb function (Luqmani et al 2006, 2009, SIGN 2000, O'Brian et al 2006).

The knee in rheumatoid arthritis

- Inflammation of the knee often leads to quadriceps atrophy and flexion contracture, which require treatment, e.g. with ice and exercises.
- A popliteal cyst (Baker's cyst) may produce swelling posteriorly in the popliteal fossa, this may rupture causing swelling and pain in the calf and may be mistaken for a DVT.
- Longstanding knee involvement may result in valgus instability, flexion contracture and reduced mobility (Isenburg et al 2004).

Foot care

- Foot involvement in rheumatoid arthritis has been shown to occur in 50–89% of patients (Michelson et al 1994, Kerry et al 1994).
- The prevalence of foot and ankle symptoms has been shown to be related to the duration of systemic illness, i.e. patients with longstanding rheumatoid arthritis have a high prevalence of foot and ankle symptoms (Michelson et al 1994).
- It is important to remain focussed on the core skills within physiotherapy relating to foot care. It may be necessary to refer onto another member of the MDT such as orthotics/podiatry services.
- Involvement of the small joints in the feet often occurs early in rheumatoid arthritis and for many patients, even mild involvement of the feet can cause a significant reduction in mobility and function (Keenan et al 1991, RCP 2009).
- In conjunction with the general impact of the disease, changes in the feet such as hallux valgus, hallux rigidus and valgus heel cause progressive functional impairment that can prevent patients from participating in work, leisure and normal daily living activities.
- Toe deformities including: claw, mallet, hammer toes and flexion of both IP joints with planter subluxation of the MTP joints may occur; toes may also cross over one another.
- Symmetric involvement of the metatarsal-phalangeal (MTP) joints may result in tenderness to palpation and can lead to widening of forefoot.
- Subluxation of MTP joints with anterior displacement of plantar fat pad can lead to patients reporting of painful feet on weight bearing, and is often described as 'like walking on pebbles' This can lead to tender calluses and in a small number of patients, ulceration.
- Other changes to the feet may include subcutaneous nodules, which tend to form over bony areas, tenosynovitis of long flexor and extensor tendons and bursitis.
- Foot care advice is important and appropriate referral to podiatry services for the management of foot problems is important.
- Foot exercises can be provided that may improve balance and proprioception.
- Foot orthoses and specialist foot wear are an effective intervention (RCP 2009).
- Gait re-education may be useful once a patient has been provided with supportive footwear.

Thermotherapy in rheumatoid arthritis

- Superficial heat and cryotherapy (ice/cold) are commonly used in patients with rheumatoid arthritis to relieve pain, stiffness, muscle spasm and swelling.

- Both can be applied by the patient safely in their own home, with no harmful effects. There is no evidence to show that heat or cryotherapy have any undesirable effects on disease progression or joint destruction (Luqmani et al 2006).

- Heat appears to be effective in relieving stiffness (Luqmani et al 2006, Hurley et al 2002, Robinson et al 2002, RCP 2009).

- The skin should be protected from dry heat sources such as hot water bottles, wheat bags, electric heat pads, or jelly pads.

- Showers or baths, a basin or bowl of hot water or a damp towel heated in the microwave provide a moist heat source (RCP 2009).

- Cold appears to be beneficial for pain relief, with cold rather than heat being useful for active joints (Luqmani et al 2006, Robinson et al 2002, RCP 2009).

- Sources of cold therapy include using a bowl of cold water (ice cubes can be added), for hands or feet, a bag of frozen peas, mouldable ice pack (wrapped in a damp tea towel) or a damp towel kept in the fridge.

- Paraffin wax baths combined with exercises have shown to provide short-term effects for hands (Luqmani et al 2006).

- Thermotherapy tends to be used as an adjunct to other treatments and as a palliative therapy to help manage the symptoms of rheumatoid arthritis (Luqmani et al 2006, Robinson et al 2002, RCP 2009).

Use of aids, gadgets, assistive devices, splints and walking aids

- It is important to remain focused on the core skills within physiotherapy relating to this area of patient management. It may be necessary to refer onto another member of the MDT such as occupational therapy or specialist hand therapist.

- Using aids/gadgets/assistive devices can help to improve function with activities of daily living (ADL), e.g. jar openers, electric can openers (Luqmani et al 2009).

- Splinting may be useful to provide pain relief e.g. resting hand splints and working wrist splints have been shown to reduce pain on activity (SIGN, 2000).

- Walking aids can reduce load on affected lower limb joints, decreasing pain and compensating for impairments in ROM, muscle strength, joint stability, coordination and endurance (Van de Esch et al 2003).

- Unfortunately, in some cases, walking aids may increase pain in the upper limbs, therefore specially shaped walking devices are available, such as gutter crutches/frames and Fisher shaped hand holds for sticks.

- Disability, pain, and age-related impairments determine the need for walking aids and non use is often associated with less need for a walking aid, or the patient being reluctant to use a visible support (Hurley et al 2002, Van de Esch et al 2003).

Tai Chi

- Tai Chi is an ancient Chinese health promoting martial art form and has been recognised in China as a therapy for arthritis for centuries.

- Studies into Tai Chi appear to show an improvement in lower limb joint range of motion in patients with rheumatoid arthritis, without aggravating symptoms.
- It is not considered helpful for improving function, grip strength, or in reducing the number of swollen or tender joints.
- Generally, patients enjoy doing it and it promotes a feeling of well being (Han et al 2004).

Passive treatments

- Passive treatments such as electrotherapy or manual therapy techniques, can be used for specific clinical impairments to facilitate the ability of the patient to exercise or increase physical ability (RCP 2009).

Electrotherapy

- Often used to relieve pain and improve function (Brousseau et al 2002).
- Symptoms of pain, discomfort and stiffness in rheumatoid arthritis are controlled by pharmacological intervention, therefore other forms of symptom relief are used as an adjunct to the provision of medication when the patient may be suffering side effects from pain relieving medication.
- There is poor evidence supporting the use of electrotherapy with rheumatoid arthritis, with TENS being viewed as being of short-term benefit for the relief of symptoms (RCP 2009).

TENS

- TENS is used for the control of pain; however the use of this treatment modality is mainly based on clinical experience rather than evidence from clinical trials.
- The benefit of TENS is that it has few side effects and can be applied by patients themselves, in their own homes as they need it (Brousseau et al 2003).
- There are conflicting views on the effectiveness of TENS on pain outcomes in patients with rheumatoid arthritis (Brousseau et al 2003).
- There is evidence that acupuncture-like TENS has shown a statistical and clinical benefit on pain and a clinical benefit on the improvement of muscle power scores over placebo, whereas conventional TENS did not appear to show any clinical benefit for pain intensity over placebo (Brousseau et al 2003, Luqmani et al 2006).

Ultrasound

- Ultrasound (u/s) is infrequently used in the treatment of rheumatoid arthritis and there are few studies which provide scientific evidence for its use within this patient group. Minor changes in grip strength, improvement in the number of painful and swollen joints and dorsal flexion of the wrist have been found following the application of u/s.
- Long-term benefits are unknown and no harmful effects have been reported.
- However, it should be remembered that self-management and empowerment is one of the management techniques in rheumatoid arthritis and in light of the poor supporting evidence for the use of u/s this makes ultrasound an unlikely choice as a treatment modality.

Low level laser therapy (LLLT)

- The effectiveness is uncertain and there appears to be little if any analgesic effect (Brousseau et al 2005, Hurley et al 2002, Heussler et al 1993).
- There is insufficient evidence to draw any conclusions about the effectiveness of laser (Brousseau et al 2005).

Electrical stimulation

- There is no evidence to justify the use of electrical stimulation with rheumatoid arthritis patients to improve muscle strength and resistance to fatigue (Pelland et al 2002).

Acupuncture

- Conflicting evidence exists for the use of acupuncture in the treatment of rheumatoid arthritis.
- Studies to date do not appear to show an improved effect on ESR, C-RP, pain, number of swollen or tender joints, or patient global assessment of pain.
- However, some clinicians use it with their patients, reporting some benefit, with no detrimental effects being reported (Casimiro et al 2005).

Manual therapy

- 'Hands on' techniques include joint and soft tissue mobilisation and manipulation.
- It is important to consider the contraindications to manual therapy such as osteoporosis or the presence of inflammatory arthropathy in the spine (Maitland 2005).
- The effect of manual therapy remains uncertain due to the scarcity of research in this area (RCP 2009).

Spondyloarthropathies

- These are inflammatory conditions affecting the spine and enthesis (attachment of tendons and ligaments into bone), which overlap and are distinct from rheumatoid arthritis.
- Patients are seronegative for anti-immunoglobulins and present at any age with young adults being primarily affected, with a slight male predominance.
- The different seronegative spondyloarthropathies have distinct clinical features (Boxes 15.1 and 15.2).

Box 15.1 Seronegative spondyloarthropathies

- Juvenile ankylosing spondylitis
- Psoriatic arthropathy
- Reactive arthritis
- Reiter's syndrome
- Enteropathic arthritis (ulcerative colitis, Crohn's disease)
- Ankylosing spondylitis

> **Box 15.2** Clinical features of spondyloarthropathies
>
> - Sacroiliitis
> - Spondylitis
> - Peripheral arthritis
> - Enthesopathy – achilles tendinitis or plantar fasciitis
> - Systemic features include:
> - Psoriasis
> - Inflammatory bowel disease
> - Iritis
> - Genitourinary inflammation

Psoriatic arthritis

- There is an association between psoriasis and inflammatory arthropathy.
- Peripheral joints as well as the axial skeletal and sacroiliac (SI) joints can be affected.
- Psoriatic arthritis can present in a number of ways:
- Symmetrical polyarthritis (rheumatoid like)
- Spondyloarthropathy (resembling AS)
- Asymmetric oligoarthritis (inflammation in 2–4 joints)
- Distal interphalangeal joints
- Arthritis mutilans (severe form of arthritis)

Reactive arthritis and Reiter's syndrome

- Typically have large joint involvement and may result from an immune reaction to infection elsewhere in the body.
- There may be a history of genital or gut infection, the commonest genitourinary trigger being *Chlamydia*.

Enteropathic arthritis

- This may accompany ulcerative colitis or Crohn's disease.
- Patients may develop ankylosing spondylitis or an acute peripheral arthritis.
- SI joint involvement may be asymmetric.

Ankylosing spondylitis (AS)

- A chronic inflammatory disease, which mainly affects the axial skeleton.
- Inflammation occurs in the synovial tissue, spinal ligaments, facet joints, and intervertebral discs.
- AS can be primary (Idiopathic) or secondary (associated with psoriasis or inflammatory bowel disease).

- Clinically, patients suffer from pain and stiffness of the spine and sacroiliac joints. Peripheral joints can also be involved and enthesitis can also be a feature (Khan 2002, Sieper et al 2002).
- Osteoporosis is common in AS, with a reported incidence of 18–62% and males being greater than females (Bessant and Keat, 2002).
- It is usually seen in the axial skeletal, often in patients with syndesmophytes, cervical fusion and peripheral joint involvement.
- The risk of vertebral compression fracture in an AS patient, occurring in a 30 year period following diagnosis is 14% and may follow a relatively minor trauma (Bessant and Keat 2002).
- In early AS, inflammatory mediators are implicated in causing osteoporosis whereas in late AS, decreased mobility may result in osteoporosis.
- Evidence is available to show that patients with AS who smoke, have poorer functional outcomes (Averns et al 1996). The costovertebral joints are affected, which leads to a reduction in mobility of the thoracic cage, AS can therefore reduce the capacity of the lungs, smoking can add to this and could make patients more prone to shortness of breath and lung infections.
- Exercise is important in the management of this aspect of AS.

Physiotherapy management of AS

- Physiotherapy is central to the management of AS and newly diagnosed patients should be seen as soon as possible after diagnosis.
- Due to the chronic status of the disease, physiotherapy management should include education about the disease and self-management techniques.

Physiotherapy aims of treatment in AS

- The aims of physiotherapy management are to:
- Prevent/minimise deformity
- Maintain range of movement
- Maintain muscle power
- Maintain function and quality of life.
- Treatment should be adapted to each individual patient and will depend on clinical findings following assessment, such as:
- Disease activity
- Pain
- Deformities
- Function/disability.
- Physiotherapy intervention will include:
- Education and self management
- Pain control
- Exercise to maintain/improve: CV fitness, posture, function, range of movement (spinal and peripheral joints), muscle strengthening (including antigravity muscles), and stretching specific muscle groups
- Checking posture, and informing patients about postural awareness and ergonomics.

Patient education

- Patients should be advised not to wear braces, which hold the spine rigid, as they can worsen symptoms. Immobility leads to increased stiffness and pain.
- Patients should be given information regarding the disease, treatment options and self management techniques, e.g. problem solving approaches, in order to improve their quality of life (Bodenheimer et al 2002).
- The patient should have overall responsibility for their management and appropriate self management information and advice will empower them and enable informed choices to be made.
- Patients should be advised about the risks associated with contact sports (e.g. rugby), or sports where there is a risk of falls (e.g. skiing or horse riding), due to the risk of spinal fracture. In impact activities (e.g. netball, jogging and step aerobics), patients should be advised about having good shock absorbing soles on trainers to help lessen the impact on joints.
- Driving may be a problem for patients, resulting in joint stiffness following long journeys, frequent stops to stretch may be useful. Good driving posture can be maintained using cushions. Head-rests need to be correctly positioned as a relatively small impact during an accident could have serious consequences. Patients who have difficulty turning their head, may need to use additional mirrors, car accessory shops will be able to help. Patients are advised to contact the DVLA and their motor insurance company if they have particular problems with rotation.
- Education has been shown to improve self efficacy, which has been described by Van der Linden et al (2002) as a prerequisite for success, with the physiotherapist motivating the patient to follow a suitable exercise programme, which will lead to a better outcome of their disease (Barlow and Barefoot 1996).
- The National Ankylosing Spondylitis Society (NASS) provides an excellent resource for advice, information, updates about the latest research and support for both newly diagnosed and established patients and their families http://www.nass.co.uk.
- Arthritis UK (formally ARC) and Arthritis Care also produce patient information and advice.

Exercise

- AS patients need to remain physically active and an exercise regimen should include a cardiovascular workout as well as specific stretches and strengthening exercises. Patients should aim to get out of breath at least once a day as this is the best form of breathing exercise.
- Ankylosing spondylitis causes inflammation around the joints causing stiffness and pain, which makes it difficult for some patients to exercise.
- Non-steroidal anti-inflammatory drugs are usually prescribed to control these symptoms.
- If joints and muscle pain is controlled by medication, patients will find undertaking exercise much easier.
- The physiotherapist may need to ensure that the patient understands why they have been prescribed the medication they should be taking.
- It is important to remain focused on the core physiotherapy skills relating to advice regarding medication and it may be necessary to refer the patient on to another member of the MDT to discuss this aspect of their management.

- Physical and medical treatments are mutually complementary (Dougados et al 2002).

- Patients should be encouraged to take part in a regular daily exercise programme, with some patients finding that exercise enables them to reduce their intake of medication (Van der Linden et al 2002).

- The Cochrane review on physiotherapy interventions for ankylosing spondylitis (Dagfinrud et al 2008) concluded that physiotherapy exercises were beneficial: exercise, either home based or supervised group physiotherapy is better than no exercise and has been shown to improve movement and physical function.

- Supervised group physiotherapy is better than home exercises and has been shown to improve movement and overall wellbeing.

- Functional disability in AS has been found to progress more rapidly in older patients and smokers, and less rapidly in those who regularly do back exercises and have better social support (Ward 2002).

- Mazen and Khan (2008) advised that, although there have been advances in the pharmacological treatment of ankylosing spondylitis, physiotherapy is still an essential part of its management and recommends that physiotherapy should be included as a vital component in the non-pharmacological management strategy for this disease. They concluded that all patients should receive instructions on posture correction and an exercise programme and be encouraged to perform a programme of exercises in water if possible.

- The provision of physiotherapy and in the most severe cases, inpatient rehabilitation has been shown to be of benefit to patients with ankylosing spondylitis.

Range of movement exercises

- Reduction in all planes of movement throughout the spine can occur in AS, due to the stiffening effects of the disease process.

- Exercises should ensure that the joints are moved through the entire range of available movement.

- The exercises may have to be modified to accommodate the patient's posture and restricted range.

- It is important to keep patients motivated and to this end incorporate pieces of equipment into the patients routine.

- Breathing exercises should be a regular feature of range of movement exercises, as chest expansion can be limited due to the costovertebral and sternocostal joint becoming involved.

- Jaw stretching exercises should also be encouraged.

Strengthening exercises

- Pain leading to inactivity and postural deformity can lead to weak muscles (Cooper et al 1991).

- Muscle strengthening is necessary to maintain a correct posture.

- The extensor muscle groups of the cervical, thoracic and lumbar spine, lumbar side flexors and thoracic rotators should be strengthened in addition to the abdominal muscles.

Aerobic exercises

- Aerobic exercise conditions the heart and lungs by increasing the oxygen available to the body and by enabling the heart to use oxygen more efficiently.

- Aerobic exercise will also increase resistance to fatigue, increase general stamina and improve mood and therefore improve quality of life and enable patients to carry out their work and maintain an active lifestyle.
- Due to the disease process, many patients have difficulty carrying out impact exercises on land, although low impact exercises are possible, the hydrotherapy pool is an excellent place in which to undertake aerobic exercise, as the impact is significantly reduced.
- Increasing respiratory rate and chest expansion helps to mobilise the thoracic joints.

Aquatic therapy exercises

- Aquatic therapy is an excellent form of treatment for ankylosing spondylitis.
- To further assist or resist buoyancy, floats can be utilised to increase a stretch or make a movement more difficult. Bats or flippers can be used to increase surface area or lengthen a lever to increase resistance to help strengthen muscles.
- Speed of movement through the water can also be used to increase the resistance of the exercise.
- Breathing exercises and team games such as relay races can be incorporated to add variety and improve cardiovascular fitness.
- Water aerobics can also be performed and patients often find this type of exercise more comfortable in water then on land.
- Refer to the aquatic therapy chapter for more information about treatment ideas.

Muscle stretching

- Muscle stretching is an important part of exercise regimen in ankylosing spondylitis. Prior to stretching, adequate warm-up should take place, or stretching can be done after a shower/bath following the application of heat (Bruckner and Khan 2005).
- Bulstrode et al (1987) describe the contract–relax method of muscle stretching as being useful for lengthening tight muscle tissue with this being suitable to be carried out on land or in a pool.
- Muscles can also be stretched by using a slow prolonged stretch, the stretch being held for a minimum of 15 seconds (Bruckner and Khan 2005).
- Stretching should be pain free and the stretch should be felt in the appropriate part of the muscle being stretched.

Pain control in AS

- As with other inflammatory arthritis heat can help to relieve pain and stiffness.
- Some patients may benefit from a hot bath or shower first thing in the morning and/or before bed, stretching exercises can be done at the same time.
- Hot water bottles or electric blankets may also be useful in bed.
- Ice or cooling can also be used on inflamed areas.
- Soft tissue massage may help relieve muscle tension.
- Pain in AS can be aggravated by inactivity and is often reduced by exercise and patients will often report being woken in the early morning by joint stiffness and pain.
- Exercise, therefore plays an important role in the pain management of AS.

Tai Chi for AS

- Lee et al (2007) have suggested that Tai Chi improves disease activity and flexibility in patients with ankylosing spondylitis following a regular programme of 1 hour of exercise two times per week.

Systemic lupus erythematosus (SLE)

- SLE is often symmetrical non-erosive and usually affects the knees, wrist and proximal interphalangeal joints.
- Clinical features include disorders of the skin, pulmonary and cardiovascular systems, renal function, haematological conditions, neurological problems, fatigue and myalgia.
- Joint subluxation and soft tissue contractures may cause deformities and tendon rupture may occur as a result of tenosynovitis.
- Muscle strengthening and low impact aerobic exercise should be encouraged.
- Caution should be taken when exercising during a flare (Liang 1994).
- Tench et al (2003) demonstrated that exercise helps to reduce fatigue.

Septic joints

- The most serious diagnosis of hot swollen joints is septic arthritis, which can be fatal. Delayed or inappropriate treatment can cause joint damage.
- Patients who present with an acute history of a hot swollen and tender joint should, even in the absence of fever, be treated as a septic joint unless established as otherwise.
- These patients should be referred to A&E urgently or for urgent specialist assessment by a rheumatologist or orthopaedic surgeon for immediate appropriate treatment (Coakley et al 2006).

The references for this chapter can be found on www.expertconsult.com.

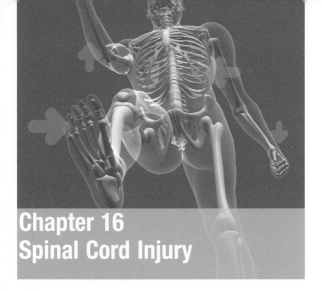

Chapter 16
Spinal Cord Injury

- Patients with a spinal cord injury (SCI) are usually managed within a specialist unit, by an interdisciplinary team.

- Patients with a SCI may present at a local hospital, e.g. most new cases present to the accident and emergency (A&E) department of a district general hospital, whilst patients with an established injury may be admitted to a local hospital during a period of acute deterioration or require ongoing input following discharge from a specialist unit.

- Physiotherapy plays an essential part in the management of patients from the acute phase through to end stage rehabilitation.

- Interventions include the teaching of physical skills and coping techniques that someone with a SCI will need, to regain their independence within the community.

- Many of the techniques employed are not specific to SCI rehabilitation, but are methods widely used within cardiorespiratory, musculoskeletal, orthopaedics and neurology rehabilitation, albeit applied to the SCI population.

- Thorough assessment and re-assessment is the key to developing an appropriate and effective treatment plan.

- It must be remembered, however, that along with disturbance of motor function and sensation, many other body systems may be affected and careful consideration of the impact of therapy upon these systems is required.

Aims of rehabilitation

- A spinal cord injury is considered to be one of the most devastating conditions that can occur following a trauma.

- In seconds an individual is catapulted from a familiar life as an able-bodied person into a previously unknown situation and an environment of, in most cases, permanent disability.

- Rehabilitation therefore needs to address not only the physical aspects, but also the psychological aspects that occur following a spinal cord injury.

- Whilst in the acute stage the individual will for various reasons often not fully understand the enormity of the changes to their life.

- During mobilisation, rehabilitation and community re-integration the impact of loss of muscle power, sensation, movement, bladder, bowel, temperature control and sexual function in daily life will become clear.

- Adjustment to the injury is a lifelong process in which constant changes occur in the patient, their circumstances and needs; support thus needs to begin soon after injury (Bromley 2006).

- Rehabilitation aims to provide the individual with the knowledge, physical skills and coping strategies that are required, whilst developing their ability to regain the control of their life that may have been lost after the initial injury.

Goal planning

- Goal planning aims to place the patient at the centre of their rehabilitation programme, whilst increasing their engagement in rehabilitation activities (Kennedy et al 1991).

- It is based on the patient being an active participant in their rehabilitation and aims to recognise and utilise the patient's strengths in order to meet their own identified needs.

- Goals are set with the rehabilitation team, specific measurable and realistic targets being defined to be achieved in an agreed time.

- Regular review and monitoring of success can become an empowering process.

- Areas of unmet needs can be recognised and addressed and the roles and contribution of the various health care professionals can be clarified.

- The need to address all areas affected by the SCI throughout rehabilitation is essential if the process is to be considered as one of learning and development of new skills and knowledge.

Functional goals of rehabilitation

- A knowledge of the anticipated functional outcome and physical independence in activities of daily living allows targets to be set to assist the patient achieve their physical goals.

- It also provides a structure for the team to work towards in conjunction with each patient and supports the goal planning framework.

- Goals are strongly influenced by the level of the spinal cord injury and the remaining innervated muscles (Appendix 16.3, number 6, p. 397).

Factors that may affect rehabilitation

- The extent and speed of progression through rehabilitation and the final goals achieved will be influenced by:

- Age
- Level of lesion
- Completeness/incompleteness of the lesion
- Any associated injuries
- Previous medical history
- Degree of spasticity
- Morphology of the individual
- Psychological factors, e.g. motivation, locus of control, depression, etc.
- Pain.

Acute physical/medical management

Road side/initial management of acute trauma

- The highest proportions of patients with a SCI will have been involved in a fall or road traffic accident.
- At the scene of the injury, initial attention is focussed on maintaining the airway, breathing and circulation (ABC).
- In an actual or suspected SCI, a jaw-thrust/chin lift technique is used to maintain a patent's airway rather than extension of the neck (ACS 2006).
- Once considered safe, extrication and transfer to the closest accident and emergency (A&E) department is conducted with 'full body spinal protection' established.
- This utilises a cervical collar, spinal board and head restraint (Harrison 2007).
- All unconscious or multitrauma patients with the potential for SCI are treated prophylactically as if they have injured their cord.
- The management of the individual will commence immediately to address the multisystem impairments that are secondary to SCI and to prevent avoidable complications.
- Conservative management is followed initially, using postural reduction with or without traction to align the vertebral column.
- Respiratory support is provided if required, regular turns are instigated for the management of the skin and a regimen of treatment for the care of the paralysed bladder and bowel is commenced.
- Patients may be sedated or require admission to the intensive therapy unit (ITU) for multisystem management.
- A variety of medications may be used to control the effects of a damaged spinal cord, including those to alleviate pain, treat infections or anticoagulation therapy to prevent the formation of a deep vein thrombosis.
- It is no longer standard practice to offer high-dose methylprednisolone for spinal cord swelling (Short et al 2000), but this may still be seen in some district general hospitals.

Management of the spine

- The duration of bed rest depends on the type and cause of injury, the degree of spinal instability, the method of management, i.e. conservative or surgical and medical stability.

- The principles of management of the spine are to:
- Enhance neurological recovery
- Avoid neurological deterioration
- Achieve biomechanical stability of the spine at the site of the impairment, preserving spared neural tissue until healing occurs (Bromley 2006).
- The decision to manage the injury conservatively or surgically is multifactorial and dependent upon experience and ability of the medical team.
- There appears to be no difference in outcome between surgical and conservative management, although surgery may be associated with greater complications El Masry & Jaffray (1992).
- Patients with non-traumatic injuries are usually mobilised as soon as they are medically stable.

Conservative management

- Patients with traumatic injuries may be treated with a minimum of 6 weeks bedrest. An X-ray and computerised tomography scan (CT) of the spine will decide whether further bedrest is indicated. The total bedrest period may be 10–12 weeks in an uncomplicated case.
- Dislocations are usually treated with postural reduction, using pillows for the thoraco-lumbar lesions and neck roll and skull traction for the cervical lesions (Figures 16.1 and 16.2).
- Skull traction is usually maintained for 6 weeks, and is dependent thereafter on a CT taken to check the position and degree of bony callus formation.
- If further bed rest is indicated, the position of the neck will typically be maintained by using a neck roll or hard collar.
- If Halo-traction with a vest is used, the patient can be mobilised earlier, but the Halo traction will be maintained for at least 12 weeks post-injury.

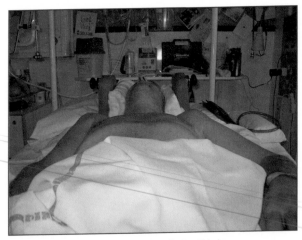

Figure 16.1 Cervical spine immobilisation using head blocks.

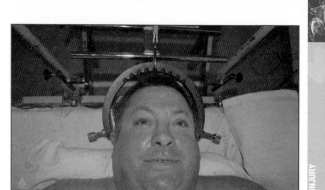

Figure 16.2 Cervical spine immobilisation with skull traction.

Surgical intervention

- Surgical management of a traumatic injury will greatly reduce the period required on bedrest.
- The type and length of internal fixation used will vary depending on the site, number of levels involved and severity of the injury.
- The length of the fixation should be kept to a minimum by the surgeon and usually should extend just one segment above and below to prevent additional complications, e.g. reduced range of movement in the spine caused by the implant.
- The postoperative bedrest period can vary, but is typically 1 week.

Physiotherapy assessment and treatment planning

- The overall purpose of physiotherapy for patients with spinal cord injury is to improve health-related quality of life through improving their ability to participate in activities of daily life (Harvey 2008).
- The accurate identification of the factors impacting on the person's ability to participate is achieved through assessment and re-assessment and is the key to successful management.
- Assessment tools are numerous and should be used to monitor and measure progress.
- The International Classification of Functioning, Disability and Health (ICF) can be used to facilitate the process. The reader is referred to Chapter 16 in Volume 1 (World health Assembly, 2001).

Acute physiotherapy management and rehabilitation

- The initial bed rest phase will be experienced by all individuals with a spinal cord injury.
- The duration will vary greatly dependent on cause, impairment and management.

- This period demonstrates a period where intervention is deemed essential to influence respiratory and life-threatening conditions.
- This is also an opportunity for many patients to commence rehabilitation and education, albeit in a limited capacity.
- The physiotherapeutic aims of acute management of an individual with a spinal cord injury are:
- Maintain and progress respiratory function
- Joint management and prevention of contractures
- Maintain muscle strength and strengthen partially innervated muscles
- Development of compensatory movements in some instances (e.g. 'trick' elbow extension)
- Prevention, early identification and management of complications.

Maintenance and progression of respiratory function

- Pulmonary complications in spinal cord injury are common and are directly correlated with mortality. The higher the level of neurological injury, the more complications are likely (Bromley 2006).
- Respiratory physiotherapy aims include:
- Improve ventilation and gas exchange
- Reduce airway obstruction – 'plugs'
- Promote sputum mobilisation and expectoration
- Improve force and endurance in both inspiratory and expiratory muscles
- Maintain chest wall compliance
- Develop ventilatory reserve to cope with increased activity and infection.
- Prophylactically patients should be offered breathing exercises, preferably using an incentive spirometer to provide 'biofeedback'. (assisting re-education of preserved respiratory musculature)
- Mechanical ventilation is considered when the vital capacity drops below 1 litre, and is essential below 500 mL (CSCM 2005). The use of intermittent positive pressure breathing (IPPB) should be considered for preventative treatment of patients with low vital capacities. It is also a useful tool to teach the ultra high lesion how to 'rescue breathe' with their upper accessory muscles when off the ventilator by manipulating the 'sensitivity' dial.
- Abdominal binders should be used by patients without abdominal innervation when upright. This prevents the typical postural drop in vital capacity seen in the majority of SCI patients (Prigent et al 2010).
- Sputum clearance techniques should be taught to the patient or their family/ carers when assistance is required. A peak cough flow (PCF) of 160 L/min is deemed essential for clearing airways, with values greater than 270 L/min ensuring a reduction in respiratory infections in the neurologically impaired (ATS 2004). This is difficult to achieve for many patients without innervation of the abdominal muscles and those with low vital capacities. When this is the case, a manual-assisted cough or use of the cough assist machine is recommended (BTS 2009).
- Respiratory deterioration can occur due to any number of reasons, e.g. ascending neurology, respiratory muscle fatigue, abdominal distension, over sedation, excessive IV infusion, respiratory infection, aspiration or even enforced smoking cessation (Dicpinigaitis et al 2006).

- When deterioration does occur, fatigue will be an issue, a 'little and often' approach is suggested.
- Close liaison with the medical team is necessary, the physiotherapist is encouraged to use a combination of humidified oxygen, postural drainage, breath augmentation, e.g. IPPB, manual hyperinflation or cough assist machine, and sputum clearance techniques, e.g. assisted cough timed with suction, for those whom can't clear to the mouth.
- Early implementation of Non-Invasive Ventilation (NIV) or mechanical ventilation is advised with rising PaCO$_2$, prior to respiratory arrest, to protect the healing spinal cord (Gardner et al 1986).
- Early tracheostomy is advocated for those difficult to wean from invasive ventilation (Harris 2007).
- Suction must be approached with caution in tetraplegia during the period of spinal shock. Unopposed vagal tone due to the parasympathetic dominance evident in this patient population predisposes the patient to bradycardia and potentially sinus arrest (RCP 2008). Pacemaker insertion should be avoided due to the fact this presentation typically resolves naturally as spinal shock passes and a pacemaker would contraindicate any future MRI scans. It is better managed with pre-oxygenation and prophylactic sympathomimetics such as glycopyrrolate. It does not contraindicate chest physiotherapy, as omission would invariably lead to respiratory failure.
- Weaning from ventilation is a team approach and should be gradual due to respiratory muscle fatigability.
- An approach of progressive ventilator free breathing has been shown to be twice as effective as the typical approach of decreasing pressure support, as used in the general population (Peterson et al 1994).

Joint management

- The outcome of the rehabilitation depends very much on maintaining adequate range of movement (ROM) and muscle length in the affected joints during the bed rest period.
- Prolonged periods of bed rest, pain, spasm, lack of regular repositioning and unopposed muscle activity can lead to muscle contracture and joint stiffness.
- The results of contracture development may include functional dependence, inhibited goal achievement, pain, pressure sores, difficulty to seat, increased carer load, increased spasms, respiratory compromise and a poor body image.
- In some cases it may be necessary to try to increase the 'normal' ROM in a joint to enable the patient to achieve certain functional goals later on, e.g. increased external rotation of the hip with knee and hip flexion ('tailor position') for dressing, or increased elbow extension with wrist and shoulder extension for weight bearing without triceps innervation.
- Positioning:
- Sustained stretch through positioning can help prevent length-associated changes and contractures in muscle.
- A 24-hour positioning programme should be devised for both the acute and rehabilitation patient and discussed with the nursing staff.
- Thorough assessment should help to identify the assistance required to facilitate and maintain these positions and the length of time tolerated (Figures 16.3, 16.4 and 16.5).

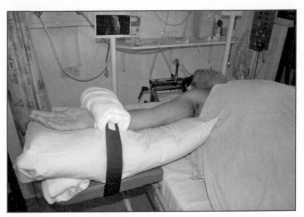

Figure 16.3 'Unilateral crucifix' used to achieve shoulder abduction and external rotation, with elbow extension and forearm supination in tetraplegia.

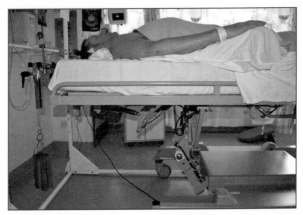

Figure 16.4 The contralateral upper limb should be placed with the shoulder by the side, elbow extended, forearm pronated, with elevation distal to the elbow being delivered by a 'ski-jump' pillow to minimise dependant oedema. Care should be taken not to allow the shoulder to fall into protraction and extension.

- Passive and active movements:
- Passive/active assisted movements must be applied in a controlled and rhythmic manner, fully supporting joints, as paralysed structures can easily be damaged.
- Wherever a patient has some control of movement, guided active participation should be encouraged.
- Adequate analgesia needs to be provided.

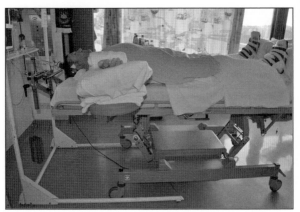

Figure 16.5 Use of pillows or pressure-relieving ankle foot orthosis (PRAFOs) should be encouraged to maintain a plantargrade ankle.

- Education of the patient and family in how they can assist the process should be part of the treatment consideration.
- Close liaison with the occupational therapist is advocated to manage the special requirements of the upper limb ensuring there is co-ordination of goals and treatment.
- In order to maintain full and pain-free range in the shoulder, mobilisation of the scapula and accessory movements to the shoulder and clavicular joints are indicated prior to physiological ranging.
- While mobilising the shoulder, great care must be taken not to move the cervical spine.
- The following movements should be carried out:
- Depression of the shoulder, required for lifting activities, maintained by daily bilateral stretches of the upper trapezii
- Bilateral shoulder adduction prevents shortening of the rhomboids
- Pectoral stretch
- *Full shoulder flexion, including above 90°, unless pain is caused at the fracture site*
- Elbow flexion involves stretching of long head of triceps from 90° shoulder flexion or full elevation
- Elbow extension with full wrist extension with the arm by the side of the body. A C5/6 will not be able to lock the elbow when attempting to take weight through the arms without this. If a tenodesis grip is being encouraged and developed the fingers must be allowed to flex during this stretch
- Elbow extension with supination and pronation. Loss of supination compromises the lifting position for transferring. Loss of pronation compromises the potential for hand–mouth activities and a successful tenodesis grip.
- In patients with unstable lesions of T10 and below being managed conservatively or awaiting surgery, hip flexion is initially restricted to 30° in order to avoid excessive movement of the lumbar spine.
- The movement must always avoid pain at the fracture site.

- Full knee flexion is maintained with unilateral tailor position (full external rotation of the hip with limited hip flexion and full knee flexion). Rotation of the pelvis must be monitored during this movement.
- Further lower limb movements should be carried out as follows:
- Accessory movements to the metatarsal joints help to prevent deformity of the foot, which might otherwise cause pressure problems when wearing shoes and during standing.
- Adduction across midline with a straight leg.
- Abduction to the edge of the bed only (max. 45°).
- Mobilise the patella before flexing the knee.
- Extension of the hip (hip stretch) is necessary for all incomplete lesions with the potential to walk and complete lesions with the potential to use callipers, but should not be commenced without prior discussion and agreement with the consultant.
- This is achieved by placing the patient in side lying after 2–3 weeks post-injury, depending on the fracture.
- When carrying out the movement, the pelvis must be stabilised, the knee flexed to 90° with the hip in neutral rotation with no abduction or adduction.
- Particular vigilance is needed for patients with T12/L1 levels because of possible unopposed active hip flexion.
- Hamstring stretch is not usually carried out until 6 weeks post-injury because of the pull on a healing spinal cord.
- This should not be initiated without prior discussion with the consultant.
- If carried out while the patient is still on bedrest, the straight leg raise is restricted to 60°.
- There are a range of other options available to a physiotherapist to maintain joint range and function:
- Splinting
- Bio feedback
- Functional electrical stimulation
- Accessory joint movements
- Soft tissue release
- Spasticity management (medication, positioning and ranging to avoid increase in tone).

Maintenance of muscle power and strengthening of partially innervated muscle groups

- Post spinal cord injury a number of problems can often be identified with muscle strength within the same individual: complete paralysis, partial paralysis of a muscle and neurologically intact muscles which can be functionally weak and/or deconditioned.
- The appropriate intervention for the partially paralysed muscle or the neurologically intact muscle is the development and instigation of a strengthening programme.
- A strengthening programme can commence during the acute phase using all remaining partially innervated or intact muscles, e.g. high cervical lesions may undertake sling suspension or assisted exercises, whereas weight training/ Thera-Bands may be appropriate for paraplegics.

- With all patients care must be taken to ensure excessive effort does not cause movement of the fracture site, encourage spasticity or develop unwanted compensatory strategies.

Development of desired compensatory movements

- The time spent in the acute phase on bedrest can be used to commence the development of appropriate compensatory movements, the most notable being trick extension of the elbow (elbow extension without triceps activity) and tenodesis grip.

Trick extension of the elbow

- This movement can be taught to C5 or C6 spinal cord injured patients without triceps activity to prevent shortening of the biceps tendon and to aid functional upper limb movement.
- To achieve trick extension the patient must learn to relax biceps in combination with lateral rotation and protraction of the shoulder and allow gravity to extend the elbow.
- Shoulder flexion without elbow flexion ('straight arm raise') is also a skill that should be promoted for function.
- Development of this skill does not hinder recovery of triceps activity.

Tenodesis grip

- The tenodesis grip should be developed in individuals with a C6 or C7 spinal cord injury.
- It utilises flexion of the wrist by gravity and passive extension of the fingers to open the hand around an object whilst in forearm pronation. Active wrist extension places passive tension on the long finger and thumb flexors, enabling an object to be picked up. The efficacy of this movement can be improved by allowing the finger flexors and thumb web space to shorten.
- Early development of the tenodesis grip through shortening of the finger flexors continues to be controversial.
- Unlike trick extension of the elbow, development of tenodesis grip can limit recovery of the finger extensors due to the shortening of the finger flexors and this can hinder the development of a 'normal' grip and release pattern where recovery has been demonstrated. This can be managed nonetheless where evidence of neurological recovery exists by splinting and re-education.

Identification and management of complications

- A physiotherapist will maintain close, regular contact with the patient throughout the period of acute management and rehabilitation and therefore is often able to identify complications at an early stage.
- The complications most frequently encountered and managed by physiotherapy will be discussed.

Deep vein thrombosis (DVT)

- DVTs most commonly occur in legs, but can also appear in the arms.
- If a DVT is suspected or diagnosed, passive movements to both legs or arms are discontinued until therapeutic anticoagulation is achieved.

Pulmonary embolus (PE)

- Passive movements to the legs or arms may dislodge an undiagnosed DVT.
- If a patient complains of sudden, sharp chest pain and breathlessness passive movements must be stopped immediately and the medical team informed.

Heterotrophic ossification (HO)

- The physiotherapist is often the first member of the team to identify the development of bone in the connective tissues, most commonly around the hips, knees and elbows.
- Often the first indication of ossification is a different end-feel to a joint or raised infection markers.
- There may be swelling, redness and increased temperature in the affected joint or muscle group. One cause of HO is thought to be minute trauma to tissues that have experienced rough, jerky handling.
- The range of movement is greatly at risk in the affected area and it is crucial to maintain at least functional range, i.e. minimum 90° at hips and knees to achieve a good sitting position.
- Initially passive movements are discontinued until the inflammation has subsided, and then recommenced with care, ensuring that there are no forced movements.
- As the initial tissue reaction settles range of motion is increased through positioning and passive movements.
- Regular monitoring of the range of movement is important.
- Drug therapy using bisphosphonates may sometimes be indicated.

Swelling

- Following spinal cord injury swelling tends to occur for two reasons:
- Overstretching of ligaments and joint injury in the unprotected joint.
- This tends to be due to poor positioning, i.e. hyperextension of the knees whilst on bed rest or during activities such as standing and gait re-education where the joint is not fully protected due to weakness, e.g. weakness of the hamstrings resulting in knee hyperextension.
- Careful positioning with adequate support to the legs will prevent this during the bed rest phase, whilst consideration to positioning and the appropriateness of an orthosis needs to be considered during standing and gait re-education.
- Postural/gravitational oedema.
- This tends to be due to poor vasomotor control, altered muscle tone and excessive administration of intravenous fluids.
- It can occur in either the hands or feet.
- If it is not managed and dispersed, collagen deposits can change into fibrous tissue and limit joint movement.
- Management is essential through elevation, passive movements and application of compression garments such as elastic stockings.
- If splints are used, they should be reviewed to prevent pressure areas forming.

Spasticity

- If excessive spasticity develops, passive and active movements, stretches and mobilisations may have to be modified and/or increased.

- Prolonged passive stretching and reflex inhibitory postures may be useful to break a dominant pattern, e.g. hipflicks and 'frog' position.
- If the individual is mobilising, then weight bearing through standing and/or walking can help.
- The degree of spasticity should be monitored and communicated to the other members of the team.
- Drug therapy is often useful to manage this.

Pain and painful shoulders

- Pain is a common complication following SCI which can limit participation in rehabilitation, the ability to perform functional activities and impacts on quality of life.
- Kennedy et al (1998) found that 'pain at 6 weeks post injury is the strongest predictor of pain at one year post discharge.'
- It therefore can have a significant impact on the person with spinal cord injury at all stages post injury.
- The location, intensity, time since onset of spinal cord injury, duration and cause are highly variable.
- Correct identification of the cause of pain, e.g. nociceptive or neuropathic and early management is important.
- Shoulders have been widely documented as being a common site for pain following spinal cord injury.
- The incidence of shoulder pain in acute tetraplegia has been reported to range from 51% to 78% (Crowe et al 2000, Mackay-Lyons 1994, Waring and Maynard 1991, Lee and McMahon 2002) and as high as 85% during rehabilitation (Salisbury et al 2003).
- Pain has been reported to be a potential barrier to recovery of upper limb function and independence (Mackay-Lyons 1994).
- Education, correct positioning and frequent changes in positioning of the arm are important factors in preventing shoulder pain.
- Close liaison with the medical team is essential for appropriate analgesia provision.
- Patients should be encouraged to move the arms actively as much as possible and as early as possible.
- Maintenance of accessory movements and involvement of the scapula during passive and functional tasks (even when carried out by a carer) is essential to pain-free range.

Mobilisation

- In spinal cord injury rehabilitation, mobilisation usually refers to the period when the patient moves from bed rest to the wheelchair in preparation for active rehabilitation.

The first mobilisation

- The initial mobilisation of an individual requires the co-ordinated approach of the whole team to ensure the process is a safe and smooth transition.

- The process will be started by the medical team when the individual is deemed stable and fit to mobilise and a date for first mobilisation into the wheelchair will be defined. In some instances mobilisation may need to occur with a collar or brace applied.
- Nursing staff will usually start to sit the patient up in bed, gradually increasing the duration and degree of elevation over a period of a few days prior to actual mobilisation.
- It is the role of either the physiotherapist or occupational therapist to provide a suitable wheelchair for first mobilisation.
- Measurements, i.e. hip width, thigh and calf length and back height will need to be taken to ensure the correct size wheelchair is provided.
- The type of wheelchair is dependent upon the level and completeness of injury, which will depict the degree of support required and if other aspects are required, e.g. tilt in space and head rest.
- A cushion with suitable pressure-relieving and postural support properties will also be required.
- Re assessment of an individual's definitive seating needs will need to be undertaken once the early rehabilitation has been completed.
- It is usually the role of the physiotherapist and nursing staff to undertake the first mobilisation.
- Typically an abdominal binder is applied to those without abdominal innervation, graduated pressure stockings and ephedrine is taken 30 minutes prior to mobilisation to aid orthostatic hypotension.
- The physiotherapist needs to ensure correct posture and adjust the wheelchair as required once the patient is hoisted into it.
- It is the responsibility of all attending staff to monitor the patient closely, especially for symptomatic signs of low blood pressure.
- Mobilising the individual who requires ventilator support offers additional challenges which must be managed safely. Often a third person is required to manage the tracheostomy, ventilator tubing and ventilator.
- First mobilisation may only last up to 20 minutes, with postural hypotension or concerns over skin condition being the limiting factor.
- If the patient complains of dizziness, the legs should be raised and the chair tipped backwards until the symptoms subside.
- The duration of mobilisation should gradually be increased over the following days or weeks until the patient is able to manage sufficiently long enough in the wheelchair to participate in active rehabilitation. During this period, the patient will also wean from the use of ephedrine.
- Subsequent mobilisations are usually undertaken by the nursing staff.

Skin management

- An appropriate pressure-relieving cushion must be provided for mobilisation and the skin on the ischial tuberosities, greater trochanters and sacrum in particular needs to be monitored closely, ideally, immediately on returning to bed.
- Patients need to be taught how to relieve pressure from the ischial tuberosities.
- The most common method is forward leaning.

- Side leaning can also be utilised, as can a vertical lift, although this is not recommended due to the increased pressure put on the shoulder complex.
- With each method the ischial tuberosities need to clear the cushion and the position must be held for 2 minutes (each side if side leaning) at least hourly.
- Patients with a high level of injury who are unable to safely use one of the techniques described can change the tilt of their chair to redistribute the pressure.
- Initially the patient will require assistance with pressure relief and require prompting from the nursing staff to carry this out.
- The patient should however progress to completing the task independently as soon as they are able. Verbal independence is imperative in those without the physical ability.
- Skin management must be carefully considered and monitored throughout rehabilitation during all activities and tasks, positioning and seating.

Psychological impact

- It is at this stage that the true impact of the individual's spinal cord injury often becomes apparent to them as they first become aware of an altered ability to balance.
- The response to this is highly variable and for some this stage poses a particular emotional challenge and presents particular problems to the staff.
- Involvement of a psychologist should be encouraged and sought with consent of the patient, whilst the team need to support the patient through this stage.

Rehabilitation following mobilisation

- Whenever physical independence in functional activities cannot be achieved, the physiotherapist must ensure that the patient has the knowledge to direct all necessary procedures and that the carers have been shown how to assist or carry out any handling skills that may be required.
- It is essential that the rehabilitation process prepares the patient as far as is practically possible for the future lifestyle that they wish to pursue.
- This will necessitate regular goal planning, problem solving and close communication between all team members.
- Independence is not only related to physical competence, it is more to do with the ability of an individual to direct and control their life situation.
- Physiotherapy should utilise an individual's own coping skills to maximise their full potential, physical or otherwise.
- Risk assessment of each of the rehabilitation tasks is paramount and continuous, to ensure that the patient is progressed in a safe manner avoiding possible complications or injury.

Limitations

- The medical team may place certain limitations on the initial rehabilitation phase due to the stability or healing of the fracture site, associated injuries, infection or problems related to a disease process.
- These limitations may take the form of limiting specific activities, e.g. weight bearing through a fractured limb or through provision of a collar or a brace.

- Clarity about any limitations in place and for how long these apply will need to be sought prior to the early stages of rehabilitation.

Activities restricted by a collar

- Tetraplegic patients, who have had their fracture conservatively treated, will usually wear a collar until the neck is strong enough to control and hold the head adequately.
- The type and duration of collar used is at the discretion of the consultant.
- Some patients may have a soft collar, others may have a more restrictive one, e.g. a Philadelphia collar.
- Rehabilitation will be guided by the biomechanical restrictions of a collar.
- Any exercise where movement of the head plays an important part in achieving the activity cannot be completed and therefore should not be attempted, e.g. balancing on a plinth, lifting in long-sitting, rolling, unassisted lying to sitting and advanced wheelchair skills involving back wheel balance.
- Although the soft collar does not restrict rotation, this should not be encouraged initially.

Activities restricted by a brace

- A brace is intended to stop forward flexion and rotation of the trunk.
- A correctly fitted brace will automatically dictate which activities are restricted: i.e. activities which require leaning forward beyond vertical when long sitting, e.g. legs-up transfer, lifting in long-sitting, and dressing on the bed.
- Activities which require flexion or rotation of the trunk itself will also be impossible to carry out, e.g. bath and floor transfers, balancing, rolling and advanced wheelchair skills involving back wheel balance.

Balance training

- Balance training is essential to enable the paralysed person to gain confidence in the sitting position and should be worked on in both long sitting (if able) and short sitting.
- This is achieved rapidly for lower lesions, but may require much perseverance in tetraplegia.
- Postural awareness using the visual feedback of a mirror is progressed to unsupported sitting or dynamic exercises or games.
- The patient must develop a good functional sense of balance before other functional tasks can be pursued.

Strengthening

- A strengthening programme should be based upon an accurate assessment of muscle strength and task analysis and should consider the importance of specificity of training to facilitate carry over to the task.
- It is also important to consider endurance, not just strength.
- There are a number of ways in which a muscle can be strengthened:
- Assisted, gantry suspension or use of a mobile arm support for functional activities
- Resisted exercises, e.g. using weights, pushing up a slope, squats, sit to stand, lifting

- Aquatic therapy and swimming
- Functional electrical stimulation (FES) and use of a FES bike
- Speed and endurance training
- EMG and bio feedback for very weak muscles.

- Strengthening of the neck muscles is particularly important for posture and function in those with a cervical or upper thoracic injury and should be introduced initially using isometric exercises, if still using a collar, following discussion with the consultant.

- Strengthening of the back extensors for those with a lower spinal cord injury is also of great importance and should be commenced during the rehabilitation phase.

- It is important to monitor the effects of strengthening, particularly resistance training, upon any identified spasticity and adjust accordingly.

- The patient must also be able to monitor closely their position whilst carrying out the programme to ensure the correct muscles are being trained and poor posture is avoided. This may require supervision.

- It is inevitable that many individuals will demonstrate muscle imbalance, but the effects on posture must be minimised and the appropriate stretches used to enable postural maintenance.

- Individuals may develop shoulder pain, due to muscle imbalance and the long-term use of the joint as a weight-bearing joint.

- Exercises to strengthen the rotator cuff help prevent the development of long-term complications and should be instigated from an early stage.

Matwork

- Rolling, lying to sitting, moving across the bed and lifting form the basis of many bed-based functional activities such as dressing, positioning and getting in and out of bed and can also be considered as the building blocks for activities such as transfers and moving within the chair.

- These skills will generally be mastered in paraplegia, especially those with abdominal innervation, with greater ease and speed than those with tetraplegia.

- These tasks will often need to be broken down into smaller component parts until the whole task can be completed.

- The reader is referred to the recommended reading for further information and diagrams.

Transfers

- Not all patients will be able to transfer independently and those with lesions above C6 are unlikely to achieve the level of function to enable them to transfer independently.

- However, persons with a higher level of injury may be able to participate in a level transfer and will often be given the opportunity to explore this, even if for emergency purposes only.

- Transfers may be practised from an early stage in the rehabilitation process.

- Progress to independent transfers or those requiring the assistance of nursing staff, other members of the team or family occurs when deemed safe and appropriate.

- The use of various pieces of equipment such as sliding boards may be trialled during the development of the patient's ability to transfer and their suitability for long-term use assessed.
- The basic safety principles that cover any patient's ability to transfer are:
- Castors should be positioned in a forward direction to improve the forward/backward stability of the chair
- The patient should bring their bottom forward in the chair to avoid scraping the skin when transferring over the wheel, or other skin protection precautions should be taken
- Avoid knocking or bumping the limbs
- Vertical forces should be applied to the lift to avoid the chair moving sideways
- Positioning the chair at an angle to the transfer surface helps to clear the wheel when lifting
- The influence of spasticity should be considered and how this will interfere with the transfer.
- For lower tetraplegics and most paraplegics, physical independence can be progressed through the learning of advanced transfers.
- These require the ability to lift across significant height differences, e.g. bath transfers and on and off the floor.
- The ability to lift one's own wheelchair in/out of the car, back wheel balance, and negotiate kerbs and stairs are all taught if practical.

Bed transfers

- These are usually the first transfers that the patient will attempt and involve movement across equal heights.
- The patient may use legs down or legs up techniques dependent on their ability to maintain balance, the strength in their arms and trunk and their ability to move their legs either from the bed or from the chair.
- For full independence in this transfer the patient must also master the ability to place their legs on and off a bed independently.
- If the patient is unable to produce a strong lift then the chair may be placed at 90° to the bed to facilitate a forward lift.
- A variety of transfer boards are available and should be trialled with those who are unable to achieve sufficient lift, or demonstrate additional complications such as spasms.

Car transfers

- Car transfers are regarded as an advanced transfer and pose a number of challenges, e.g. negotiating the large gap between the car seat and the wheelchair and the confined space available for assistance or manoeuvring.
- They are, however, often taught relatively early in the rehabilitation process, where appropriate and safe, to enable the patient to commence visits out with family and friends and when applicable, weekend leave.
- Transfers therefore often start with teaching relevant family and friends how to assist the transfer into the passenger side of the car and then progress to independent transfers into the drivers' side if returning to driving is a possibility.
- Sliding boards can be used to provide the necessary assistance for those patients with a weaker ability to lift and the patient should be taught how to

use the confines of the car to provide points of balance support, e.g. using existing hand holds, resting their head against the support of a seat or reclining the seat to facilitate positioning once in the car.

- The position of the legs for the transfer is dependent on personal preference and the presence of factors such as spasticity and therefore a variety of positions can be trialled.
- In most cases it is easier for the patient to place both the legs into the car or one leg in and one leg out before the transfer.
- Consideration needs to be given to the method the patient will employ to dismantle the wheelchair and lift it in and out of a car.
- This will need to be developed once the patient has gained sufficient confidence to transfer independently.
- The exact method of dismantling and placing the chair in the car will depend on the type of chair and may impact on the final wheelchair choice.

Toilet and shower seat transfers

- This transfer is dependent on the access to the toilet, the space available and the presence of any adaptations, i.e. hand rails.
- The use of a sliding board may be difficult in the space available and therefore this transfer may be problematic.
- The ability to move in the wheelchair towards the toilet before the transfer and a good strong lifting technique are required.
- Transfers can be practised at a variety of angles to the toilet, i.e. next to, at 90° and 180° with the aim to provide as many options for toileting as possible.
- The position of the feet needs to be trialled, but many opt for feet on the floor.
- Dressing pre- and post-toileting often occurs in the wheelchair due to the extra stability it provides and therefore the individual must be very careful not to knock or scrape their skin.
- Transferring through 180° from the chair to toilet seat may be a technique that can be learnt by the more able patient allowing a transfer to take place in more confined spaces.
- The transfer from wheelchair to toilet seat is similar to the process required when getting into and out of a shower, although in addition to the above, the patient must be aware of the need to ensure areas to be used for gripping are dry to avoid slips and falls.

Bath transfers

- In order to achieve a bath transfer the patient must be able to perform a good strong and controlled lift that allows them to raise their bottom higher than the supporting hands.
- The patient needs to practise lifting and tucking simultaneously, which involves the contraction of latissimus dorsi in long sitting to lift the pelvis.
- They will need to be made aware of the safety issues associated with transferring in a wet environment and the added risk of damage to the skin when transferring, due to it having been soaked for a prolonged period.
- To prevent pressure-related issues the patient should sit on a cushion when in the bath to avoid prolonged contact with the firm surface.

Floor transfers

- Floor to chair or a controlled chair to floor transfer is usually only achieved by paraplegics and very low tetraplegics.

- It is used for many functional activities, e.g. to get back in the chair following a fall, to participate in activities on the floor and to enable stair climbing on their bottom.

- The ability to carry out this transfer is greatly affected by the range of motion and flexibility of the shoulders and lower limbs, body proportions, upper limb strength, balance and motivation.

- The task is initially broken down into component parts, decreasing the distance from the wheelchair using a stool.

- Once this has been mastered, progression towards the full distance can be made.

- To get onto the floor the patient needs to lift the head up and bring the body forwards, this is followed by controlled eccentric muscle action to lower the bottom to the floor.

- Lifting back onto the chair requires the patient to bring their head forward onto flexed knees enabling sufficient tuck to be able to pivot the bottom upwards towards the chair seat.

- Great care must be taken to ensure that the skin is not knocked on the way down or back up.

- The height of the transfer required can be reduced slightly by removing the cushion from the chair prior to the transfer; however, a method for replacing the cushion once in the wheelchair must also be taught.

- The type of transfer will be influenced to some degree by the type of wheelchair, i.e. rigid frame chairs promote sideways transfers and folding chairs lend themselves to forward or backward transfers.

Wheelchair mobility, skills and selection

- 'Wheelchair mobility is fundamental to the independence of people who are unable to walk' (Harvey 2008).

- It is therefore vitally important to maximise the ability through correct selection of the wheelchair and achievement of mobility and advanced skills where appropriate.

- It is important to commence wheelchair skills at a very early stage initially encompassing the basic activities of moving forwards, backwards, turning, slopes and teaching relatives safe pushing, up and down kerbs, how to fold, lift in and out of a car.

- For those with a higher level of injury a power wheelchair will usually be used for mobility using hand control (C4 and C5), head switches, chin control, mouth or breath control and recently the development of systems to use eye control.

- The choices available for manual wheelchair selection are vast and encompass tilt in space wheelchairs, manual wheelchair with power-assist wheels, rigid or folding frame wheelchairs.

- The appropriate selection is multifactorial and includes factors such as level of injury, completeness of injury, pain, spasticity, premorbid lifestyle, anticipated post injury lifestyle, wheelchair service provision, achievement of skills such as car transfers and potential for a return to driving.

- A range of chairs should be trialled where available and judged on comfort, ease of manoeuvrability, storage, use, ability to carry out activities of daily living, impact on transfers and independence i.e. ability to get wheelchair in and out of a car.
- A manual wheelchair will be required as a reserve, should a power chair fail.

Activities of daily living

- Activities of daily living such as dressing, feeding, drinking, grooming, typing, computer work and cooking tend to be activities that are commenced by the occupational therapist.
- They are dependent on co-ordination, the appropriate range of movement, balance and muscle strength and interaction and therefore close liaison and joint working between the occupational therapist and the physiotherapist is essential.
- The ability to achieve these activities is dependent on the level and completeness of injury and whilst those with a high level of injury may not be able to achieve these activities physically, they should be verbally independent in instructing these skills.
- Various types of splints, environmental controls, software and adaptations can be used to enable the individual to be as independent as possible.
- Information regarding return to work and driving should be provided when applicable.

Standing

- Standing is used in the early rehabilitative phase to help train the vasomotor system and manage orthostatic hypotension.
- Long-term standing following spinal cord injury has long been advocated two to three times a week for 60 minutes for the following reasons:
- Aids bladder and bowel function
- Joint and contracture management
- Spasticity management
- Balance training
- Psychological well being
- Bone density.
- However, the evidence to support the theory and practice is inconclusive.
- Many patients do enjoy the activity and continue to stand following discharge, generally using a tilt table if they have a high level of injury or a standing frame.
- There are a number of different types of frame commercially available for those requiring assistance to stand, e.g. 'Grandstand' or 'Easy Stand' to the more traditional Oswestry standing frames.

Gait training

- Ambulation can be taught to complete paraplegics and well-motivated low tetraplegics.
- However, it remains of functional benefit to only a few.

- Few physiotherapist working outside of a spinal unit will come across this method of gait training and ambulation.
- Further reading is available providing more information on this subject (Bromley 2006, Harvey 2008).

Cardiovascular fitness

- Increasing cardiac and ventilatory demand in a controlled manner is essential in SCI to minimise morbidity and mortality in the future (Harvey 2008).
- Guidelines established by the American College of Sports Medicine recommend those with SCI exercise for at least 20 minutes, three to five times a week at an intensity corresponding to 50–80% of maximum exercise capacity (Figoni 1997). This intensity is suggested by Franklin (1985) to be around 70–85% of maximal heart rate.
- The type of exercise undertaken depends on a patient's neurology, their interest and availability of space and equipment.
- At the National Spinal Injuries Centre we offer FES cycling, arm ergometry, the 'Rolling Road' (a treadmill for wheelchairs), functional timed wheelchair propulsion tasks, sports and circuits based on the model used for aerobics classes in any local gym.

Incomplete spinal cord injuries

- The incidence of incomplete SCI varies according to the literature and could be higher than suggested due to the many incomplete injuries that are not admitted to a spinal injuries unit from where the statistics are collated.

Incomplete syndromes

- It is important to remember that no two lesions and injuries are the same.
- The pathology of each lesion will be different due to the complex nature of the spinal cord.
- There are, however, certain types of lesions that are referred to as syndromes (Table 16.1).

Functional outcomes

- Functional outcome is difficult to predict and is dependent on many factors including age, type of injury, length of time since injury and pre-morbid status.
- Waters et al (1995) suggested that the majority will walk with or without aids and 76% of incomplete paraplegics will be community ambulators.

Physiotherapeutic management

- The management of the incomplete spinal cord injured patient differs significantly from that of the patient with a complete lesion.
- As with most patients undergoing rehabilitation for a neurological condition, the ultimate goal is normal movement.
- Often this is not achievable and compensations and orthoses are required to achieve the final goal.
- It is important to recognise the need for early intervention to be directed towards minimising the secondary effects of spinal cord injury.

Table 16.1 Incomplete spinal cord syndromes

Syndrome	Central cord syndrome	Brown–Séquard syndrome	Anterior cord syndrome
Cause	Most common type of incomplete spinal cord injury (Shaw 1995) Usually affects older people who sustain injuries in falls or road traffic accidents and usually also present with cervical spondylosis	Transverse hemisection of the spinal cord, whereby half the cord is damaged laterally (Sullivan 1989 cited by Edwards 2006) Lateral damage to one side of the cord sometimes caused by penetration injuries such as stab and gunshot wounds	Results from damage to the anterior part of the spinal cord Traumatic – forced flexion, compression injuries which may occur in diving or road traffic accidents (Foo et al 1981 cited by Edwards 2006) Non-traumatic – herniated intravertebral disc, infarction secondary to anterior spinal artery thrombosis or rupture of aortic aneurysm
Clinical presentation	Bilateral loss of pain temperature, light touch and pressure with varying degrees UL's disproportionately more affected more than LL's Flaccid paralysis at level of the lesion due to disruption of the anterior horn cell Recovery tends to be LL's, bladder/bowels, UL and hands (Roth et al 1990)	Motor loss occurs on the same side due to destruction of the corticospinal tracts Flaccid paralysis at the level of the lesion due to damage of the anterior horn cell Loss of pain and temperature on the opposite side to the lesion due to destruction of the spinothalamic tracts Loss of position sense, vibration and tactile discrimination on the same side as the lesion	Motor loss Loss of pain and temperature sensation Preservation of tactile and proprioception due to intact dorsal columns
Functional outcome (Burns and Ditunno 2001)	57–86% ambulate independently 97% under 50 years 41% over 50 years	Almost all will ambulate successfully	Poor motor recovery

> **Box 16.1** Principles to be followed during rehabilitation of a patient with a SCI
>
> - Minimise secondary effects
> - Loss of body schema
> - Altered muscle tone and movement dysfunction
> - Weakness
> - Muscle imbalance
> - Prevent length-associated changes in musculoskeletal system
> - Shortening/lengthening
> - Change in phenotype and muscle characteristics
> - Alteration of mechanical resistance
> - 'Restoration' of normal movement
> - Promotion of plasticity through the creation of an enriched environment
> - Careful consideration of the development of compensatory movements and use of external devices/orthoses
> - Consider the impact of pain, fatigue and psychological factors

- Patients who do not demonstrate complete cord transection on scan and therefore have the chance of some sparing should be treated, at least initially, as an incomplete injury.
- There are many ways to achieve the final goal, the above principles should be considered throughout the acute and rehabilitation period (Box 16.1).

The high cervical lesion (C4 and above)

- For many, the rehabilitation of an individual with a high cervical lesion can be challenging.
- Physical independence in many activities of daily living and care may be unachievable. The patient needs to be able to communicate their wishes and describe all the aspects of their care from ventilator settings, need for suction, correct positioning in the bed or chair, to bladder, bowel and skin care.
- Developing the ability to instruct carers is an essential part of regaining control over their life.
- Throughout rehabilitation physiotherapy management is directed at:
- Maintaining and maximising respiratory function
- Teaching breathing using accessory muscles to enable the person to manage for very short periods should the ventilator become disconnected, e.g. during transfers
- Establishing means of communication
- Identifying postural and seating needs in the wheelchair and bed
- Identification of equipment, e.g. powered chair
- Strengthening of innervated muscles and minimising effects of muscle imbalance
- Establishing independent neck range and strength
- Reducing and managing spasticity
- Maintenance of joint range for hygiene, care-related activities and body image
- Education of patient, family and carers.

- A patient with a high SCI should be given the opportunity to explore possible leisure opportunities and sports.
- Using equipment, knowledge and assistance a ventilated person with a complete C3 injury can achieve assisted skiing, whilst a patient with a C2 injury can learn to paint using mouthsticks.
- The duration of admission for patients with this level of injury is often longer to enable them to be discharged safely to the appropriate environment with the appropriate equipment, education and level of care.
- An example of a complex patient pathway for a high cervical lesion is included in Appendix 16.1.

Sport

- Sport has long been recognised as being important in the rehabilitation and re-integration of patients with spinal cord injury.
- Therapeutically it assists balance retraining, co-ordination, strength, wheelchair skills and endurance.
- It can be particularly beneficial to the self confidence of those who enjoyed sport pre-injury and also to those introduced to sport in a wheelchair for the first time.
- Sport provides a challenge or focus away from the formal rehabilitative process and can be enjoyed by individuals of all spinal injury levels ranging from Boccia and blow darts for very high lesions to swimming, table tennis and wheelchair basketball for the lower lesions.
- Activities such as scuba diving, sailing and skiing can be trialled following discharge.

Community re-integration and discharge

- Returning to the community, for the first time is a challenging time for the person with SCI.
- The security of the hospital environment with availability of health care professionals to manage concerns and the familiarity of other wheelchair users is replaced by a world where disability and the needs of a wheelchair user may be unfamiliar.
- Anxieties in relation to home and family life, relationships, access, employment, care provision, finance, attitudes and isolation are all real threats.
- The patient should be prepared for the transition from the hospital to the community as a continuation of their rehabilitation goals.
- Review of access in the home environment, frequent community visits, continued social networking, links with local peer groups and community services, awareness and preparation of social support systems, and provision of written material and information may all be of benefit (Whalley Hammell 1995).

Ageing with spinal cord injury

- Medical advances preventing complications, such as renal failure, have influenced the survival prognosis of individuals with a SCI.
- The challenges associated with ageing are now becoming more evident requiring different approaches to be developed through research.

- It is important that these patients are supported by professionals who can recognise and understand age-related changes, implementing strategies that include use of adaptive equipment, review of functional techniques, environment and care input to prevent deterioration and to promote independence.
- McColl et al (2002) list five changes that patients with SCI undergo with ageing:
- The long-term effects, e.g. shoulder pain, chronic bladder infections
- Secondary health conditions of the original lesion, e.g. post-traumatic syringomyelia
- Other pathologies, e.g. cancer
- Degenerative changes, e.g. joint problems
- Environmental factors, e.g. societal, cultural, that may potentially complicate the experience of aging with a SCI.
- These factors have potential to compromise the ability of someone with a SCI to remain independent and be able to participate in their communities in later life.

The references for this chapter can be found on www.expertconsult.com.

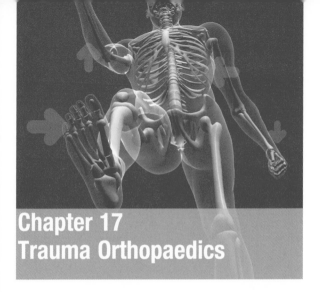

Chapter 17
Trauma Orthopaedics

Inpatients

- Trauma orthopaedics does not have to be complicated. There will be many different challenges that will not be encountered in other areas of physiotherapy.

- With a little preparation and knowledge about traumatic injuries and fixation, the management of patients in this setting becomes much easier and also much more enjoyable.

- Following the assessment set specific, measurable, appropriate, realistic and timely (SMART) goals and treatment plans in conjunction with the patient.

- From the first treatment session, the patient's discharge should be planned.

- Where will they go after discharge?

- What assistance will they need?

- What follow-up will be required?

- The majority of patients require physiotherapy outpatient treatment, which may be in a trauma outpatients setting, in the patient's home or in an outpatient department near to the patient's home.

- Wherever they are treated, the physiotherapist will need a detailed referral including details of the injury, the operation, post operative instructions, past medical history, neurovascular status, previous and current range of movement (ROM) and power, previous and current mobility, physiotherapy treatment received, any complications of surgery or treatment, drug history at discharge and any follow-up dates to visit the surgeon. Most trauma wards have a template for this information.

- Understanding a patient's injuries will influence the treatment plans and also the referral to outpatient physiotherapy.

Fractures

- Knowing how to describe a patient's fracture can sometimes be complicated; however, breaking this down into sections will make it far simpler.
- The description of a fracture should enable any physiotherapist to have a good appreciation of a fracture without reference to an X-ray.
- The following questions will provide the information that will provide a clear description of any fracture.

Open and closed fractures

- If a fracture is exposed to the environment, then it is considered to be an open injury.
- This can be caused by the bone penetrating the skin from the inside or from something penetrating the skin from the outside.
- If the injury is not open to the environment, it is considered to be closed.
- Open fractures will obviously have wounds associated with them and also have a much higher risk of infection and this is crucial information for outpatient physiotherapists.

Intra-articular or extra-articular?

- Does the fracture involve the joint surface or not?
- Intra-articular fractures can have a slower rate of healing and will also have a greater effect on joint movement.
- Do not need to mention if the fracture is in the middle third of the bone.

Types of fractures

- The type of fracture a patient has sustained will be a major determinant of the stability of the fracture, the subsequent treatment choice and weight bearing status (Table 17.1).
- The majority of fractures only contain two fragments and are classified as 'simple' fractures.
- If the bone has been fractured into more than two fragments, then it is classified as being 'multi-fragmented', also known as 'comminuted'.
- In some cases it is beneficial to include the number of fragments, e.g. a proximal humerus fracture, can be written as a two-part fracture (simple surgical neck fracture); a three-part fracture (surgical neck and greater tuberosity fractures); or a four-part fracture (surgical neck, greater and lesser tuberosity fractures).

Table 17.1 Types of fractures	
Type of fracture	Subdivisions
Simple	Transverse, oblique, spiral
Wedge	Bending, spiral
Multifragmented	Segmental, irregular

- It is important to know the different types of fractures and their subdivisions and worth having an orthopaedic textbook available to assist with this (McRae 2006). The main types of long bone fractures encountered will be simple transverse, oblique or spiral.

- Basically, a transverse fracture will be more stable than an oblique fracture, which is usually more stable than a spiral.

- In some cases, a transverse fracture will be stable enough to put weight through without causing any displacement.

The bones involved and location of the fracture

- Name the specific bone that was fractured.
- Describe whether left or right and where the fracture is on the bone.
- For long bone fractures, divide the bone into thirds – proximal, middle and distal.
- Name the section where the main part of the fracture occurs.
- If a fracture extends over two sections, this can be recorded as being at the junction, e.g. middle/distal.
- There are several bones throughout the body where it is more beneficial to describe specifically where the fracture occurred: e.g. 'distal' phalanx, 'transverse process' of the vertebra, 'posterior' rib, 'neck' of the talus; 'distal pole' of the scaphoid.

Angulation

- Angulation occurs when the two main fragments of the fracture are still in alignment, but are at an angle to each other. This is quite common, e.g. radial fractures (Figure 17.1).
- The direction of angulation is described according to the direction the fracture site is pointing (consider the two fragments forming an arrow pointing in the direction of angulation), e.g. Colles fractures may have a 'dorsal' angulation.

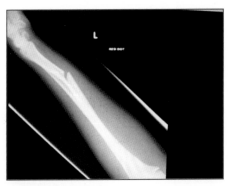

Figure 17.1 Forearm fracture dorsal angulation.

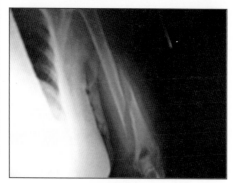

Figure 17.2 100% laterally displaced humeral fracture.

Displacement

- Displacement occurs when the two main fragments of the fracture are no longer in alignment with each other.
- This can occur when the muscles pull the fragments in opposite directions.
- The displacement is described according to the direction of displacement of the distal fragment, e.g. medial or lateral; posterior or anterior; volar or dorsal; varus or valgus (Figure 17.2).
- The extent of the displacement is described by the approximate percentage that it is displaced (Figure 17.3a, b).
- Each bone will have its own classification systems, e.g. Schatzker classification system for tibial plateau fractures.
- These classification systems may not be known to the outpatient physiotherapist; therefore, although it is reasonable to include them in a referral, also include a full description of the fracture.

Principles of fracture fixation

- When a patient is admitted with a fracture, the surgeon will make a decision whether to treat them operatively or non-operatively.
- If they choose to fix the fracture, they will base the decision on four principles that will give a patient the best chance to return to their premorbid state (Table 17.2).

Healing process

- The healing process of a bone begins the moment it is fractured.
- Depending on where a fracture is located and the surgeon's choice of treatment, the bone will either heal by direct or secondary bone healing.
- The main difference between the two types of healing processes is that there is no callus formation with direct healing.
- Direct healing (absolute stability), occurs if the fracture is intra-articular, extra bone in the joint would be detrimental to movement and therefore, the surgeon will aim for direct healing. For this to be achieved, there must be no movement

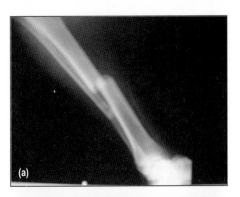

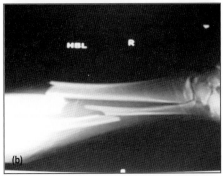

Figure 17.3 (a) Closed transverse fracture of the middle third of the (R) tibia with a 100% anterior displacement. (b) Also present is an associated 'closed oblique fracture of the middle third of the right fibula with 80% anterior displacement'.

Table 17.2 Four principles used to choose method of fracture fixation	
1. Stability	The type of fixation used will be based on the stability needed to allow the correct type of healing to occur (i.e. relative versus absolute stability)
2. Preserve soft tissue	Soft tissue is essential in the healing process, so it is necessary to preserve this when inserting metal work
3. Anatomical reduction and fixation	Anatomical reduction is needed to allow muscles and joints to function properly and unless alignment, length and rotation are correct, the patient will have irregular movement and gait
4. Early ROM	The fracture should be stabilised sufficiently to allow early ROM, to encourage healing and prevent long-term stiffness

at the fracture site (absolute stability), and is achieved surgically by inserting a locking plate.

- Secondary healing (relative stability), used for extra-articular fractures and is achieved via operative and non-operative management. Movement will occur at the fracture site, resulting in callus formation, as the bone undergoes several phases from the inflammation stage right through to the remodelling stage.

• Many patients ask about the healing process and the physiotherapist should familiarise themselves with both of these processes.

Factors affecting bone healing

• There are many factors that will influence fracture healing.
• These can be found in any orthopaedic textbook, but some of these factors are set out in Table 17.3.

Table 17.3 Factors influencing fracture healing

Factor	How it affects bone healing
Age	In general, younger patients will heal quicker and have a greater ability to remodel than older patients
Smoking	There is a lot of research to suggest that people who smoke are more at risk of complications, e.g. delayed or non-union and increased healing times of the fracture and wound
Diet	Bone and soft tissue healing requires a large amount of calories, proteins and minerals
Systemic diseases	Diseases such as osteoporosis and diabetes will delay the healing process as they significantly reduce the number of proliferating cells
Degree of trauma	The more extensive the injury is, the more disrupted the surrounding soft tissue and the slower it will heal
Degree of immobilisation of the fracture	Fractures require some form of immobilisation to heal; therefore, if there is repeated disruption of the repairing tissue it will affect healing
Intra-articular fractures	Reasons for impairing healing include: Synovial fluid has collagenases which retard bone growth Joint movement can cause the fragments to move and hence, slow healing
Vascular injury	Bones need nutrients to heal and these nutrients are delivered to the bone via the blood supply from arteries, periosteal circulation and soft tissue If this is disrupted, bone healing is affected
Loss of bone apposition	Bone needs to be in relative contact to heal Therefore, if there is separation or interposition of soft tissue it will affect bone healing
Infection	Colonisation of bacteria can cause necrosis and oedema at the fracture site, which will slow and even stop bone healing

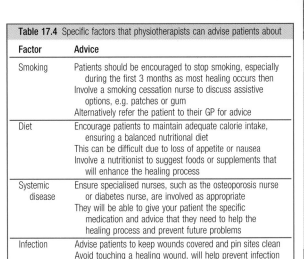

Table 17.4 Specific factors that physiotherapists can advise patients about

Factor	Advice
Smoking	Patients should be encouraged to stop smoking, especially during the first 3 months as most healing occurs then
	Involve a smoking cessation nurse to discuss assistive options, e.g. patches or gum
	Alternatively refer the patient to their GP for advice
Diet	Encourage patients to maintain adequate calorie intake, ensuring a balanced nutritional diet
	This can be difficult due to loss of appetite or nausea
	Involve a nutritionist to suggest foods or supplements that will enhance the healing process
Systemic disease	Ensure specialised nurses, such as the osteoporosis nurse or diabetes nurse, are involved as appropriate
	They will be able to give your patient the specific medication and advice that they need to help the healing process and prevent future problems
Infection	Advise patients to keep wounds covered and pin sites clean
	Avoid touching a healing wound, will help prevent infection

- There are other factors that can affect bone healing such as steroid use, hormones, cancer and radiotherapy.
- The physiotherapist should be familiar with these and the background information relating to the factors in Table 17.3 as a patient's surgeon will discuss many of these factors with them, but patients often ask their physiotherapist for clarification.
- Although not expected to be an expert on these factors, a physiotherapist should be able to encourage a patient to give themselves the best opportunity to recover as quickly as possible.
- Therefore, a little knowledge of each of these factors will help provide answers to a lot of a patient's concerns.
- The patient will not be able to influence most of the factors listed in Table 17.3; however, there are a few specific points that require advice from a physiotherapist (Table 17.4).

Types of fixation

- Once the surgeon has decided on the type of fixation as outlined in Table 17.4, they will choose the type of metalwork to achieve the best fixation.
- There are many types of fixations that will be encountered that are used with different types of fractures (Table 17.5).

The influence of fixation on the physiotherapy intervention

- The type of fixation that a patient has will inform whether or not the patient's joint can be moved or they can weight bear on the operated limb.
- The same fracture can be fixed in different ways and this will influence the physiotherapy management (Table 17.6).

Table 17.5 Types of metalwork, fixation types and fractures associated with these

Metalwork	Type of fixation	Example
Wires	Kirschner wires – to hold the fracture together Circlage wires – wraps around the bone to hold it together Tension band wiring – used to compress the fracture together (relies on active joint movement to work properly)	Extra-articular distal radius fracture Periprosthetic proximal femur fracture Patella fracture
Screws (minimally invasive)	Lag technique – to compress the fracture Positional technique – to hold the bones in the correct position	Medial malleolus fracture Sacroiliac joint disruption
Plates and screws	Neutralisation plate – to hold the bone in place and prevent bending and twisting at the fracture site Bridging plate – when there is a gap in the bone such as a multifragmented fracture, used to cross the fracture site and hold the bone out to length Compression plate – used to apply compression across the fracture site Locking plate – to ensure no movement occurs at the fracture site (absolute stability)	Distal fibula fracture Midshaft humerus fracture Radial shaft fracture Intra-articular tibial plateau fracture
Intramedullary nail	Antegrade – inserted from the proximal end of the bone Retrograde – inserted from the distal end of the bone	Tibial shaft fracture Distal femur fracture
External fixation	Pins and rods – to hold the bone out to length especially whilst soft tissue recovers Ilizarov – a more robust type of external fixator that holds the fracture site rigid. The system has the flexibility to be either more rigid or less, depending on whether more half pins are used (more rigid) or how much tension is applied through the wires	Open tibial shaft fracture or multifragmented distal radius fracture Generally used for non-unions or mal-unions of distal tibias in the trauma setting Both can be used if the soft tissue will not tolerate internal fixation

Table 17.6 Range of fixation methods used for distal radius fractures and effect on physiotherapy intervention

Fixation	Stability	Cast	Movement allowed
Kirschner wire	Weak	Non-removable	No movement allowed but can use fingers and thumb to do light functional tasks with fingers
External fixator	Weak	No cast but pins in radius and index metacarpal	No movement available at wrist and limited in fingers but can do very light functional tasks with fingers
Locking plate fixation	Strong	Removable	Movement allowed and functional tasks allowed but no lifting heavy objects

- In terms of weight bearing, metalwork that sits on the outside of the bone (plates, external fixators) tends to be a weight-sharing device, whilst metalwork that sits inside the bone (intramedullary nail) tends to be a weight-bearing device.
- Patients are more likely to be allowed to take some weight through their operated limb with an intramedullary nail than with a plate or external fixator (excluding Ilizarov frames).
- The surgeon should confirm this in their post operative instruction.

Other considerations

Pain

- Pain will play a major role in a patient's rehabilitation following a traumatic injury and their subsequent management.
- How this is managed will shape the style and duration of the rehabilitation programme and subsequent discharge.
- If pain is poorly controlled, patients will refuse to be treated or only allow minimal input.
- Too much pain relief leads to drowsiness, nausea, faintness and even a loss of function.
- Either way will lead to a suboptimal rehabilitation programme meaning a delayed discharge.
- A physiotherapist will not be expected to set up a pain relief regimen, but will be expected to know when a patient needs more or less pain relief.
- Most trauma centres have pain specialists or acute pain teams that may need to be involved with individual patients.
- Patients may need background pain relief, e.g. paracetamol, codeine or tramadol to help with the pain caused by the injury or surgery.

- For more severe pain, they may need fast-acting pain relief such as Oramorph.
- Patient-controlled anaesthesia (PCA) and patient-controlled epidural anaesthesia (PCEA) machines may be another option that patients can use to gain adequate pain relief.
- Rehabilitation may cause increased pain; therefore, it is often prudent to ensure patients have extra pain relief prior to a treatment session.

Neurological issues

- Patients may have incurred associated injuries to the spinal cord, peripheral nerves or a head injury.
- Temporary or permanent neurological damage is often encountered in patients following involvement in a high-energy accident.
- Recovery time can be very slow, taking many months to show tangible signs of improvement.
- Neural integrity and extent of damage is determined in a number of ways, from magnetic resonance imaging to direct vision during surgery.
- Most surgeons will adopt a 'wait and see' approach if neural damage is considered temporary or occasionally patients may undergo nerve conduction studies to provide information about neural status.
- If neural function is altered, it is the responsibility of the physiotherapist to ensure it does not lead to complications, such as muscle shortening.
- Patients in bed for long periods require correct positioning to avoid muscle shortening and long-term complications (Table 17.7).
- Early intervention prevents more debilitating problems in the future.
- Casts or splints can be useful in these circumstances which should be ordered via plaster room technicians or occupational therapists as soon as possible.
- If sensation is affected, monitor their skin condition whilst using these.
- Educate a patient and their family about the possible complications and encourage them to be actively involved in preventing them.
- Teaching regular passive stretches and providing equipment to assist this is crucial, e.g. a bandage to self stretch ankle dorsiflexion.
- Lower limb neurological deficits can be helped by orthoses, e.g. a 'foot up' splint will assist a patient achieve a better 'heel-toe' gait pattern, by maintaining dorsiflexion during the 'swing through' phase.
- Despite orthoses, patients need educating about correct gait patterns, ensuring they comply with their weight-bearing status.

Table 17.7 Example of the consequences of delayed intervention

A patient suffers an acetabulum injury and bruised sciatic nerve following a fall, which leads to a temporary foot drop

The foot drop is not corrected early enough and despite the nerve recovering the patient has shortened plantarflexors

The long-term shortening of the plantarflexors leads to gait issues, due to the lack of dorsiflexion and inability to generate power during 'push off'

Table 17.8 Examples of complications that can occur following a traumatic injury

Complication	Signs and symptoms
Infection	Redness and pain around the incision site. Can sometimes have a bad aroma Possibly raised temperature and increased CRP. Night sweats are possible
Wound breakdown	Redness around the wound and persistent oozing
Pulmonary emboli	Breathlessness, drop in oxygen saturation
Deep vein thrombosis	Pain, swelling and redness in the affected area
Fat embolus	Breathlessness, agitation, tachycardia, pyrexia, cyanosis
Compartment syndrome	Severe pain especially with passive stretches; swelling and tight compartments on palpation; sensory, vascular or power disturbances
Implant failure	Sudden increase in pain whilst moving

Complications

- There are many short-term and long-term complications that can arise from traumatic injuries (Table 17.8).
- Table 17.8 is not an exhaustive list and further reading is recommended.

Starting treatment

- Often it is quite difficult to know where to start when faced with a complex patient.
- Whatever the injuries it is useful to take some time after completing the assessment to plan SMART goals and the immediate treatment session.
- It is essential to include the patient in this process, as goals must be patient-centred and achievable.
- With patients that have painful injuries or following surgery, it is crucial to consider the pain when planning early treatment sessions.
- Break the management down to simple components that will enable effective treatment of even the most complex of patients.
- Treatment sessions will involve ROM, power, joint position, function and discharge planning.

Chest treatment

- Patients may need chest management for routine chest complications or for complications due to general anaesthetic and specific chest trauma.
- Chest trauma is often encountered on a trauma ward and it is a good idea to know about the common types of injuries, e.g. rib fractures or flail segment, pneumothorax, haemothorax, lung contusion or surgical emphysema.

- For information about the assessment and treatment of these conditions the reader should consult a respiratory text.
- The most common chest injury is rib fractures, with the main issue being pain.
- The pain team should be involved as soon as possible, as without adequate pain relief it will be difficult to deliver an effective treatment, which can lead to pulmonary complications in a third of patients with rib fractures (Zeigler 1994).
- Spinal cord injured patients will need chest treatment and the reader is referred to the chapter on spinal cord injuries for information on chest and other management.

Treatment considerations

- When planning a patient's treatment consider the entire hospital admission period and not just the post-stabilisation period.
- It is not unusual for a patient to be waiting in bed for up to 2 weeks for their operation, allowing swelling to subside or a specific surgeon to operate.
- Bed rest leads to many complications such as chest problems, muscle weakness and shortening, decreased fitness and possible pressure areas.
- Any injured joints should be resting in optimal positions, with or without a cast, to protect against muscle shortening.
- Think about preventing complications, a lot of treatment needs to be delivered before stabilisation of the injury has been completed.
- Once stabilisation of the injury has been achieved, treatment will largely depend on the surgeon's instructions.
- Once treatment goals have been set, rehabilitation can begin (this will include the prevention of complications), towards achieving the planned discharge from hospital.
- The following sections outline the basis for treatment goals and plans. These can be used irrespective of the type of management the surgeon advocates.

Range of motion

- ROM is affected in some way in all patients.
- It is very beneficial to start ROM early after an injury, to help the healing process and prevent long-term restrictions; therefore, consult the surgeon to ensure this is possible.
- Determine why a patient's range is reduced, are there any factors that physiotherapy can influence (Table 17.9).
- Always check the surgeon's instructions before commencing joint movement. Although early ROM is a principle of fixation, there are reasons why movement may be delayed.
- Wounds may need to be completely dry or healed before any movement is allowed or a patient's bone quality or fixation may not be strong enough to withstand movement, e.g. osteoporosis or Kirschner wires in situ.
- Manual treatment, such as passive or active assisted ROM, is very effective initially and can help to alleviate a patient's anxiety (Hengeveld and Banks, 2005).
- However, patients need to know how to work on their ROM independently. Active ROM or active assisted ROM using aids such as a bandage or a sliding board should be taught.

Table 17.9 Factors affecting ROM and physiotherapy interventions

Factor	Physiotherapy influence
Swelling	Due to the inflammatory response to the injury and subsequent surgery RICE treatment and gentle movement are very beneficial Cryocuff to cool and compress the injured area
Pain	Ensure adequate pain control before starting any ROM treatment Gentle ROM can decrease a patient's pain and relieve muscle tightness or spasm, joint stiffness and anxiety
Soft tissue tightness	Usually due to lack of movement and poor joint position, a risk for patients enduring several days of bed rest ROM exercises and stretches are used to lengthen tightened structures and to regain normal length
Anxiety	Passive ROM or CPM can start to move joints, leading to decreased pain and increased patient confidence to move their affected limb

- Techniques such as passive intervertebral movements (accessory or physiological) can maintain movement in joints that have not been injured and proprioceptive neuromuscular facilitation techniques, e.g.contract–relax, can be used to improve functional movement.
- For patients who are very anxious or cannot do any movement for themselves, use of equipment such as continuous passive movement (CPM) machines may be necessary.
- Teaching the patient to use their injured limb functionally will help to improve range, e.g. walking with a proper 'heel–toe' gait pattern will help to mobilise the ankle and knee and lengthen the surrounding muscles.
- Showing a patient how to use their injured arm to eat and comb their hair will encourage movement in their upper limb joints.
- Ensure the postoperative instructions are followed whilst teaching these functional exercises.
- Be cautious when moving joints that have associated wounds or incisions as excessive movement can cause wound breakdown.
- It is crucial that wounds heal properly, avoiding complications from infection.
- Some surgeons instruct that movement of the affected joint is left for up to 2 weeks, to ensure adequate healing before movement is begun.

Muscle power

- Improving muscle power can be difficult in the early stages of rehabilitation due to reduced ROM, swelling and pain.
- Gentle strengthening exercises should be started, when permitted, as soon as possible after fixation, to prevent further muscle weakening and to promote healing.
- Active and active assisted ROM, isometric and isotonic contractions are very useful in the initial stages.
- Resistance training with weights or Thera-Band is restricted during the early healing phase, but may be permitted if the fracture has a stable configuration and strong fixation.

- Patients with weakness due to neural problems, e.g. foot drop due to sciatic nerve bruising, will fatigue easily.
- Exercises should be undertaken on a 'little and often' basis with little or no resistance and progressed as function returns.

Function

- In addition to the musculoskeletal treatment consider function, mobility and discharge planning.
- As in many other acute specialties the physiotherapist will often be the first person to mobilise a patient.
- Think about the patient's injuries and how they will affect their function and mobility. What functional tasks can they do?
- When should they be mobilised?
- What is their weight-bearing status?
- What restrictions do they have?
- How did they mobilise premorbidly?
- How many people will be required to mobilise the patient?
- What equipment will be needed?
- What does the patient have attached, e.g. catheter?
- Assessment should provide most of the answers and therefore it should be possible to organise the environment and have any equipment in place before mobilising the patient.
- Ensure that there is sufficient space and follow correct manual handling procedures to ensure there is as little risk attached to the process as is reasonably practicable.
- Initially when teaching a patient how to move in bed, get out of bed or stand up, use equipment that is available to make the task as easy as possible, e.g. electronic beds to sit the patient up, overhead rings, stand hoists or rota stands.
- As the patient progresses ensure that the rehabilitation mimics their home environment as much as possible, e.g. standing up from a low bed.
- Once the tasks are mastered then it will be necessary to work with other multidisciplinary team (MDT) members to ensure the patient has any equipment they may need at home to enable them to function safely.

Mobility

- The priorities should be the safety of everyone involved and adherence to the postoperative weight-bearing instructions.
- It is advisable to start with a mobility aid to ensure the safest possible mobility, even if it is considered that the patient could use a less supportive aid, e.g. get a young patient with an ankle fracture to mobilise with a frame, progressing onto crutches.
- The patient's injuries will tend to dictate what equipment they will need to mobilise with. The assessment findings will determine this before commencing treatment, e.g. a patient with a pelvic and a distal radius fracture will need a gutter frame or gutter crutch for their injured arm, just as a patient with bilateral lower limb injuries will need a wheelchair and sliding board.
- For patients living in multistoreyed accommodation, they will need to be taught the safest way to mobilise up and down stairs. This may involve using two crutches, a rail or going up and down on their bottom.

Gait

- Unless a patient is non-weight bearing, the aim should be to achieve a 'heel–toe' gait pattern.
- The physiotherapist should ensure that they are familiar with the phases of gait. Always follow postoperative weight-bearing instructions.
- Refer to the assessment chapter in the first volume of this book for outlines of weight-bearing status.

Discharging a patient

- Discharge planning starts during the assessment.
- In summary, once a patient has been taught a routine of exercises, is mobilising safely and independently and the home environment is prepared they can be discharged from the acute inpatient setting.
- Prior to discharge ensure that they have a comprehensive home exercise programme with written instructions and an outpatient physiotherapy follow-up appointment, by faxing a completed referral to their relevant outpatient location.
- Most of the referral will have already been filled out during the assessment, but will require the addition of information about the patient's current neurovascular status, ROM, power, a summary of treatments given and any future appointments they have with the surgeon.

Summary

- Working in an acute trauma orthopaedic unit may involve working with complex multitrauma patients.
- Treatment of these patients involves breaking their treatment sessions down into planned, manageable sections.
- A good treatment programme depends on the physiotherapist having a good understanding of a patient's injuries and the surgery, a good assessment and treatment plan and an awareness of when to progress treatment appropriately.

Trauma outpatients

Referral

- Trauma patients will be referred in a number of different ways for physiotherapy outpatient treatment.
- It is best if the patient's physiotherapy can be performed as close to their home as possible, to enable them to attend regular and frequent treatment appointments.
- This may mean that an outpatient department could receive referrals from accident and emergency departments, trauma clinics or inpatient units from across the country, or even the world.
- A consequence of this is that there will be differing levels of communication that accompany referrals regarding prior treatment given medically or therapeutically, the patient's expected progression and any planned outcomes.
- If the information provided is missing specific details it may be necessary to contact the referrer to ensure that you have the information that you need before commencing treatment.

- The referrer should have provided a reasonable baseline of information, so that it is possible to treat the patient according to their plan.
- X-rays or scans can be requested for information and these may be received as film images or accessed via digital systems, a radiology report may accompany the patient's referral in some cases.

Communication with the referrer

- If the patient returns to the referring clinic for further assessment regarding their progress, or for tests, e.g. X-rays, a letter can be provided that they can take with them or one can be sent to the clinic, which can request any additional information required.
- Any response can be posted or brought back by the patient. It may be necessary to contact the consultant via their secretary or the clinic, if the need for information is pressing.
- The patient's GP can be an additional source of information, as they should receive reports from the clinic.
- Clinic and GP communication should be used regarding onward referral, problems with analgesia and for further opinions regarding the patient's signs and/or symptoms.

Urgent communication with the referrer

- At the beginning of the treatment session it is important to reiterate that if anything untoward is found during the assessment of the patient, the priority for treatment may be getting the patient referred to the right person for their management, e.g. in the event that a patient is identified as having a deep vein thrombosis (DVT), grossly infected wound, evidence of compartment syndrome or a highly unstable joint.
- This may take a few phone calls and it is important to do this at the earliest opportunity following the assessment.
- It is important not to delay the appointments of the other patients due to be seen, therefore it may be necessary to enlist assistance from another physiotherapist or the receptionist to cover patients or make the necessary calls.
- A more experienced member of staff should provide support during this process.

Goal setting

- Following the assessment of the trauma outpatient, it is essential to create a list of problems that the patient and physiotherapist have identified as needing to be treated.
- This list, which should be written down, may seem extensive and will need prioritising to define the way in which the patient will be treated.

Problems likely to be encountered

- The main problems likely to be encountered are:
- Psychological issues
- Acute inflammation
- Pain

- Swelling
- Wound complications
- Decreased ROM
- Hypermobility of joints
- Decreased muscle strength
- Decreased muscle length
- Decreased proprioception
- Poor gait pattern
- Neurological signs and symptoms.

- These problems may be interconnected, but for discussion purposes in this chapter, they have been divided up into subsections.
- All the problems need to be managed within the individual treatment goals set for the patient and within their management plan defined by the medical team. The patient's past medical and drug history will need to be considered alongside the problems before any intervention takes place.
- If a patient sustains an intra-articular fracture, they are less likely to get full range of movement back in that joint, especially if the fracture is fixed internally.
- This needs to be explained to the patient early on in their rehabilitation so that you are both working towards the same expectation.
- You may need to refer the patient back to their surgeon if they are not progressing as you would expect, asking the surgeon how much progress they were expecting them to make and treat the patient accordingly.

Psychological issues

- The psychological impact of a traumatic accident, whether it is a simple wrist fracture or a complex polytrauma, needs to be considered before any treatment is commenced.
- If a patient is highly distracted by their emotions, then they are less likely to be compliant with treatment. It is, therefore, important to allow a patient to express these emotions during the session.
- If a patient has said something that suggests they are potentially holding back a lot of emotion, do not be afraid to ask about it, as often all the patient needs to do is talk and all you need to do is listen.
- Physiotherapists are not trained in counselling, but a good understanding of how a patient is feeling will significantly improve the therapist–patient relationship.
- In addition a conversation may provide details that will be essential if other MDT members need to become involved in the patient's management.
- The reader is referred to the chapter on rehabilitation which covers other aspects of the patient's psychological state. Common examples of post-trauma emotions are outlined in Table 17.1.
- Patients may be unduly anxious about their pain, describing symptoms in general terms and indicating global areas of discomfort when asked to show where they are experiencing symptoms.
- It may help to encourage them to participate in their treatment, e.g. teaching how they can reduce swelling using ice or by applying massage to the area.

Acute inflammation

- The management of acute inflammation is a priority in the treatment plan when dealing with soft tissue injuries.
- The main symptoms of acute inflammation are redness, increased temperature, pain, swelling and loss of function.
- The use of protection, rest, ice, compression and elevation (PRICE) is advocated by the ACPSM in their clinical guidelines for practice during the first 72 hours of management (CSP, ACPSM 1998). This document provides detailed advice about the use of PRICE and is essential reading for any physiotherapist managing acute inflammation associated with an injury.

Pain

- Pain is the main problem that will be encountered when dealing with trauma patients. It can greatly hinder the patient's physical and psychological progress.
- It is important to consider why the patient is experiencing a particular pain, in the particular location after a specific injury.
- Once the acute inflammation has been managed, pain will need to be controlled.
- Pain can be due to structures inside and around the joint.

Excessive activity

- Pain can often be caused by the patient trying to do too much, too soon or overdoing activities.
- This can sometimes be due to frustration related to the healing process, and can present with a boom and bust lifestyle.
- It is important in these situations to talk the patient through the process of pacing and finding a baseline of activity that they can do every day.
- This change will require discipline and the patient will need strong support throughout the process (Butler and Moseley 2003).

Discomfort from internal fixation

- If a patient has had an internal fixation for a fracture, the stabilising metalwork can sometimes cause significant discomfort, which will lead to it being surgically removed.
- In the author's experience, in most cases metalwork will be left in situ for up to a year before it is removed, but in cases when it is essential, this will be carried out earlier.
- If there are any concerns about a patient's metalwork, e.g. it is very prominent, then advice should be sought from a more experienced physiotherapist, who can assist in making the decision whether the patient needs to be referred to the trauma doctors for a surgical opinion.

Pain modulation

- The drug history gathered during the assessment will indicate what the patient is taking for analgesia.
- Many patients fail to take medication as it has been prescribed for them.

- This can be due to a number of reasons:
- Because they think they are better
- They may dislike taking tablets
- They do not see the need for them or think they are bad for them.
- Often a patient will not feel that they need pain relief because they are not doing their exercises as instructed.
- Once the exercises have been corrected patients often complain of pain, which is when the physiotherapist needs to reinforce the need to use analgesia.
- Physiotherapists generally do not prescribe medication, therefore advising patients to take medication prescribed for them or raising concerns about medication with the medical team or the patient's GP are the appropriate courses of action.
- If the patient is unhappy or has questions about their medication they should consult a pharmacist or their GP.
- General advice should be to tell the patient to follow the instructions that they have been given and that the recommended dosages are not exceeded.
- If the patient is on high-dose prescriptions of analgesia, then this should be managed by their GP. These patients can benefit from encouragement to use other modalities to help with pain relief, e.g. ice, soft tissue mobilisation or electrotherapy.
- Contemporary physiotherapists use a number of treatment modalities for pain, e.g. ultrasound or TENS, which can be beneficial for certain injuries.
- Consider precautions and contraindications for each of these modalities, especially as trauma patients often have wounds and/or internal metalwork (Robertson et al 2006).

Swelling

- Swelling is very common with any injury, whether it is a soft tissue injury or a fracture.
- The management of acute swelling should follow the PRICE guidance.
- Chronic swelling can be a problem as it causes limitations to movement, pain, functional problems, gait disturbance, as well as concern for the patient that they might be continuing to cause damage, adding to their injury.
- Before starting to treat swelling, it is important to consider why it is there, e.g. if a patient has had an ankle fracture, and has started weight bearing on it and the ankle continues to be swollen. This is a normal occurrence post injury, especially in the lower limbs, where it is difficult to get rid of swelling due to gravity.
- It is essential to be aware of problems such as deep vein thromboses and infection, which will present with swelling, but usually with heat, redness and tenderness. These will require emergency medical attention.
- In order to help patients understand why their limb keeps swelling, the following analogy can be useful.
- An uninjured body part is like a new balloon straight out of the packet; it is hard to blow up, as the rubber is tight. The injured body part is like an old balloon, which has been inflated for a few days, the rubber has been stretched and is easier to blow up. Therefore it is important to try to stop the limb from swelling initially, to avoid the structures from becoming stretched.

- There are various ways of controlling the swelling, e.g. by using Tubigrip or a compression sock, such as a flight sock, which the patient will need to wear all day (Clarke et al 2006).
- The support will provide external elasticity to stop the limb from swelling, allowing the body's own elasticity to 'retighten'.
- Another way to reduce swelling is by elevating the limb above the level of the heart on a regular basis throughout the day.
- The use of contrast baths or ice can be very effective in helping to decrease chronic swelling (Robertson et al 2006).
- Soft tissue techniques, such as effleurage can help to mobilise the swelling and remove it from the limb, allowing the soft tissues to recoil back to normal size.
- The patient should be encouraged to carry out treatments themselves as often as possible throughout the day.
- This will take effort and discipline, so the patient needs to be convinced that the treatment will benefit them, as it is important that the patient is compliant.
- The swelling could be being exacerbated by the patient overdoing activities, which will need to be identified during the subjective assessment.
- In this case, using pacing could help to reduce the swelling.

Complications

- After a patient has had an operation to reduce and fix their injury, they potentially will have a significant wound that will need monitoring.
- As a patient will visit physiotherapy regularly after their surgery, it will be possible to see changes that occur and will need to act to ensure that the patient is managed correctly.
- A wound that is red, hot, swollen and oozing will need to be shown to a senior physiotherapist and referred to a doctor for antibiotics.
- It is better to err on the side of caution and if there are any concerns, refer the patient to the trauma team or their GP.
- Once the wound has healed, it is important to keep the scar mobile to prevent it becoming tethered to the structures under it, which may be painful and restrict range of movement.
- Regular massage with and without moisturiser will help to mobilise the scar from the underlying tissues.
- The reader is referred to Chapters 4 and 14 for more information on scar and wound management.

Decreased ROM

- Decreased ROM is the most common problem after a traumatic accident.
- It may be due to a number of causes, e.g. pain and swelling or decreased muscle strength.
- Regaining full ROM after an injury is a priority, requiring guidance from the trauma medical team.
- Improving ROM will decrease joint hypomobility and enable muscle strength to be increased.
- The operation notes should provide clear guidance from the surgeons about how much ROM can be forced. If unsure, it is best to get advice from a senior clinician or the medical team.

- Passive ROM exercises, e.g. pendulum shoulder exercises, can be very useful after the initial injury (e.g. a nerve palsy).

- Physiotherapists can use passive physiological movement exercises (PPM) to re-educate a patient's movements and to help increase range.

- Passive accessory and physiological movements were developed by a physiotherapist, Geoffrey Maitland, and are used widely in clinical practice by many physiotherapists (Maitland et al 2005).

- The use of PPM, often in combination with soft tissue mobilisation and passive accessory mobilisations (PAMs) can be very useful for improving decreased ROM.

- For decreased movement in the spine, passive physiological inter-vertebral movements (PPIVMs) and passive accessory intervertebral movements (PAIVMs) can be used with great success (Maitland et al 2005).

- Mobilisations with movement (MWMs), natural apophyseal glides (NAGS), sustained natural apophyseal glides (SNAGS) are also effective at increasing range. These are particularly useful for treating patients post fracture, with associated soft tissue healing, so as not to aggravate the injury or increase symptoms (Mulligan 2010).

- Active ROM exercises should be given to the patient to do on a 'little and often' basis and are done in conjunction with ice, heat or analgesia, whichever is appropriate for the patient.

- It is important that the patient understands why they are doing the exercise and that they are not doing any harm by performing controlled movements. This understanding helps to increase the patient's compliance.

- Patients can be taught active assisted exercises, e.g. using a towel wrapped around a foot to enable the patient to pull on this to assist the movements of inversion and eversion at the ankle, or using a walking stick in both hands to help with shoulder movements.

- Initially after surgery, e.g. tension band wiring, surgeons may wish to limit the amount that ROM is pushed.

- In this situation it may be better to do active movements without any additional assistance.

Hypermobility of joints

- With traumatic injuries such as dislocations, especially recurrent ones, there may be an issue with hypermobility, rather than hypomobility.

- Some patients may have hypermobility syndrome, which can be assessed using a Beighton Scale (Grahame et al 2000).

- If a patient presents with a first time dislocation, they may have been immobilised in order to enable the joint to stiffen up. It is the role of the physiotherapist to get them moving again and to strengthen the supporting muscles, i.e. the rotator cuff, to increase the stability of the joint.

- It is likely that the patient may redislocate the joint and if this becomes a recurrent problem the consensus opinion is that surgery will be required to provide a longer-term solution.

Decreased muscle strength

- Decreased muscle strength is often a finding of the assessment and may be a result of immobilisation, pain or injury to the muscle.

- If the assessment has found very little muscle activity, it can sometimes be helpful to perform some gentle soft tissue mobilisation to the muscle, which may have the effect of enabling it to contract more effectively.

- In the initial stages of treatment, it is possible to use active or active assisted exercises to build up strength, until the patient can achieve Grade 4 muscle power.

- Resistance at this stage can come in the form of weights or Thera-Band, which may be used to strengthen throughout available range. Body weight can be used as a resistance, e.g. press-ups against a wall, heel raises or single leg dips.

- It is important that these exercises are completed with no or minimal pain, so that the patient maintains their compliance.

- Exercises can be modified by changing the use of holds or slowing the movement down, relevant when trying to increase control at a joint.

- It is important to also consider a patient's proximal and core strength and incorporate training into their treatment. The use of pelvic and shoulder stabilisers can greatly change a patient's ability to perform a movement and reduce their symptoms, e.g. gluteus medius can be strengthened to prevent the knee dropping into a valgus posture during single leg dips.

Decreased muscle length

- In association with joint immobility and loss of range the muscles surrounding joints can become shortened.

- Stretching techniques can be used to increase muscle length; however, it is important that the patient understands exactly how they should stretch and why they are doing it.

- There is evidence to show that muscles respond in different ways to different types of stretches, e.g. sustained stretches or ballistic stretches.

- A sustained stretch of up to 1 minute, repeated four times for each muscle group, may be the most beneficial method for lengthening tightened muscle groups (Bandy and Irion 1994, Herbert and Gabriel 2002, Gremion 2005).

- It is important that stretches are carried out on a regular basis and that they are performed correctly in order to achieve the desired outcome.

- Proprioceptive neuromuscular facilitation techniques, e.g. contract–relax, muscle energy techniques and myofascial release can also be used to increase the length of tight muscle tissue (Voss et al 1985, Chaitow, 2003, 2006).

Decreased proprioception

- Decreased proprioception in a limb can be responsible for re-injury if not included in the rehabilitation process.

- Following an ankle sprain, proprioceptive feedback is often disrupted, resulting in episodes of unexpected loss of control of the ankle on uneven surfaces which can lead to further ligament and/or bony injury.

- It is important to educate the patient about the role proprioception plays in preventing further episodes of the ankle 'turning'.

- Single leg standing, initially with eyes open, progressing to eyes closed, is a simple exercise that can be given to patients with ankle or knee problems.

- More demanding exercise may be required, e.g. single leg stands on wobble boards, throwing and catching objects, or passing a football round a stationary leg whilst standing on a wobble board.

- Progression can be achieved by combining activities and making the surface more unstable. The introduction of the Nintendo Wii Fit board has meant patients can receive information about their balance and test it through games.

- Sports players may need to achieve higher-level proprioception, therefore jumping, hopping and running on either flat or uneven surfaces may need to be added to their rehabilitation. They should be confident in doing this before returning to their sport.

- Proprioception in the upper limb can be improved by the use of weight-bearing activities, e.g. press ups against a wall or on the floor, useful after a shoulder dislocation.

- Difficulty can be increased using gym balls, e.g. legs supported on a ball and the patient weight bearing through their affected arm. This can be progressed by placing the hand onto a wobble board or cushion.

Poor gait pattern

- Pain and decreased range of movement cause the most issues with gait.

- In practice, patients view getting off crutches as a positive factor and tend to want to do this too early, resulting in them acquiring an antalgic gait pattern.

- A faulty gait pattern can result in secondary back, hip or neck pain due to the increased strain these areas are put under.

- It is better for the patient to walk well with crutches than badly without them, and the patient must be made to understand this.

- Following a fractured ankle dorsiflexion is often reduced in range and walking with crutches ensures that the patient achieves a 'foot flat' position during the weight-bearing phase of gait and then stretches into dorsiflexion when moving into the 'toe off' phase.

- Progressing to one crutch will require the patient to use the crutch on the opposite side to the injury, this will ensure a normal reciprocal gait pattern is achieved.

- When weaning the patient off the single crutch the process should gradually build up the amount of distance they do without it.

- It is important that the patient is assessed before they return to running or jumping. If they are unable to do this comfortably and with a reciprocal pattern, they require further work on their strength and/or mobility.

Neurological signs and symptoms

- Neurological symptoms are common after a traumatic accident.

- Nerve injury due to impact or stretch may leave the patient with decreased sensation, muscle strength and function, e.g. a patient with a humeral shaft fracture may have a radial nerve palsy, due to the nerve's close proximity to the bone.

- Nerve damage can also cause either sensitisation (increased sensitivity) or desensitisation (decreased sensitivity) of areas supplied by the nerve.

- If the patient has had decreased range of movement in the limb for a long time, or they have been holding themselves in an antalgic position, the nervous system can become symptomatic.

- Symptoms can appear after the injury and healing process are well established and the patient may describe symptoms that are different to their injury pain. The symptoms may be widespread and described as a toothache or linear and described as sharp shooting pain or by more unusual descriptions, such as feeling a tight wire running down the leg.

- It is important to assess the patient fully at this point for decreased range at the relevant spinal area and to undertake a neurological test (Petty 2006).

- First point of treatment is to address the cause of the problem, e.g. correcting and re-educating posture or gait pattern.

- The patient should be encouraged to move the limb, respecting their symptoms, this facilitates normal movement in the nervous system and increases cardiovascular activity, which will in turn improve blood flow to the nerves.

- In cases where the patient has severe limiting nerve pain they will need to be referred to a doctor to be assessed for neuroleptic medication such as gabapentin and amitriptyline.

Other complications to consider

- After a traumatic accident, additional complications can occur, such as complex regional pain syndrome (CRPS), which can cause increased pain, swelling and redness around a joint.

- Treatment will involve massage, gentle increased loading of the area, education and reassurance to help the patient to use the joint as normally as possible (Gifford 2002).

- Mal- or non-union, myositis ossificans and osteophyte or exostosis development in or around a joint are problems that are encountered during the treatment of trauma patients.

- It is important to consider these if a patient fails to respond to treatment as expected, in the appropriate timeframe.

Progression of treatment

- The rate and amount of progression during treatment varies with each individual patient.

- The more complicated the fracture or soft tissue injury, the longer it will take to heal; in addition, the type of fracture will be influential, e.g. transverse fractures heal faster than spiral fractures (Atkinson and Coutts 2005).

- Other medical conditions such as diabetes will extend the healing time and, in some cases, people take a long time to heal, irrespective of their age and health.

- In early management the physiotherapy will focus on maximising function and movement of the injured area/s within the boundaries of the trauma team instructions, e.g. treatment will aim to regain movement in an ankle following a fracture and internal fixation whilst they are non-weight bearing.

- When permitted to weight bear the patient should have the range of joint mobility to enable them to walk with minimal restriction from tight articular structures.

- Progression should encompass instructions from the trauma team or GP, which will be used in conjunction with clinical reasoning that takes into account the holistic knowledge obtained during assessment and subsequently, relating to the patient.
- This approach should ensure that appropriate progression of rehabilitation occurs, enabling patients to return to their normal lifestyle wherever possible.

The references for this chapter can be found on www.expertconsult.com.

Page numbers followed by "f" indicate figures, "t" indicate tables, and "b" indicate boxes.

Index